Heart and Lung Transplantation

Hikaru Matsuda • Shigeru Miyagawa
Yasushi Shintani
Editors

Heart and Lung Transplantation

Historical Developments, Clinical Achievements, and Future Perspectives

Springer

Editors
Hikaru Matsuda
Professor Emeritus, The University of Osaka
Suita, Osaka, Japan

Shigeru Miyagawa
Department of Cardiovascular Surgery
The University of Osaka Graduate School of Medicine
Suita, Osaka, Japan

Yasushi Shintani
Department of General Thoracic Surgery
The University of Osaka Graduate School of Medicine
Suita, Osaka, Japan

ISBN 978-981-96-8809-8 ISBN 978-981-96-8810-4 (eBook)
https://doi.org/10.1007/978-981-96-8810-4

This Springer imprint is published by the registered company Springer Nature Singapore Pte Ltd.
The registered company address is: 152 Beach Road, #21-01/04 Gateway East, Singapore 189721, Singapore

Foreword 1

Recently, the dawn of research on organ transplantation as a method of longevity has been recognized. If this method is further developed, it will be easy to transplant lungs, heart, and other important internal organs from one to another. When there is a patient with a serious senile disease such as atrophied kidney and simultaneously there was another patient who was suffering serious injury and inevitably die, the kidney of the injured patient could be removed and replaced with that of an old man. (1914)

This is a passage from a book of short essays titled *Though the Window of the School* written in 1914 by Dr. Aihiko Sata, President of Osaka University (1905–1924), who invited Dr. Haertel from Germany in 1922 and appointed Dr. Yoshio Ozawa as his successor of the First Department of Surgery.

In the early days after becoming a professor, Dr. Ozawa conducted the experiments, which were not successful, in the operating room of the former First Department of Surgery with Dr. Yoshiaki Takeda as the assistant. He transplanted a heart from one dog to the neck of another dog, as Nobel Prize-winning surgeon Carrel had done. It is not clear whether Dr. Ozawa heard about this experiment from Dr. Aihiko Sata, who had met Carrel at the Rockefeller Center and heard about it firsthand, or whether Dr. Ozawa himself had heard about it when he was studying surgery in Germany. Anyway, the history of organ transplantation experiments at the Department of Surgery of Osaka University should be said to have started with the most difficult organ to transplant at that time.

In 1964, when heart transplantation was starting to become a hot topic in Japan, I moved to Los Angeles to learn cardiac surgery, responding to a letter from Dr. Jerome Kay. At that time, the levels of cardiac surgery in Japan and the United States were quite evident, and the gap between Japan and the United States in the discussion of heart transplantation at academic conferences was so great that it was enough to surprise the trainees in cardiac surgery from Japan.

I invited Takao Sonoda (later professor of urology), who had just completed his studies in the United States and was on his way back to Japan. They made passionate speeches about their desires to pursue heart and kidney transplantations as their research theme upon returning to Japan. The following year, Dr. Sonoda informed me that the Department of Urology of Osaka University had decided to make renal transplantation a research project of the department.

When I returned to Japan in the summer of 1966, I suggested to Dr. Manabe who had just been appointed professor, that the department should now begin preparations for heart transplantation. However, his reply was surprising, "Well, don't be in such a hurry." I was very much disappointed and I prepared for the coming day by performing allogenic valve transplants with the help of the Department of Forensic Medicine. However, Professor Manabe changed his mind so rapidly.

After so-called Wada transplantation was performed in August 1968, public opinion was beginning to coalesce around the Wada transplant, with praise and criticism eventually turning into slander. At a meeting of the Board of Trustees the day before the annual meeting of the Japanese Association of Thoracic Surgery in 1968, Professor Ichiro Akakura of Keio University said, "It is outrageous that some journalists are distributing pamphlets slandering and condemning what Professor Wada has done without knowing why, and I would like to hear directly from Professor Wada". At his prompting, Professor Wada gave a detailed explanation of the first heart transplant surgery in Japan. Professor Manabe, who stood up after him, clearly came from the standpoint of supporting heart transplantation medicine and said, "We cannot leave this issue as it is". I would be very happy if we could make some kind of statement here in support of heart transplantation. However, this proposal was not taken up by the chairperson, and the meeting was adjourned.

I believe that this was a great opportunity for the Japanese academic society to take charge of this issue. If the society did not look right or left at this time, but had firmly stated that heart transplantation is an extremely useful procedure for the treatment of severe heart disease and must be developed and implemented in future, heart transplantation in Japan, as well as other types of organ transplantations, would have been treated quite differently from that in today and the transplantation of hearts would have been more effective. If he had stated and announced that the transplantation surgery in Japan must be developed and implemented in the future, heart surgery and other transplantation surgeries in Japan would be treated quite differently from that today, and we would never be so behind the other countries.

Nobuo Miyazaki, a heart transplant patient under the care of Professor Wada, died the next day. The media was even more critical of his death, but Miyazaki's 83-days survival period was one of the best among nearly 100 heart transplants performed in the world that year.

The path that heart transplantation has taken in Japan since then has been a series of unfortunate events that readers of this book will no doubt be familiar with, and for patients who would not have been saved without this treatment, it was indeed a miserable time.

It was during these days as I was served as the Chirman and Professor of the First Department of Surgery since 1978 to 1991, that I visited Professor Lower in Richmond in 1984. He told me that if understanding of brain death was so poor in Japan, why not resuscitate and use the arrested heart? He was the first in the world to have tried this technique before Barnard, and as you know, it is gaining attention again today due to the shortage of donors. Of course, it is possible to use this method if the understanding of brain death is not yet advanced. However, at that time, the removal of the heart from a brain-dead body was already common in the world. What would happen if a heart transplant were to go backwards and be performed using an arrested heart and fail?

Thinking about this, I could not immediately accept Lower's advice. At the time, the situation in Japan was such that a heart transplant from a brain-dead patient would become feasible after some more years of discussion, and I had no idea that it would take another 15 years to realize a heart transplant in Japan. In retrospect, this was indeed a significant opportunity. If we had followed Lower's advice and successfully performed the transplant using an arrested heart, we would have been able to resume heart transplantation in Japan 15 years earlier. All of this would have been possible if we had succeeded in using an arrested heart.

Fifteen years is too long a time to take the risk of not succeeding, and I wonder how many people could have been saved in 15 years. But if we had not succeeded, it would have taken many more years to resume heart transplantation in Japan.

There is no way to know which was the correct answer. However, if I had known at the time that it would take another 15 years to perform a heart transplant from a brain-dead body, I would have decided to use an arrested heart. This would have been another great opportunity not only for us but also for all Japanese patients who necessitated heart transplantation.

On February 28, 1999, the first successful heart transplant was performed at Osaka University Hospital by Professor Matsuda, and the second one was performed on May 12 at the National Cerebral and Cardiovascular Center by Vice Director of the hospital Dr. Kitamura (later President). The readers of this book are already well aware of the subsequent developments in the field of heart transplantation in Japan. It has been more than 60 years since the initial experimental study performed by Professor Ozawa of the first Department of Surgery, and the first and the second successful heart transplant in Japan was performed by the descendants of the First Department of Surgery Dr. Matsuda and then Dr. Kitamura. This book summarizes the history of research and practice of organ transplantation performed in the First Department of Surgery of the Osaka University Medical School, and the most difficult heart transplantation has been a major subject among them since the beginning. This may have been due to the character of Professor Ozawa, who dared to take on challenges.

This message is a brief description of the milestones in the development of transplantation medicine in this department, mainly in the predawn period.

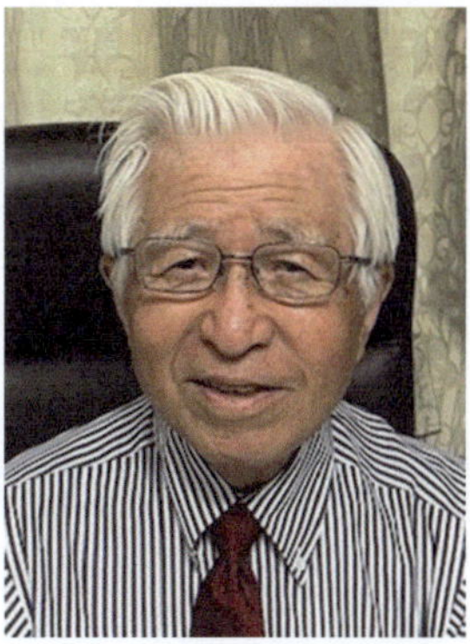

Osaka, Japan Yasunaru Kawashima

Foreword 2

The beginnings of heart transplantation in Japan is a story of perseverance, courage, and a strong will to save Japanese patient lives who were suffering from severe heart disease. The initial heart transplant surgery performed in 1967 was not successful and it seemed to have set the country backward in the pursuit of heart transplantation due to moral and ethical debates. Finally, in 1997 Japanese law recognized brain death which resulted in donors with a beating heart to allow heart transplantation to proceed.

As Japan was now opening their doors to heart transplantation, Dr. Yasunaru Kawashima of Osaka urged the International Society for heart and lung Transplantation (ISHLT) board of directors to plan its 2000 Scientific Annual Meeting in Japan in hopes of focusing the Japanese public's attention on the value of heart transplantation. The ISHLT board acknowledged its responsibility to bridge a gap in the ISHLT's international purpose to spread the science of transplantation throughout the world. I had the honor of representing the ISHLT as the Program Chair of the 2000 Osaka Meetings which were a resounding success. I worked closely with Dr. Kawashima who led the local Japan Organizing Committee along with Drs. Hikaru Matsuda and Ryota Shirakura. Together, we welcomed more than 1200 physicians, surgeons, and allied health personnel to Osaka for the ISHLT scientific sessions. Furthermore, the meeting forged a bridge for Japanese transplant physicians to collaborate with heart transplant physicians and scientists throughout the world.

Prior to 1997, many Japanese nationals were transported to the United States for heart transplantation. As a humanitarian effort, 5% of our patients in the United States could be from foreign countries many of whom were from Japan. A large number of heart transplant surgeries were performed at my institutions (UCLA and Cedars-Sinai Medical Centers) where I provided care for them. After being stabilized and watched carefully for a few months the Japanese heart transplant patient was then transported back to Japan, where they were provided outstanding care from Japanese transplant physicians trained in the United States. Over the years, Dr. Takeshi Nakatani from the National Cardiovascular Disease Center has sent many Japanese physicians to train with me and others in the United States which has resulted in well-trained transplant physicians in Japan. When comparing the long-term survival of Japanese heart transplant patients cared for by Japanese transplant physicians, long-term survival exceeds that of international averages. In my discussions with Dr. Shinichi Nunoda of Tokyo's Women Medical College and from the Japan Heart Transplant Registry, the Japanese heart transplant patients have an astounding 89% 10-year survival compared to 50% in the rest of the world according to the ISHLT registry. No doubt, dedicated care provided to these patients with meticulous rejection surveillance, close management of comorbid diseases, high medication compliance, and frequent clinic visits contributed to these outstanding results.

In the last 10 years the number of heart transplant surgeries in Japan has been increasing to more than 100 heart transplant surgeries performed in 2023. However, despite the relaxed laws overseeing organ donors in Japan and recent increases in annual heart transplant surgeries, there remains a severe organ donor shortage in Japan. The Japanese population is about one-third of that of the United States but does not come close to performing one-third of the 4000 annual heart transplants performed in the United States. Countless more lives could be saved in Japan with increased deceased organ donation.

For the future, I look forward to many more contributions from the Japanese transplant physicians and healthcare providers. The remarkable success of long-term outcomes should be emulated throughout the world to extend the lives of all heart transplant recipients. The history of heart transplantation in Japan has formed a strong foundation by which Japanese heart transplant physicians will continue efforts to save more lives and ensure a high quality of life after heart transplant surgery.

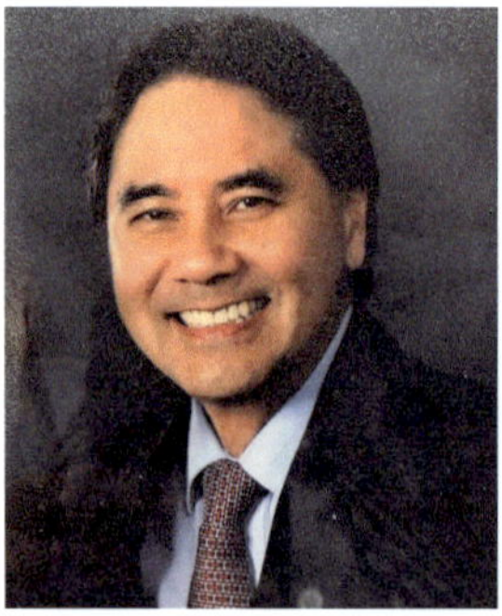

Los Angeles, CA, USA

Jon Kobashigawa

Foreword 3

Bridging the gap between organ (heart) and tissue (homograft, allograft) transplantation.

A quarter of a century has passed since heart transplantation began in Osaka, Japan, in 1999. As of August 31, 2023, the total number of heart transplants had reached 780 in Japan, with an increasing number of centers performing more than 100 transplants per facility. The National Cerebral and Cardiovascular Center (NCVC), under the leadership of myself, Junjiro Kobayashi, Deputy Director, and Tomoyuki Fujita, Division Director of cardiovascular surgery, reached 100 transplants on July 12, 2017, the earliest in the country. However, there is still a clear shortage and the waiting period is currently estimated to be up to 8 years. Most patients are placed on a left ventricular assist device (LVAD) and await transplantation, and even then, the mortality rate during the 10-year waiting period is more than 25%.

I, as a chairman, recall with nostalgia that when the law was revised in 2010, the Organ Transplant Office of the Ministry of Health, Labor and Welfare (MHLW) drafted a proposal for priority rights for pediatric recipients and that Takeshi Nakatani and Norihide Fukushima, both from the former First Department of Surgery (FDS), participated as committee members, which was subsequently approved by the Japanese Society of Medical Sciences.

Now, recalling the theme of this issue "The former FDS of Osaka University Medical School and Organ Transplantation," there were nearly 10 graduates who joined the FDS in the first term (graduated in 1965) in the year when Professor Hisao Manabe was appointed in the FDS, Osaka University, and a few of them majored in cardiac surgery. The major research themes in cardiac surgery from that time were heart transplantation and artificial hearts. Among my classmates, Hajime Hirose, who became later a professor of thoracic surgery at Gifu University School of Medicine, went to South Africa to study heart transplantation under Dr. C. Barnard, and Hisateru Takano, who became later Deputy Director of the NCVC Research Institute and Director of the Advanced Medical Center, went to the United States to study artificial heart under Professor Tetsuzo Akutsu at the University of

Mississippi. I studied under Dr. J.H. Kay at the University of Southern California—St. Vincent's Hospital, Los Angeles, USA, where Prof. Kawashima also studied previously. It was 1969 when coronary artery bypass surgery had just started in the United States. For this reason, my main research project shifted to surgical treatment for ischemic heart disease. After returning to Japan, I felt I was also given the freedom to participate in heart transplantation project when I was appointed Professor in 1981 at the opening of the Third Department of Surgery at Nara Medical University. I remember working late into the night to prepare a manual for heart transplantation with Associate Professor Choken Oyama and Lecturer Kanji Kawachi (later Professor of Thoracic Surgery at Ehime University), both of whom were from the former FDS, Osaka University. As a result, our application for permission to perform heart transplantation was approved in December 1993 as one of the nine facilities in Japan. As you may know, the recommendations for the initiation of heart transplantation in Japan were made for the Osaka University-NCVC combined team and for Tokyo Women's Medical University. However, without this approval at the Nara Medical University as a heart transplant facility, I would not have been invited by Dr. Haruhiko Kikuchi, President of the NCVC (from the Department of Neurosurgery, Kyoto University) at that time. I felt it was important that effort should not be spared and that enthusiasm should be accompanied by determination.

I remember well that in October 1997, President Kikuchi asked me to promote heart transplantation program in NCVC and also improve the results of coronary artery bypass surgery, where many of the staff were seconded from the FDS of Osaka University. At the NCVC, Takeshi Nakatani, a trainee of the former FDS of Osaka University, was working hard to establish a heart transplant team, and a heart failure ward, beds for patients with LVADs, and an ICU (sterile room) for transplant recipients were established at a rapid pace. We once had a heart transplant procedure practice in an animal experiment with the surgeons at NCVC and I found that they were all excellent surgeons, so I had no major concerns or worries. Among them, Toshikatsu Yagihara from the former FDS and Kunio Miyatake from the First Department of Internal Medicine of Osaka University gave me advice from the time of my arrival and helped me a lot with my surgery. At the time of my appointment as a Deputy Director at NCVC, both men were also head of the Department of Cardiac Surgery and the Department of Cardiology, respectively, and I had the feeling that the cardiac surgeons from the FDS of Osaka University were "trusted" at the NCVC, where there was a group of physicians from various academic backgrounds. At the NCVC, the surgeon's opinion was respected in the choice of surgical methods, and I performed the Lower-Shumway method in the first case of heart transplantation in 1999, the original bicaval anastomosis method in the second case, and the modified bicaval anastomosis method in the third case. This is reported by our NCVC team in the *Annals of Thoracic Surgery* in 2001. Currently, the modified bicaval anastomosis method is used in more than 90% of heart transplant cases in Japan, including pediatric heart transplant cases. It is one of the honors that the method has since been frequently used, supported by many reports that it is easy to adapt in size-mismatched cases.

There is also a growing interest in the utilization of the post-cardiac arrest heart (DCD), which is being actively practiced in the UK and Australia. Professor H. Matsuda from the former FDS is also advocating its promotion. However, I feel that sufficient discussion is needed on the interpretation of "death" as "cardiac death" in hearts that are resuscitated using the organ care system. Discussions should begin immediately, starting with consensus building in academic societies, followed by discussions involving the MHLW.

An essential part of the establishment in heart transplantation is the artificial heart. Here, too, the achievements of those from the former FDS are worthy of special mention. As mentioned above, my classmate Hisateru Takano devoted his life to the development of the artificial heart from the time of Professor Manabe of the FDS. Initially, in collaboration with Toyobo Co. Ltd., he completed the so-called "Takano Pump," an extracorporeal pneumatic-driven pulsatile flow pump. Without it, heart transplantation in Japan would never have started. In my time, implantable pulsatile or continuous flow LVADs made in the United States had already started to appear, but the "Takano Pump," renamed the Nipro Pump, was essential. Unfortunately, this pump was only approved for domestic use and was not approved for use in foreign countries. Nowadays, the mainstream is centered on implantable continuous flow pumps, which can be easily miniaturized, and catheter-type pumps and ultra-compact continuous flow artificial hearts developed by Yoshiyuki Taenaka (Deputy Director of NCVC Research Institute) and Eisuke Tatsumi (Director, Artificial Organs Department at NCVC), both from the former FDS, can be used for a variety of different purposes. However, the "Takano Pump" was indispensable for the beginning and establishment of heart transplantation program in Japan.

I have also focused on tissue transplantation of heart valves and blood vessels using cryopreservation methods. Beta-propiolactone treated human allogeneic valves (homografts) were used by Professor Yasunaru Kawashima and colleagues at the former FDS, Osaka University, mainly for reconstruction of the right ventricular outflow tract in tetralogy of Fallot and other disorders. These preservation methods, however, have been abandoned thereafter because of its excessive tissue damage. In 1990, I obtained a research grant from the Ministry of Education, Culture, Sports, Science and Technology. With this grant, I set up a small cryopreservation bank in the laboratory of Nara Medical University and began our research. In December 1992, an Englishman living in Nara was killed in a traffic accident, and a homograft was donated first for clinical application. About 30 valve surgeries were performed using cryopreserved homografts. I then moved to the NCVC, where I spent a year developing the NCVC Tissue Transplantation Guidelines, and in 1999 the NCVC Tissue Bank was approved. To me the new tissue bank was magnificent compared to that at Nara Medical University, and the key to its success was that it has been established as a tissue bank of NCVC rather than that of the surgical department only. For the initial operating costs, I applied for the MHLW Scientific Research Fund and conducted it as a "research" project until the national approval for advanced medical treatment (*senshin iryo*) in 2002.

On the other hand, in 2001, I combined the existing academic groups into one and established the Japanese Society for Tissue Transplantation. Together with Professor Shuji Shimazaki of Kyorin University and others from the Department of Emergency Medicine at Osaka University, who had been performing allogeneic skin grafting for burns, we developed various guidelines for tissue transplantation. These were recognized and approved by the MHLW, and in accordance with these guidelines, tissue transplantation can now proceed without legislation. As mentioned above, the procedure initially started out as "advanced medical treatment" and over the next 20 years developed until it was approved as an insured medical treatment in all fields in which it currently participates heart valves, blood vessels, skin, bone, amnion, and pancreatic islets. The guidelines of the Japanese Society for Tissue Transplantation have been translated into English and submitted to the WHO, forming the basis for tissue transplantation in Japan. On October 8, 2008, the Japanese Society for Tissue Transplantation and the East-West Tissue Transplant Network received the Health Culture Award and the MHLW Award. There are few academic societies that have received awards from the MHLW.

Currently, efforts are being made to close the contact between organ and tissue transplantation. First, the harvest of homografts for tissue transplantation from donor hearts unsuitable for heart transplantation is permitted through the establishment of mutual trust and cooperation between organ transplant coordinators (accredited by the Japan Organ Transplant Network) and tissue transplant coordinators (accredited by the Japanese Society for Tissue Transplantation). In addition, we have applied to obtain the permission from the MHLW, led by Satsuki Fukushima, Director of the Department of Cardiac Surgery at the NCVC, for the donation of valves and blood vessels from the hearts removed from heart transplant recipients, which can be cryopreserved or used as fresh tissue transplants. This method has been used in other countries for a long time and is called "recycle use" or "reuse." In Japan, most heart transplant recipients have advanced cardiomyopathy, and it is known that there are no pathological abnormalities in the aortic (valve) or pulmonary (valve) arteries of these patients. This finding has made donation from transplant recipients possible.

On the other hand, many recipient patients in Japan have been placed on a long-term LVAD and often suffer from aortic valve regurgitation. Therefore, the pulmonary artery (valve) is the best choice for donation from the recipient heart. Pulmonary artery homografts are very useful for the Ross operation and other congenital heart disease surgery. I consider it the best procedure for young women of childbearing potential, as they can exercise and conceive after the Ross operation and there is no need for warfarin or oral medication, and it has been proven to be quite successful. Pediatric cardiac surgeons have also found the pulmonary artery homograft very useful in the Norwood operation. Moreover, a new surgical procedure called "Partial Heart Transplantation" has recently begun utilizing the fresh homografts. Donation of homografts from the cardiac transplant recipients is quite appropriate for this purpose. As is well known, organ and tissue transplantation are legally integrated in foreign developed countries, but in Japan they are separated. However, if the medical and healthcare communities are united, they can work together. I hope that an organ and tissue transplant system that does not lag the international community will be established and that the trend of helping each other will expand. I am convinced that the contribution of the graduates of the former FDS of Osaka University is very significant in many areas of transplantation medicine.

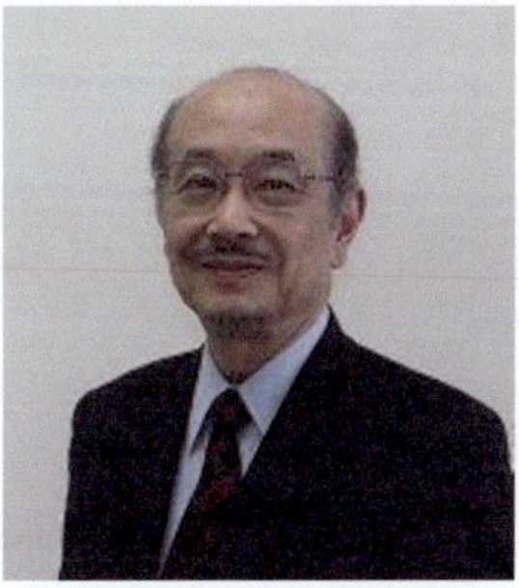

Osaka, Japan Soichiro Kitamura

Preface

In 2022, we celebrated the 100th anniversary of our department, the First Department of Surgery of Osaka University Medical School, since Professor Fritz Härtel was invited from Germany in 1922. Also, considering the quarter-century milestone since the breakthrough of brain-dead donor (BDD) heart transplantation was performed in our department in 1999, we decided to organize the publication of a book on the historical development and current status of heart and lung transplantation performed by our group. Although our achievements are limited in terms of the number of transplants performed, we thought it is important to review the historical development in order to consider the next steps for organizing the frontline strategy of heart and lung transplantation in Japan.

This book, contributed by our colleagues, covers the historical steps to develop heart and lung organ transplantation from BDD, focusing on the efforts of our surgical department, which is currently one of the leading institutes for heart/lung transplantation in Japan. In addition, we invited our colleagues working abroad to make this book more international in scope. The international contributors are from Columbia University Irving Medical Center (New York, NY), Texas Children's Hospital (Houston, Texas), University of Pittsburgh (Pittsburgh, PA), Stanford University (Stanford, CA), and Hannover Medical School (Hannover, Germany).

After a historical overview of our activities to revitalize heart transplantation, we describe our research on organ preservation and mechanical circulatory support. In particular, mechanical circulatory support with ventricular assist devices (VADs) has been actively pursued with the introduction of implantable VADs prior to the introduction of heart transplantation, establishing the strategy of bridge to heart transplantation.

In clinical achievements of heart and lung transplantation from BDD, we have performed 184 heart transplants, including 3 combined heart and lung transplants, and 83 lung transplants from BDD. In heart transplantation, the 5-, 10-, and 15-year survival rates are 93.8%, 89.0%, and 79.7%, respectively, with the longest survival being 24 years. All three patients of combined heart-lung transplantation are alive up to 16 years post-transplant. For lung transplantation from BDD, the 5- and 10-year survival rates are 76.6% and 70.6% for single lung transplantation, and for bilateral lung transplantation, the 10-year survival rate is as excellent as 80.8%.

The "Future Perspectives" is the main part of this book and discusses recent advances in organ preservation, exploring the mechanism of immune response and immunotolerance. In lung transplantation, its specific immune system and CLAD (chronic lung allograft dysfunction) are discussed in this part. As one of the newly developed strategies to overcome the donor shortage, use of donors after cardiac death (DCD), particularly of controlled DCD, is rapidly growing in international programs, and updates will be presented from Stanford for heart and Pittsburgh for lung transplantation. Simultaneous heart and abdominal organ transplantation has controversial issues in terms of medical and surgical burden including donor shortage, and the current status of combined heart and kidney transplantation is presented from NY.

The development of VADs continues to be an important issue in cardiac transplantation, and the fastest-growing area is pediatric use. In pediatric cardiomyopathy, the EXCOR Berlin Heart has been introduced in Japan and its contribution is well appreciated. In complex congenital heart disease, the latest cutting-edge information from Houston will be presented. Finally, xenotransplantation will be covered with the latest information from basic research on the development of genetically modified pigs.

We hope that this project will serve as a primer for medical students and young surgeons interested in heart and lung transplantation, as well as useful information for researchers interested in organ transplantation and related scientific fields.

This book is a tribute to the late Professor Yoshio Ozawa and the late Professor Hisao Manabe. I would also like to express my deepest gratitude to my mentor, Professor Emeritus Dr. Yasunaru Kawashima, who guided us from the beginning to establish the system for heart and lung transplantation, and to Professor Emeritus Dr. Ryota Shirakura, my friend, who devoted himself to establishing the support system for the smooth start of heart transplantation as described here.

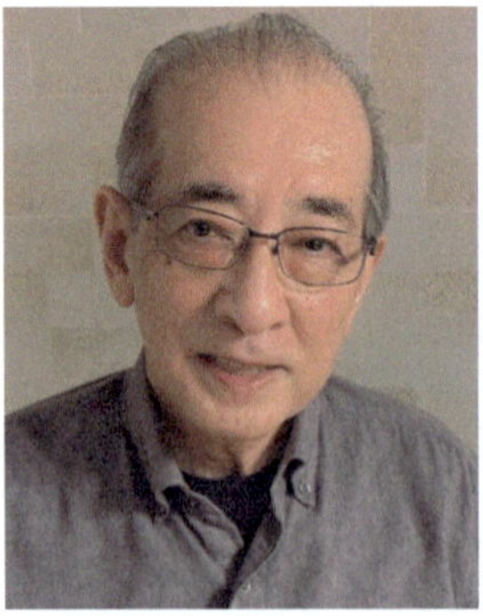

Osaka, Japan Hikaru Matsuda

Contents

About the Editors and Contributors

About the Editors

Dr. Hikaru Matsuda is a Professor Emeritus at the University of Osaka. He has served as the charirman and professor of the First Department of Surgery, the University of Osaka from 1991 to 2005. During his professorship, the first heart transplantation under legislation from brain-dead donor in 1999 and also performed the first lung transplantation from brain-dead donor in 2000 with Dr. Shin-ichiro Miyoshi. He also dedicated in the introduction of implantable ventricular assist devices in Japan during early 1990s. Currently, working of adult congenital heart disease and introduction DCD.

Prof. Shigeru Miyagawa Since July 2021, Dr. Shigeru Miyagawa has led the Department of Cardiovascular Surgery at the University of Osaka as Professor and Chairman. Along with continuing to perform a wide range of cardiovascular surgeries and train young surgeons, he has made significant contributions to regenerative medicine research for heart failure through an iPS cell-based approach and medical device development. Recently, he pioneered AI- and IoT-driven surgical technologies and is working to introduce the next generation of artificial hearts in Japan. In the field of transplantation, he promotes donation after circulatory death (DCD) to address organ shortages. His accomplishments exemplify translational research that bridges innovative science and patient care.

Dr. Yasushi Shintani has been Professor and Chair of General Thoracic Surgery at the University of Osaka since 2019 and also serves as Director of the Respiratory Center at its affiliated hospital. He specializes in surgery for respiratory diseases and lung transplantation, including lung cancer, emphysema, and mediastinal tumors. His department is a nationally designated center for both brain-dead and living-donor lung transplantation. In his research career, the research focuses have been on tumor microenvironments, cancer metastasis, ischemia-reperfusion injury, and lung regeneration. Dr. Shintani has authored over 200 peer-reviewed papers and is a recognized leader in both thoracic oncology and transplantation medicine.

About the Contributors

Dr. Yasunaru Kawashima is the honorary president of the National Cerebral and Cardiovascular Center and the professor emeritus at the University of Osaka. From 1978 to 1991, he was the chairman and professor of the First Department of Surgery at the University of Osaka, and he started to organize the platform for heart transplantation reaching to settle the new legislation in 1997. He dedicated himself to promoting heart transplantation in Japan as a lifetime work. He is also well known as a world-famous congenital heart surgeon.

Dr. Soichiro Kitamura is a disciple of Professors Manabe and Kawashima at the First Department of Surgery, Osaka University and is an internationally renowned cardiac surgeon. He is particularly known as an authority on pediatric coronary artery bypass surgery utilizing the internal thoracic artery. At the National Cerebral and Cardiovascular Center (NCVC, Suita, Japan), he played a pivotal role in initiating and spreading of heart transplantation in Japan, inventing the modified bicaval anastomosis which has become the most utilized technique for orthotopic heart transplantation worldwide. Dr. Kitamura is currently a President Emeritus of the NCVC and has also dedicated to advancing tissue transplantation with homograft valves in Japan.

Dr. Jon Kobashigawa is the director of the Advanced Heart Disease Section and the Heart Transplant Program at the Cedars-Sinai Medical Center in Los Angeles, California. He has been a professor of medicine at Cedars-Sinai since 2010. As an internationally renowned leader in heart transplantation, he is dedicated to promoting heart and lung transplantation as a past president of the International Society of Heart and Lung Transplantation (ISHLT). In 2023, he received the ISHLT Lifetime Achievement Award. Furthermore, he has supported the development of Japan's heart transplantation system since its start.

Contributors

Iki Adachi Texas Children's Hospital, Michael E. DeBakey Department of Surgery, Baylor College of Medicine, Houston, TX, USA

Yasuhiro Akazawa Department of Cardiovascular Medicine, The University of Osaka Graduate School of Medicine Suita, Osaka, Japan

Junsang Cho Texas Children's Hospital, Michael E. DeBakey Department of Surgery, Baylor College of Medicine, Houston, TX, USA

Hiroshi Eguchi Department of Pediatric Surgery, The University of Osaka Graduate School of Medicine, Suita, Osaka, Japan

Satsuki Fukushima Division of Adult Cardiac Surgery, National Cerebral and Cardiovascular Center, Suita, Osaka, Japan

Soichiro Funaki Department of Thoracic Surgery, Hyogo Medical University Nishinomiya, Hyogo, Japan

Masaki Hirose Department of Pediatrics, The University of Osaka Graduate School of Medicine, Suita, Osaka, Japan

Masayoshi Inoue Division of Thoracic Surgery, Department of Surgery, Kyoto Prefectural University of Medicine, Kyoto, Japan

Hidekazu Ishida Department of Pediatrics, The University of Osaka Graduate School of Medicine, Suita, Osaka, Japan

Ryo Ishii Department of Pediatrics, The University of Osaka Graduate School of Medicine, Suita, Osaka, Japan

Toshinori Ito Osaka Center for Cancer and Cardiovascular Disease Prevention, Osaka, Osaka, Japan

Shigemitsu Iwai Department of Pediatric Cardiovascular Surgery, National Cerebral and Cardiovascular Center, Suita, Osaka, Japan

Satoshi Kainuma Division of Adult Cardiac Surgery, National Cerebral and Cardiovascular Center, Suita, Osaka, Japan

Chizu Kamon Department of Transplantation Medicine, The University of Osaka Hospital, Suita, Osaka, Japan

Takashi Kanou Department of General Thoracic Surgery, The University of Osaka Graduate School of Medicine, Suita, Osaka, Japan

Takashi Kido Department of Cardiovascular Surgery, The University of Osaka Graduate School of Medicine, Suita, Osaka, Japan

Motoki Komori Department of Pediatric Cardiovascular Surgery, National Cerebral and Cardiovascular Center, Suita, Osaka, Japan

Kaori Kubota Department of Transplantation Medicine, The University of Osaka Hospital, Suita, Osaka, Japan

Akira Maeda Department of Pediatric Surgery, The University of Osaka Graduate School of Medicine, Suita, Osaka, Japan

Takafumi Masai Osaka Keisatsu Hospital, Osaka, Japan

Hikaru Matsuda Professor Emeritus, The University of Osaka, Suita, Osaka, Japan

Goro Matsumiya Department of Cardiovascular Surgery, Chiba University Graduate School of Medicine, Chiba, Japan

Katsuyoshi Matsunami Graduate School of Biomedical and Health Sciences (Pharmaceutical Sciences) Hiroshima University, Hiroshima, Japan

Masato Minami Ashiya Municipal Hospital, Ashiya, Hyogo, Japan

Shigeru Miyagawa Department of Cardiovascular Surgery, The University of Osaka Graduate School of Medicine, Suita, Osaka, Japan

Shuji Miyagawa Department of Pediatric Surgery, The University of Osaka Graduate School of Medicine Suita, Osaka, Japan

Yuji Miyamoto Otemae Hospital, Osaka, Japan

Shinichiro Miyoshi Koseikai Memorial Hospital, Osaka, Japan

Jun Narita Department of Pediatrics, The University of Osaka Graduate School of Medicine, Suita, Osaka, Japan

Yoshifumi Naka Department of Cardiothoracic Surgery, Cornell University Medical Center, New York City, New York, USA

Tomoyuki Nakagiri Department of Cardiothoracic Transplantation and Vascular Surgery, Hannover Medical School, Hannover, Germany

Motonobu Nishimura Kawasaki Hospital, Kobe, Hyogo, Japan

Meinoshin Okumura National Hospital Organization Osaka Toneyama Medical Center, Toyonaka, Osaka, Japan

Hiroomi Okuyama Department of Pediatric Surgery, The University of Osaka Graduate School of Medicine, Suita, Osaka, Japan

Shunsuke Saito Department of Cardiovascular Surgery, The University of Osaka Graduate School of Medicine, Suita, Osaka, Japan

Taichi Sakaguchi Department of Cardiovascular Surgery, Hyogo Medical University, Nishinomiya, Hyogo, Japan

Yasushi Sakata Department of Cardiovascular Surgery, The University of Osaka Graduate School of Medicine, Suita, Osaka, Japan

Yoshiki Sawa Osaka Keisatsu Hospital, Osaka, Japan

Fusako Sera Department of Cardiovascular Surgery, The University of Osaka Graduate School of Medicine, Suita, Osaka, Japan

Masafumi Shibata Department of Cardiothoracic Surgery, Stanford University, Stanford, CA, USA

Norihisa Shigemura Division of Cardiothoracic Transplantation, University of Pittsburgh, Pittsburgh, PA, USA

Yasushi Shintani Department of General Thoracic Surgery, The University of Osaka Graduate School of Medicine, Suita, Osaka, Japan

Ryota Shirakura The University of Osaka, Suita, Osaka, Japan

Yasuhiro Shudo Department of Cardiothoracic Surgery, Stanford University Stanford, CA, USA

Kota Suzuki Division of Adult Cardiac Surgery, National Cerebral and Cardiovascular Center, Suita, Osaka, Japan

Koji Takeda Department of Cardiothoracic Surgery, Columbia University Irving Medical Center, New York, NY, USA

Masaki Taira Department of Cardiovascular Surgery, The University of Osaka Graduate School of Medicine, Suita, Osaka, Japan

Koichi Toda Department of Cardiovascular Surgery, Dokkyo Medical University Saitama Medical Center, Koshigaya, Saitama, Japan

Yuji Tominaga Department of Pediatric Cardiovascular Surgery, National Cerebral and Cardiovascular Center, Suita, Osaka, Japan

Yasumasa Tsukamoto Department of Transplant Medicine, National Cerebral and Cardiovascular Center, Suita, Osaka, Japan

Takayoshi Ueno Division of Health Sciences, The University of Osaka Graduate School of Medicine, Suita, Osaka, Japan

Takuji Watanabe Department of Cardiovascular Surgery, The University of Osaka Graduate School of Medicine, Suita, Osaka, Japan

Yasushi Yoshikawa Division of Cardiovascular Surgery, Tottori University Faculty of Medicine, Yonago, Tottori, Japan

Daisuke Yoshioka Department of Cardiovascular Surgery, The University of Osaka Graduate School of Medicine, Suita, Osaka, Japan

Alice V. Vinogradsky Department of Cardiothoracic Surgery, Columbia University Irving Medical Center, New York, NY, USA

Part I

Historical Review

Heart and Lung Transplantation in Japan: How Prepared and What to Do Now

1

Hikaru Matsuda and Ryota Shirakura

Abstract

Brain-dead donor (BDD) organ transplantation has been accepted worldwide as the last line of treatment for end-stage organ failure. Heart transplantation (HT) is the key to this because it basically requires BDD. In Japan, HT was resumed under the transplantation legislation in 1999 at Osaka University and National Cardiovascular Center, almost 30 years after the first case at Sapporo in 1968. Initially, the number of BDD was very limited, but after the revision of the law settled in 2010, the annual number of HT from BDD increased to nearly 100 per year, and the cumulative number has reached 958 as of April 2025 in the national base. Lung transplantation (LT) from BDD in Japan also started in 2000 with two single LTs by Osaka University and Tohoku University groups with success. Thereafter, the number of LT from BDD has increased, reaching a total of 1037 as of April 2025. This review describes the historical development of heart and lung transplantation from BDD in the view of how people worked to the breakthrough for the new era of organ transplantation, and introduces our achievements during the early phase of organ transplantation from brain-dead donor at Osaka University.

Keywords

Brain death · Heart transplantation · Lung transplantation · Brain-dead donor · DCD · Living-related donor · View of life and death · Istanbul declaration · Donor pool expansion

H. Matsuda (✉) · R. Shirakura
Yoshiken-kai Shion Hospital, Osaka, Japan

The University of Osaka, Suita, Osaka, Japan
e-mail: hmatsudahuhs@gmail.com; shirakura.r@gmail.com

H. Matsuda et al. (eds.), *Heart and Lung Transplantation*,
https://doi.org/10.1007/978-981-96-8810-4_1

1.1 Introduction

Organ transplantation from brain-dead donors (DBD) is well established worldwide. In Japan, due to cultural and religious reasons, there has been a social attitude against organ transplantation from heart-beating donors (DBD). The first case of heart transplantation (HT) performed at Sapporo in 1968 caused serious negative effects on the pursuit of subsequent organ transplantation from BDD. In 1999, almost 30 years after the Sapporo case, HT was resumed, spending a long social debate on the issue of brain death as human death. This report attempts to review the historical background and the steps taken to resume HT from DBD, and also to analyze the current status of organ transplantation in Japan.

1.2 Background

The first human-to-human HT was performed by Christian Barnard in Cape Town, South Africa, in December 1967. The following year, more than 100 heart transplants were performed worldwide, including a Japanese case. The first HT in Japan was performed by Professor Wada in Sapporo in 1968, the year after the world's first case, and this Japanese case was the 30th in the world. However, the initial result of HT in the world was not as expected, and the number gradually decreased in the following years. The reason for this poor initial result was mainly due to the immature immunosuppressive therapy. The first Japanese patient died of infection 83 days after transplantation, but the survival time was longer than other HT in the world at that time.

In detail, Professor Wada's HT was performed in a closed environment within the surgical department of Sapporo Medical College, and there were many uncertainties regarding the determination of brain death and the indications for transplantation. At that time, when the understanding of brain death in Japan was still immature and the view of life and death was reluctant to accept brain death as human death, the media coverage tended to criticize Sapporo's case. The negative impact of this first case on society was so severe that HT was blocked for a long time, and it took 30 years before HT was resumed in February 1999 [1].

Another important point to be mentioned about the background of organ transplantation in Japan is the existence of living-related organ donation. In particular, partial liver transplantation from living donors has been the main strategy overwhelming BDD liver transplantation. In 2022, 336 living donor liver transplants and 86 BDD liver transplants were performed [2]. Under the strictly limited BDD, this living-related organ donation strategy has been an important alternative in liver and kidney transplantation. However, this issue of living-related organ donation is rather controversial from the international point of view, as the 2018 version of the Istanbul Declaration on Organ Trafficking and Transplant Tourism states that efforts to initiate or enhance deceased donor transplantation are essential to minimize the burden on living donors [3].

1.3 Experimental Works

Professor Yoshio Ozawa was the second chairman following Professor Fritz Härtel, who was invited from Germany in 1922, but he was the actual founder of the First Department of Surgery at Osaka University (OU). During his tenure from 1930 to 1959, animal experiments were conducted on organ transplantation, especially lung transplantation (LT) in the 1950s. As a remarkable achievement, Professor Ozawa attempted to treat right ventricular wall injury by direct suturing in a patient in 1937. This was the first case of direct treatment of cardiac injury and led to the great controversy with Dr. Tohru Sakakibara of Okayama. One year earlier, Dr. Sakakibara had performed the first successful cardiac surgery using gauze compression hemostasis for the right ventricular injury. The debate focused on compression hemostasis versus direct suturing as the treatment of choice for cardiac injury. This controversy continued for several years, overwhelming academic concerns, and was actually encouraged to start cardiac surgery in Japan.

In the following era, some experimental work on heart preservation was done in the 1970s. Shigekazu Okamoto had the idea to reanimate the cadaver heart by coronary reperfusion. A canine model consisted of 60 min of warm ischemia after exsanguination, and coronary reperfusion was performed with warm whole blood using three different strategies; in-situ perfusion using cardiopulmonary bypass circuit, ex vivo perfusion of extracted heart, and ex vivo model of heart and lung block. After reperfusion, the functional and metabolic status of the heart was examined, and as a result, the first model, in-situ reperfusion, was superior to the other two models. These experimental works suggested the possibility of using cadaver heart, non-heart-beating donor (NHBD), for HT. This in-situ reperfusion was the method used by Dr. Barnard in the world's first case. Okamoto's work was published in 1984 [4], and the results also suggested that this method could be an alternative to BDD as NHBD, which was not realistic at that time in the 1970s.

Later, the above method was followed by researches led by Shirakura and his colleagues in the 1990s [5, 6], providing 24-h cold storage of canine heart from NHBD. In lung preservation, Akashi [7] also reported the unique strategy of protecting the cadaver lung from warm ischemia by introducing lung ventilation with room air. However, the clinical application of such a strategy was not done because the preparation for transplantation from BDD had advanced nationwide in the 1990s. Interestingly, the above-described method of NHBD has become the current important strategy as DCD (donor after circulatory death) to expand the donor pool.

1.4 Preparation to Start Heart and Lung Transplantation

In the 1980s, transplant-related academic societies began to move toward the resumption of HT, and the establishment of a system began to take shape, albeit gradually. In the field of HT, the Japanese Society of Heart Transplantation was founded in 1983 by Drs. Kawashima, Koyanagi, and Taira, which developed criteria for accreditation of institutions. At the national level, social consensus building progressed, but eventually legislation became mandatory, making it difficult for a single institution to take the lead in implementation.

After many twists and turns, the law was passed by the Diet in October 1997, and implementation soon began. A system for institutional accreditation, indication criteria, and organ allocation was also established under the commitment of the Ministry of Health, and a large convoy system consisting of three institutions approved for HT, OU, National Cardiovascular Center (NCVC), and Tokyo Women's Medical College, was initiated. In addition, the organ sharing system organized by the Japan Organ Transplant Network (JOT) was started. Regarding the institutions approved for HT, University of Tokyo, Tohoku University, and Kyushu University were registered from 2002 to 2003 before the revision of transplantation law in 2010.

Along with these nationwide actions, we need to establish the support system for the possible candidates for HT even if the legislation is not settled. In this setting, we introduced the ventricular assist device (VAD) for long-term support over months. The initiation of clinical application of VADs was by extracorporeal pulsatile device such as Toyobo LVAD (Toyobo Inc. Osaka, Japan) which was designed for acute cardiogenic shock, but we applied this VAD to chronic heart failure in cardiomyopathy patients. Then, pulsatile implantable VADs were introduced from the USA [8]. One of the implantable VADs, Novacor wearable electrically driven pulsatile pump, was used in the first case of HT under the legislation [1]. Since then, a bridge-to-transplant strategy with VAD has been established in Japan under the very limited donor (details can be found in Chap. 4 of this book).

For LT, the system was established in collaboration with related academic societies, and institutional accreditation was granted to 4 university hospitals, Tohoku University, Kyoto University, Okayama University, and Osaka University, and the registration of recipients was started in October 1998. In the above-mentioned decision, our LT team was qualified as having strong cooperation with the heart transplantation team in the same department. These historic steps in our surgical department were made possible by years of efforts from the laboratory to the clinical arena to start organ transplantation in our hands.

1.5 Start of Heart and Lung Transplantation

After the enactment of the organ transplantation law, it took another year and a half before a legally approved brain-dead donor became available, and the first HT from BDD was performed at OU in February 1999 [1], and the second and third transplantations were performed by Dr. Kitamura at the NCVC [9]. In LT, single LT was performed at OU [10] and Tohoku University [11] in March of 2000 from single BDD.

HT and LT started smoothly, and the number of organ donations was expected to increase thereafter. However, donations from BDD were limited because the law was very strict in defining DBD. In 2010, the law was finally amended to allow donation with the consent of the family in cases where the donor did not have a living will (Table 1.1). Additionally, donation from a donor under the age of 15 became

Table 1.1 Comparison between the original and amended version of organ transplantation law

	Original Law 1997	Revised Law 2010
Donor's written consent	Must	Optional
Family's consent	Must	Must
Age limitation (donor)	Only for over 15 years	No limit[a]
Optional for recipient	Not written	Priority to family[b]
Donor from age < 15 years	Not written	Preferred to child recipient

[a]>12 weeks of age
[b]only for the kidney

Table 1.2 Summary of first cases of heart and lung transplantation done at Osaka University Hospital

	Heart transplantation	Lung transplantation
Patient; age, sex	43 years old, male	48 years old, female
Basic disease	Dilated phase of HCM	IPF
Duration of disease	Since 1991, medical treatment for heart failure	SOB started 1990, right heart developed starting oxygen therapy in 1995.
Hospitalization Waiting period	Since 1997 with inotropes 502 days (Status-1)	Since 1999/10 because dyspnea has increased. 580 days
VAD	Novacor since 1998/10	NA
Transplantation	Orthotopic HT Done on 1999/2	Single LT (left) Done on 2000/3
Donor: Matching, donor vs recipient Total ischemic time	BDD, distant (200 Km) BW: 55 vs 61 kg 3 h 24 min	BDD, distant (500Km) Predicted VC, 64%[a] 5 h 37 min
Post transplantation	Uneventful	Uneventful
Discharge Condition Follow-up	75 POD Back to daily life Survived 10 years	62 POD Back to daily life Survived 23 years

[a]donor left lung's predicted vital capacity (VC) to the recipient VC. *HCM* hypertrophic cardiomyopathy, *IPF* idiopathic pulmonary fibrosis. *SOB* shortness of breath, *POD* postoperative day, others, see text

possible, opening the door to children in need of heart and lung donation. The summary of each of the first cases of HT and LT in the OU is presented in Table 1.2. The first case of HT survived 10 years and LT case for 23 years, respectively.

1.6 After Revision of the Law

After the revision of the law in 2010, the number of brain-dead organ donations increased and finally exceeded 100 cases per year in 2023 (Fig. 1.1). The number of HTs and LTs also increased each year, as shown in this figure. By April 2025, the number of HTs from BDD has reached 958 nationwide, and the number of LTs has reached 1013. The characteristic point seen here is the high number of single-donor organ procurement as high as 4.48 (organs per donor) as a whole in 2023, and after

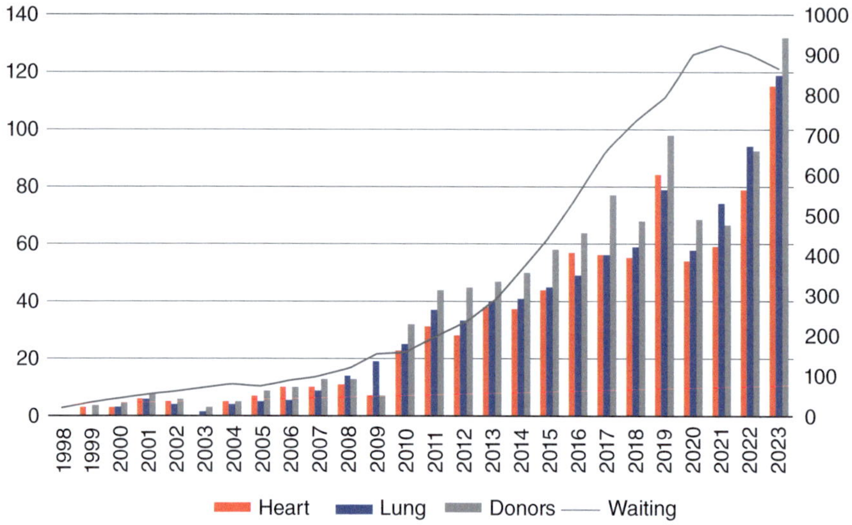

Fig. 1.1 Annual number of heart and lung transplantation, organ donation from brain dead donor (left bar in numbers), with number of patients on waiting list for heart transplantation (right bar in numbers). (Data from Ref. [12])

2010, the average number of donated organs per donor was 80.5% for heart and 85.7% for lung procurement. This result shows how people made maximum efforts to obtain as many valuable organs as possible under the severe shortage of donors. These data were obtained from the JOT website [12].

1.7 Outcome

A brief summary of the long-term prognosis of the first cases of HT and LT is presented here. Between the first case in 1999 and the revision of the law in 2010, the OU performed 19 HTs over a 10-year period. Of these, 14 patients are now surviving for more than 15 years with the longest surviving for 25 years. The case of combined heart and lung transplantation has been followed for 16 years now (see the details in Chaps. 7 and 9 in this book). Notably, in HT alone, all but one were bridged by VADs, mostly of the pulsatile type including the extracorporeal Toyobo VAD (Table 1.3).

Long-term waiting period as Stautus-1 mostly on VADs ranged from 356 to 1166 days (average 710). Here, we can see how people worked hard to prevent complications during the support by VADs to keep the waiting status as good as possible to reach transplantation [8].

In LT from BDD, as of November 2023, 78 patients had received LT and 3 had combined heart and lung transplantation at our department. The transplantation procedure was single LT in 43 patients and bilateral (double) LT in 35 patients. Of these, 8 patients have survived more than 15 years, and 6, including one heart and lung case, are still alive (Table 1.3). In terms of transplantation procedure, the late

Table 1.3 Summary of 12 patients surviving over 15 years after bridged HT by VADs

Total number	12 patients
Follow-up period	15–25 years
Status-1 period (mostly on VAD)	356–1166 days (average 710 days)
Devices used	
Extracorporeal VAD (Toyobo)	4
Novacor	4
HeartMate IP	1
Continuous flow durable VAD	3 Jarvik2000 ×2, EVAHEART ×1

Table 1.4 Comparison of the survival rates in lung transplantation (LTx) from BDD divided by the procedures at Osaka University

Procedure	Patients number	5-year survival rate	10-year survival rate
Single LTx	43	77.0%	67.0%
Double LTx	35	80.8%	80.8%
Heart/lung	3	100%	100 ($N = 2$)%

death after 15 years of survival was developed only in single LT, and bilateral (double) transplantation has been proved for its durable nature (Table 1.4).

The details of this part are also described in Chaps. 7 and 8.

1.8 How to Expand the Donor Pool

While nearly 5000 heart transplants are performed annually in the world, the number in Japan is extraordinarily low, at just over 100 per year. As shown here, the shortage of donors is serious, and the organ donation rate per million population is less than 1.0, a clear difference from the international level. A national effort to increase the number of donors to at least three per million population per year (three times to the current level) is desirable.

As the background of the social attitude to brain death, the "view of life and death" in general may be part of the reason, but the willingness to donate the organ has not been low in social studies, as over 40% of people accept. Therefore, the refinement of the national organ donation system, such as increasing the number of donor hospitals and, more importantly, donor coordinators, is very crucial to obtain the organ from the possible candidates without wasting the valuable organs. Another thing to consider is to revise the allocation system of donor hearts, which has been holding the classical scheme of status 1 and 2 without putting status 1A, resulting in the significant, not negligible number of deaths on the waiting list in HT [12]. In other words, the systematic analysis of waiting list mortality is crucial to change the allocation system [13].

Meanwhile, an internationally growing strategy to expand the donor pool is the use of DCD donors. Pioneering reports on its application for HT have been published from the United Kingdom and Australia in 2018 to 2019 [14, 15]. The strategy consists of withdrawal of life-sustaining therapy and determination of death by circulatory-determined death. Since then, it has made steady progress in Europe and the United States, and has achieved results comparable to those of DBD [16, 17].

In LT, the DCD strategy is also growing and a recent report analyzed UNOS data in the USA between May 1, 2005 and December 31, 2021 [18]. Of the 21,356 recipients who received LT, 95.4% were from BDD and 976 cases (4.6%) were from DCD. Survival analysis showed no difference in survival between the two groups. As the basic issues surrounding DCD organ transplantation, there are institutional and ethical issues in determining death. However, we believe that this method should be considered in Japan, where there is a severe shortage of donors [19, 20].

1.9 Summary

This article reviews the historical steps to establish heart and lung transplantation from BDD in Japan and points out the difficult background of the cultural background related to the "view of life and death," which opposes the acceptance of brain death as human death. After the revision of the original organ transplantation law in 2010, the number of DBDs has actually increased, but it is still very limited as below 200 per year. We need to refine the old organ donation system as well as the donor allocation system to maximize the harvest of donor organs and reduce the number of waiting list deaths. DCD, organ preservation by machine perfusion, VAD for bridge to recovery, regenerative approach, and xenotransplantation are the next targets in organ transplantation, especially for heart and lung transplantation. I hope that this review can help young researchers and people interested in organ transplantation to understand the fundamental issues to be overcome in organ transplantation.

Acknowledgments I would like to take this opportunity to thank all those who have worked hard together toward this goal, understanding that most of the colleagues involved could not be present at the actual site of transplantation.

References

1. Matsuda H, Fukushima N, Sawa Y, et al. First brain dead donor heart transplantation under new legislation in Japan. Jpn J Thorac Cardiovasc Surg. 1999;47:499–505.
2. Liver transplantation in Japan—registry by the Japanese Liver Transplantation Society. Jpn J Transplant. 2023; 58:339–355. (Abstract in English).
3. Declaration of Istanbul on Organ Trafficking and Transplant Tourism (2018 Edition) . http://www.declarationofistanbul.org/. Accessed 21 Aug 2024.
4. Okamoto S. Experimental studies on the resuscitation of cadaver hearts in dogs. The comparison of three methods utilizing normothermic coronary perfusion with whole blood Jpn J Thorac Cardiovasc Surg 1974;22:588–602. (Abstract in English).
5. Shirakura R, Matsuda H, Nakata S, et al. Prolonged preservation of cadaver heart with Belzer UW solution: 24-hour storage system for asphyxiated canine heart. Eur Surg Res. 1990;22:197–206.

6. Naka Y, Shirakura R, Matsuda H, et al. Canine heart-lung transplantation after 24-hour hypothermic preservation. Eur J Cardiothorac Surg. 1990;4:499–503.
7. Akashi A, Nakahara K, Kamiike W, et al. Attenuation of warm ischemic injury of a rat lung by inflation with room air. Transplantation. 1993;55:24–30.
8. Matsuda H. Development of ventricular assist device and heart transplantation in Japan: how people worked. Artif Organs. 2020;44:544–60.
9. Kitamura S, Nakatani T, Yagihara T, et al. Cardiac transplantation under new legislation for organ transplantation in Japan: report of two cases. Jpn Circ J. 2000;64:333–9.
10. Miyoshi S, Minmi M, Ohta M, et al. Single lung transplantation from brain-dead donor for a patient with idiopathic pulmonary fibrosis. A breakthrough after new legislation in Japan. Jpn J Thorac Cardiovasc Surg. 2001;49:398–403.
11. Fujimura S, Kondo T. The lung transplantation has come to be done in Japan. Kyobu Geka. 2000;53:986–91. (Abstract in English)
12. Number of organ donation and transplantation in Japan. Japan Organ Transplantation Network. https://www.jotnw.or.jp/data/offer03.php. Accessed 15 Aug 2025.
13. Matsuda H. Nationwide analysis of the mortality on the waiting list for heart transplantation; implication for revision of the heart allocation system in Japan. Jpn J Transplant. 2019;54:291–8. (Abstract in English).
14. White CW, Messer SJ, Large SR, et al. Transplantation of hearts donated after circulatory death. Front Cardiovasc Med. 2018;5:1–20.
15. Chew HC, Iyer A, Connellan M, et al. Outcomes of donation after circulatory death heart transplantation in Australia. J Am Coll Cardiol. 2019;73:1447–59.
16. Donors recovered in the US by Donor Type (heart). OPTN (Organ Procurement and Transplant Network). https://optn.transplant.hrsa.gov/data/view-data-reports/national-data/ Accessed 20 Jan 2025.
17. Schroder JN, Patel CB, DeVore AD, et al. Transplantation outcomes with donor hearts after circulatory death. N Engl J Med. 2023;388:2121–31.
18. Furukawa M, Noda K, Chan EG, et al. Lung transplantation from donation after circulatory death, evolution, and current status in the United States. Clin Transpl. 2023;37(3):e14884. https://doi.org/10.1111/ctr.14884.
19. Matsuda H, Shintani Y, Miyagawa S. Current international status of organ donation after circulatory death viewed from heart and lung transplantation: expanding the donor pool by cross-sectional action among transplant organs. Jpn J Transplant 2022;57:163–8. (Abstract in English).
20. Matsuda. Why is organ transplantation from cardiac death donors necessary in Japan? J Artif Organs. https://doi.org/10.1007/s10047-025-01493-z.

Part II

Organ Preservation

Heart Preservation: Myocardial Protection, Cardioplegic Arrest, Controlled Reperfusion, and Transplantation

2

Hikaru Matsuda, Shigeru Miyagawa, Yoshiki Sawa, and Ryota Shirakura

Abstract

Heart transplantation encompasses a wide range of issues, including basic medical and immunological research, ethics, and sophisticated clinical strategies, with prolonged heart preservation and prevention of ischemia/reperfusion injury being the most important issues. The heart preservation strategy is closely related to myocardial protection in routine cardiac surgery, which has a long history of development. In this article, our efforts at Osaka University were reviewed from the aspects of developing myocardial protection and strategy for vulnerable targets such as neonatal hearts, preoperatively damaged hearts, left ventricular hypertrophy, and in heart transplantation. Recognizing the role of activated neutrophils in reperfusion injury, we developed the system of leukocyte-depleted terminal cardioplegia. This strategy has also applied to clinical heart transplantation. On the otherhand, during the period before the resumption of heart transplantation from brain-dead donors, we conducted experimental studies for the possible clinical start of heart transplantation from donors after cardiac death (non-heart-beating donor) covering 24-hour cold storage. In summary, we hope

H. Matsuda (✉) · R. Shirakura
Yoshiken-kai Shion Hospital, Osaka, Japan

The University of Osaka, Suita, Osaka, Japan
e-mail: hmatsudahuhs@gmail.com; shirakura.r@gmail.com

S. Miyagawa
Department of Cardiovascular Surgery, The University of Osaka Graduate School of Medicine, Suita, Osaka, Japan
e-mail: miyagawa.shigeru.med@osaka-u.ac.jp

Y. Sawa
Osaka Keisatsu Hospital, Osaka, Japan

H. Matsuda et al. (eds.), *Heart and Lung Transplantation*,
https://doi.org/10.1007/978-981-96-8810-4_2

that our efforts described here can contribute to the current practice of myocardial preservation in heart transplantation.

Keywords

Myocardial protection · Cardioplegic solution · Controlled reperfusion · Leukocyte-depleted reperfusion · Heart transplantation · DCD · Mitochondrial change · Prolonged preservation

2.1 Introduction

In the long history of cardiac surgery, the development of the artificial heart-lung machine was the first step, and safe open-heart surgery using this extracorporeal machine led to significant advances in cardiac surgery in its early days in the 1970s to 1980s. In a new era of open-heart surgery, brain and heart protection was maintained by the introduction of hypothermia, and simple aortic occlusion under hypothermia was initiated. However, there were many cases of difficulty in weaning from extracorporeal circulation due to impaired ventricular and pulmonary function. Given the myocardial damage caused by cardiac arrest, it became an important issue for cardiac surgeons to minimize the damage to the myocardium caused by warm ischemia (stunned heart, stone heart), or in other words, to protect the myocardium as a base.

In the historical review, potassium-induced cardiac arrest was first introduced by Melrose [1] in 1975, and this concept has been the main concept until now. In the following era, the clinically relevant modifications were introduced by many cardiac surgeons and scientists, represented by Gay [2], Hearse [3], and others in the mid-1970s, and Hearse and his colleagues developed St. Thomas' cardioplegic solution in 1975. Since then, several modifications have been developed, such as warm blood cardioplegia, retrograde coronary sinus perfusion, and hot shot [4].

With the development of cardioplegic solutions (mainly potassium-based), it became clear that reperfusion injury plays an important role in addition to ischemic injury. As one of the mediators in this pathological phenomenon, neutrophil activation has been proposed as a key issue [5]. Thus, myocardial protection in cardiac surgery has evolved from the development of myocardial protection solutions to controlled reperfusion that manages reperfusion injury [6]. We have been conducting basic research and clinical applications of myocardial protection with the aim of establishing the safety of open heart surgery and developing heart preservation methods for heart transplantation. In fact, the cadaver heart reanimation method conducted in the early 1990s is the one currently used in donation after circulatory death (DCD).

The current status of myocardial protection is well advanced with the introduction of warm-blood cardioplegia, "hot-shot" as controlled reperfusion, and the development of new cardioplegic solutions. Here we reviewed our research on myocardial protection and preservation in cardiac surgery and transplantation, and look forward to further clinical development based on the leading basic research on myocardial protection in this exciting field.

2.2 Research on Myocardial Protection

In the 1980s, a new technique of myocardial protection using cardioplegia was introduced in cardiac surgery, and while the number of patients rapidly increased, postoperative cardiac dysfunction was one of the important problems to be solved. In one of the clinical studies on pediatric congenital heart disease, the changes in the structure of myocardial mitochondria in infants under the age of 2 years undergoing open-heart surgery were investigated using a potassium crystalloid cardioplegic solution [7]. The assessment of mitochondrial damage (structural damage) was performed on the biopsied myocardial specimen by electron microscopy with the permission of the family. As a result, we were able to show that mitochondrial structural damage developed after reperfusion, and in cases with prior heart failure, the damage was present before surgery and worsened after surgery.

The protection of the myocardium in children has also led to improvements in delivery methods and materials. For example, the administration of cardioplegic solutions was changed from multiple-dose to a single dose [8], and prostacyclin analogs were used as adjuvants to cardioplegia in pediatric cardiac surgery [9]. In adult cases, the clinically problematic issue was how to deal with severe myocardial injury (stone heart) after surgery in cases of myocardial hypertrophy, and we proposed an optimal dosage taking into account LV mass (left ventricular myocardial weight) obtained by ventriculography [10].

In the study of the mechanisms of ischemia-reperfusion injury, the following experimental work was carried out; prostacyclin analog [11], supplementation of nitric oxide to attenuate neutrophil activation [12], endogenous enhancement of heat shock protein 70 [13] and superoxide dismutase [14], decoy transfection against nuclear factor-kB [15, 16], diadenosine tetraphosphate (AP4A) [17], and TAT protein (TAT-BH4) that prevents apoptosis via Bcl-xL [18]. In particular, considerable evidences were obtained for the myocardial protective effects of hepatocyte growth factor (HGF) in ischemia/reperfusion injury [19–21], but it did not reach the stage of clinical application using human recombinant HGF at that time. These achievements were made before the introduction of warm-blood cardioplegia in the late 1990s, but we hope that our previous studies can be reevaluated for the refinement of myocardial protection strategies, including heart preservation in transplantation.

2.3 Development of Leukocyte-Depleted Reperfusion System

In the previous section, we presented the early stage of research on myocardial protection in cardiac surgery. As a result, the pathological phenomena after reperfusion were shown as the release of various cytokines due to neutrophil activation and endothelial damage in blood vessels [5, 6, 22, 23] (Table 2.1). Meanwhile, controlled reperfusion to resume oxygenation during cardiac arrest before releasing the aortic cross-clamp has been the main topic in cardiac surgery [24].

Table 2.1 The factors involved in neutrophil-mediated reperfusion injury

Factors	Role
C5a	Induction of neutrophil activation
P-selectin	PMN rolling
CD18 on PMN	PMN-EC and PMN-MC adhesion
ICAM-1 in EC/MC	Same as above
PECAM-1	PMN migration
Free radical	Aggravating factor for EC and MC
Elastase	Same as above

Source: Ref. [26] with permission
PMN polymorphonuclear neutrophil, *EC* endothelial cell, *MC* myocyte, *ICAM* intercellular adhesion molecule, *PECAM* platelet endothelial cellular adhesion molecule

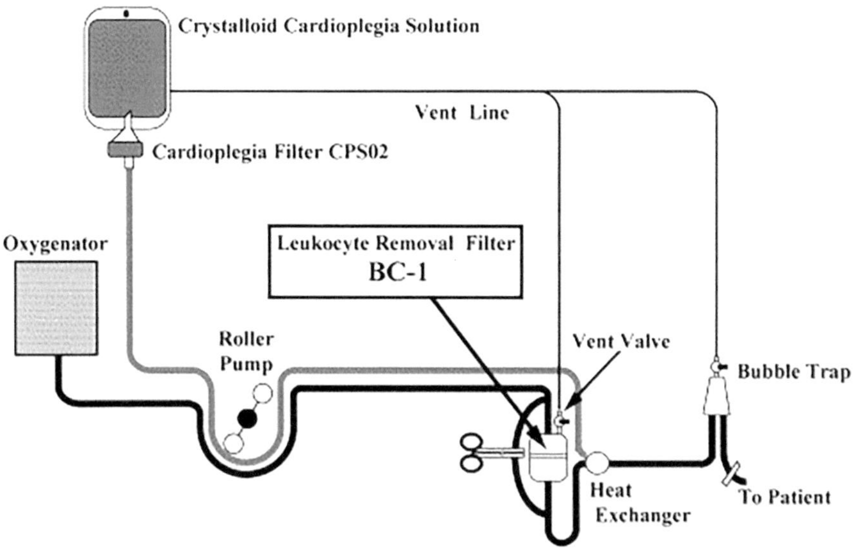

Fig. 2.1 Schematic of leukocyte-depleted blood cardioplegia procedure. *BC-1* Leukocyte Filter (Pall, East Hills, NY). (Source: Ref. [25] with permission).

In our strategy to prevent neutrophil damage during warm blood reperfusion, both pharmacological and physical removal methods were considered. Basic experiments on neutrophil removal and the search for a removal filter suitable for clinical use were conducted. Fortunately, a blood filter for clinical use (Cellsorba-80p, Asahi Medical Co., Tokyo, Japan) became available, and we planned to incorporate the filter into the myocardial perfusion circuit directly connected to the cardiopulmonary bypass circuit and apply it clinically as the method of leukocyte-depleted terminal cardioplegia (LDTC) (Fig. 2.1) [25, 26]. Clinical application of LDTC began around 1990. At the same time, international interest in this method was growing, and an attempt in neonatal cardiac surgery was reported from UCLA in 1989 [27]. Our first clinical application of this method was in the field of adult cardiac surgery, and then we proceeded to apply it to emergency surgery, cases of left ventricular hypertrophy, and the pediatric group as well.

As a result, we studied the reperfusion method in coronary artery bypass graft surgery and divided it into plain blood, crystalloid CP solution, and LTDC. While the results did not show the superiority of LDTC in scheduled surgery, we found the advantages in emergency surgery cases in terms of CK-MB leakage values and postoperative use of dopamine [28]. In other words, it seemed to be worthwhile in vulnerable myocardium such as ventricular hypertrophy. In addition, a similar study was performed in aortic valve replacement patients associated with left ventricular hypertrophy (LV mass > 300gm) [29]. In this study, the LDTC group was significantly lower in terms of myocardial cell changes and the degree of vascular endothelial damage to myocytes under electron microscopy, and there was also a significant difference in postoperative maximum CK-MB release. It has also been shown to be useful in the pediatric age group [25] (Fig. 2.2). This modality has been shown in various situations of cardiac surgery with compromised heart and prolonged ischemic time [30]. This LDTC method has also been used in heart transplantation, which started in 1999 [31]. Although the clinical application has not continued in recent practice since then for various reasons, the basic concept remains.

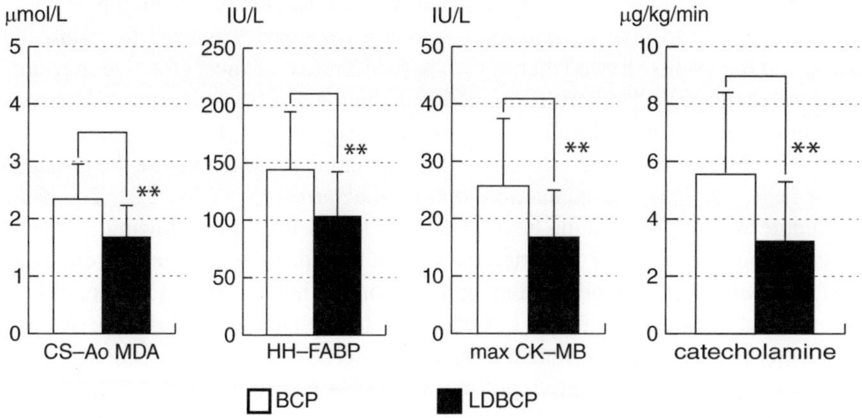

Fig. 2.2 Comparison of myocardial protective effects between blood cardioplegia (BCP)and leukocyte-depleted blood cardioplegia (LDBCP) in 50 pediatric patients. CS-Ao MDA and HH-FABP were measured at reperfusion, and others were at the first 24 h. *CS* coronary sinus, *Ao* aorta, *MDA* malondialdehyde, *HH* human fatty acid-binding protein, *max CK-MB* the peak concentration of plasma creatine kinase-MB. (Source: Ref. [25] with permission)

2.4 Prolonged Preservation of the Heart: Experimental Works

In Japan, there was a period of anguish in the preparation for heart transplantation from brain-dead donors, and it was restarted in 1999, almost 30 years after it was first done in Sapporo in 1968. The steps taken at Osaka University before the restart are reviewed in Chap. 1 of this book. During this time, instead of just waiting, we worked to select cases for possible heart transplantation and introduced ventricular assist devices from the early 1990s so that we would be ready to perform heart transplantation when brain-dead donors became available. In particular, as part of our active research into myocardial protection, we have also conducted research into heart preservation using cold storage and perfusion.

Japanese authorities, however, are very cautious to start organ donation from brain-dead donors and settlement of the legal system has been warranted. Looking back to the early experimental work in the United States before the clinical start, research on transplantation from donors after cardiac arrest had been carried out as part of the development of heart transplantation. In Japan in the 1970s, the situation to see transplantation from brain-dead donors was so difficult, and Professor Kawashima had a chance to meet Professor Lower of Medical College of Virginia, Richmond, and had a suggestion to consider the resuscitated cadaver heart [32], Professor Kawashima announced to our members that we should consider this strategy of heart transplantation instead of using brain-dead donors (see Foreword 1).

Subsequently, the important experiment was performed by Okamoto in 1974 [33]. His protocol using mongrel donors was performed in three groups after anoxia at room temperature for 1 h; heart excised for ex vivo storage, ex vivo heart-lung preparation, and in vivo reperfusion. Coronary perfusion was used to restart the heart, and the results showed that in vivo perfusion was the most effective in restoring cardiac function. The results recommended intracoronary perfusion, which was the same method used in Dr. Barnard's first case.

In the 1990s, extensive efforts were made in canine mode to explore the possibility of heart and lung transplantation after cardiac arrest [34] (Fig. 2.3). The basic procedure was to preserve the heart and lungs for 24 h by the following methods: hypotension due to blood loss, anoxia after ventilator cessation, in situ coronary perfusion with warm blood, cardioplegia to stop the heart, immersion in cold UW solution outside the body for 22 h. Orthotopic transplantation was then performed in another dog and cardiac function was assessed (Table 2.2). The results showed that cardiac function recovered well even after 24 h of cold storage after anoxic arrest [35–38]. The addition of LDTC in such a protocol enhanced the protective effects [39]. Furthermore, considering the actual clinical practice to cope with the time schedule to get the transplantation team, we established the method to preserve the heart and other organs in situ by the support of percutaneous cardiopulmonary support circuit [40, 41]. We should remember that the above-described protocol is comparable to that currently used in actual organ transplantation from DCD.

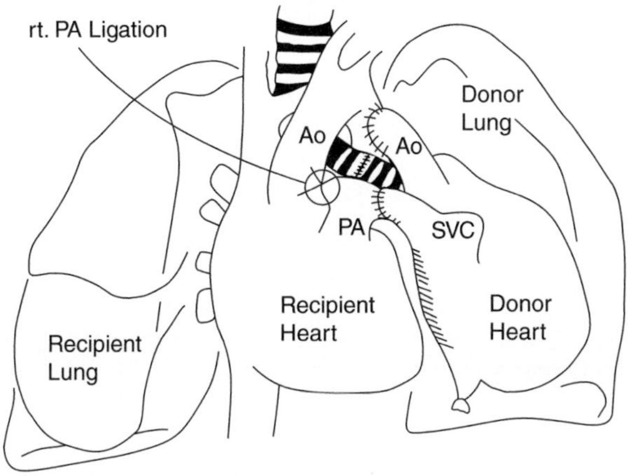

Fig. 2.3 Heterotopic heart and orthotopic left lung transplantation. *Ao* aorta, *PA* pulmonary artery, *SVC* superior vena cava. (Source: Ref. [35] with permission)

Table 2.2 Detailed protocol of preserving donor hearts in the asphyxiated model and 24 h preservation

Step	Process time
Exsanguination, pretreatment	20 min of antemortem hypotension
Respirator off	10 min of asphyxia
In situ coronary perfusion with Warm blood CP	5 min
Washout of coronary vascular bed And in situ coronary perfusion with cold CP	2 h (held at 15–17 °C)
Removal and immersion in UW solution(4 °C)	22 h
Orthotopic heart transplantation	45 min
Aortic unclamping, heart kept Non-working beating	10 min
Weaning from cardiopulmonary Bypass and observation	1 h
Measurement of cardiac function	1 h

Source: Ref. [36] with permission
CP cardioplegic solution, *UW* University Wisconsin

2.5 Normothermic Machine Perfusion

One of the recent interests in organ preservation is the manipulation of grafts under normothermic machine perfusion (NMP). This is derived from the clinical demand of DCD organ transplantation, but this concept can be extended to organ remodeling or modulation beyond the limits in DCD organ transplantation [42]. The application seems to be promising for very long-term preservation of routine brain-dead donor organs and also for pretreatment of marginal donor organs. In NMP, the approaches described above and performed in our laboratory can be applied as in vivo gene transfection, endogenous upregulation of myocyte and endothelial cell protective molecules, enhancement of mitochondrial ATP, and pharmacological manipulations.

2.6 Summary

This article focuses on a historical review of our research on myocardial protection and cardiac preservation. With regard to ischemia-reperfusion injury of the myocardium, the role of leukocyte activation is addressed and the experience with leukocyte-depleted terminal blood cardia is presented. The results of experimental study of prolonged preservation of heart and lung from non-heart-beating donors could be worthwhile in the current practice targeted into DCD.

References

1. Melrose DG, Dreyer B, Bentall HH, et al. Elective cardiac arrest. Lancet. 1955;2:21–2.
2. Gay WA, Ebert P. Function, metabolism and morphologic effect of potassium-induced cardioplegia. Surgery. 1973;74:284–9.
3. Hearse DJ, Stewart DA, Braimbridge MV. Hypothermic arrest and potassium arrest: metabolic and myocardial protection during elective cardiac arrest. Circ Res. 1975;36:481–9.
4. Buckberg GD. Warm versus cold blood cardioplegia: a self-imposed and counterproductive dilemma. Ann Thorac Surg. 1993;56:1007–10.
5. Sawa Y, Bernotat-Danielowski S, Stoll M, et al. Evidence for hypoxic myocyte derived neutrophil and endothelial cell activating factors. J Moll Cell Cardiol. 1991;23(Suppl 5):S53.
6. Sawa Y, Matsuda H. Myocardial ischemic and reperfusion injury in the field of cardiac surgery: mechanism and protection. In: Kamada T, Shiga T, McCusky RS, editors. Tissue perfusion and organ function. Amsterdam: Elsevier; 1996. p. 141–54.
7. Sawa Y, Matsuda H, Shimazaki Y, et al. Ultrastructural assessment of the infant myocardium receiving crystalloid cardioplegia. Circulation. 1987;76(Suppl V):V141–5.
8. Sawa Y, Matsuda H, Shimazaki Y, et al. Comparison of single versus multiple dose of crystalloid cardioplegia in neonate: experimental study with neonatal rabbits from birth to 2 days of age. J Thorac Cardiovasc Surg. 1989;97:229–34.
9. Matsuda H, Sawa Y, Kuki S, et al. Evaluation of prostacyclin analogue OP-4a833 as an adjunct to crystalloid cardioplegia in infants and children. Ann Thorac Surg. 1989;48:242–6.
10. Matsuda H, Maeda S, Hirose H, et al. Optimal dose of potassium cardioplegia for patients with chronic aortic valve disease: determination by left ventricular mass. Ann Thorac Surg. 1986;41:22–6.
11. Nomura F, Matsuda H, Shirakura R, et al. Experimental evaluation of myocardial protective effect of prostacyclin analog(OP-41483) as an adjunct to cardioplegic solution. J Thorac Cardiovasc Surg. 1991;101:860–5.
12. Fukuda H, Sawa Y, Kadoba K, et al. Supplement of nitric oxide attenuates neutrophil-mediated reperfusion injury. Circulation. 1995;92(9 Suppl):II413–6.
13. Suzuki K, Sawa Y, Kaneda Y, et al. In vivo gene transfection with heat shock protein 70 enhances myocardial tolerance to ischemia-reperfusion injury in rat. J Clin Invest. 1997;99:1645–50.
14. Suzuki K, Sawa Y, Ichikawa H, et al. Myocardial protection with endogenous overexpression of manganese superoxide dismutase. Ann Thorac Surg. 1999;68:1266–71.
15. Sawa Y, Morishita R, Suzuki K, et al. A novel strategy for myocardial protection using in vivo transfection of cis element 'decoy' against NFkappaB binding site: evidence for a role of NFkappaB in ischemia-reperfusion injury. Circulation. 1997;96(9 Suppl):II-280–4.
16. Sakaguchi T, Sawa Y, Fukushima N, et al. A novel strategy of decoy transfection against nuclear factor-kappaB in myocardial preservation. Ann Thorac Surg. 2001;71:624–9.
17. Ahmet I, Sawa Y, Nishimura M, et al. Cardioprotective effect of diadenosine tetraphosphate (AP4A) preservation in hypothermic storage and its relation with mitochondrial ATP-sensitive potassium channels. Transplantation. 2000;69:16–20.

18. Ono M, Sawa Y, Ryugo M, et al. BH4 peptide derivative from Bcl-xL attenuates ischemia/reperfusion injury through anti-apoptotic mechanism in rat hearts. Eur J Cardiothorac Surg. 2005;27:117–21.
19. Nakamura T, Mizuno S, Matsumoto K, et al. Myocardial protection from ischemia/reperfusion injury by endogenous and exogenous HGF. J Clin Invest. 2000;106:1511–9.
20. Ueda H, Nakamura T, Matsumoto K, et al. A potential cardioprotective role of hepatocyte growth factor in myocardial infarction in rats. Cardiovasc Res. 2001;51:41–50.
21. Ryugo M, Sawa Y, Ono M, et al. Myocardial protective effect of human recombinant hepatocyte growth factor for prolonged heart graft preservation in rats. Transplantation. 2004;78:1153–8.
22. Matsuda H, Kaneko M, Sawa Y, et al. Myocardial protection in cardiac surgery: experimental evaluation and clinical assessment of leukocyte-depleted terminal blood cardioplegia. J Moll Cell Cardiol. 1992;24(Suppl 1):33.
23. Sawa Y, Nakano S, Shimazaki Y, et al. Myocardial protective effect and its mechanism of leukocyte-repleted reperfusion in neonatal rabbit hearts. Ann Thorc Surg. 1994;58:1386–91.
24. Buckberg GD. Normothermic blood cardioplegia. Alternative or adjunct? J Thorac Cardiovasc Surg. 1994;107:860–7.
25. Hayashi Y, Sawa Y, Nishimura M, et al. Clinical evaluation of leukocyte-depleted blood cardioplegia for pediatric open heart operation. Ann Thorac Surg. 2000;69:1914–9.
26. Matsuda H, Sawa Y. The role of leukocyte-depleted reperfusion in cardiac surgery. Asia Pac Heart J. 1998;7:16–21.
27. Breda MA, Drinkwater DC, Laks H, et al. Prevention of reperfusion injury in the neonatal heart with leukocyte depleted blood. J Thorac Cardiovasc Surg. 1989;97:654–5.
28. Sawa Y, Matsuda H, Shimazaki Y, et al. Evaluation of leukocyte-depleted terminal blood cardioplegic solution in patients undergoing elective and emergency coronary artery bypass grafting. J Thorac Cardiovasc Surg. 1994;108:1125–31.
29. Sawa Y, Taniguchi K, Kadoba K, et al. Leukocyte depletion attenuates reperfusion injury in patients with left ventricular hypertrophy. Circulation. 1996;93:1640–6.
30. Hayashi Y, Sawa Y, Fukuyama N, et al. Leukocyte-depleted terminal blood cardioplegia provides superior myocardial protective effects in association with myocardial-derived nitric oxide and peroxinitrite production for patients undergoing prolonged aortic cross clamping for more than 120 minutes. J Thorac Cardiovasc Surg. 2003;126:1813–21.
31. Matsuda H, Fukushima N, Sawa Y, et al. First brain dead donor heart transplantation under new legislation in Japan. Jpn J Thorac Cardiovasc Surg. 1999;47:499–505.
32. Lower RR, Stofer RC, Hurley J, et al. Successful homotransplantation of the canine heart after anoxic preservation for seven hours. Am J Surg. 1962;104:302–6.
33. Okamoto S. Experimental studies on the resuscitation of cadaver hearts in dogs. The comparison of three methods utilizing normothermic coronary perfusion with whole blood. Jpn J Thorac Surg. 1974;22:588–600. (abstract in English)
34. Shirakura R, Matsuda H, Nakada S, et al. Prolonged preservation of cadaver heart with Belzer UW solution: 24-hour storage system for asphyxiated canine hearts.Eur Surg Res 1990;22:197–205.
35. Naka Y, Shirakura R, Matsuda H, et al. Canine heart-lung transplantation after 24-hour hypothermic preservation. Eur J Cardiothorac Surg. 1990;4:499–503.
36. Shirakura R, Matsuda H, Nakano S, et al. Cardiac function and myocardial performance of 24-hour-preserved asphyxiated canine hearts. Ann Thorac Surg. 1992;53:440–4.
37. Shirakura R, Matsuda H, Nakata S, et al. A new method to harvest multiple organs from non-heart-beating donors by use of a percutaneous cardiopulmonary support machine. Transplant Proc. 1992;24:1329–30.
38. Shirakura R, Matsuda H, Nakano S, et al. Myocardial energy metabolism in asphyxiated canine hearts preserved for 24 hours. Transplantation 1992;53:1215–1218.
39. Fukushima N, Shirakura R, Nakata S, et al. Effects of terminal cardioplegia with leukocyte-depleted blood on heart grafts preserved for 24 hours. J Heart Lung Transplant. 1992;11:676–82.

40. Fukushima N, Shirakura R, Chang JC, et al. Successful experimental multiorgan transplant from non-heart-beating donors using percutaneous cardiopulmonary support. ASAIO-J. 1998;44:M525–8.
41. Fukushima N, Shirakura R, Ohtake S, et al. Studies of multiorgan procurement system from non-heart-beating donors. Transplant Proc. 2000;32:281–4.
42. Hosgood S, Nicholson M. Current basic research in normothermic machine perfusion. Eur Surg Res. 2024; published online,;65:137. https://doi.org/10.1159/000542290.

Lung Preservation: Cold Static Preservation Solutions for Lung Transplantation

3

Shinichiro Miyoshi

Abstract

Cold static preservation formulations for lung transplantation, such as Euro-Collins, EP-TU, low potassium dextran, Perfadex, University of Wisconsin, Celsior, and ET-Kyoto solutions, were historically reviewed. Important findings obtained include the following:

1. The optimal temperature is 10 °C.
2. Extracellular fluid type is superior to intracellular fluid type solution.
3. Buffer, dextran 40, and glucose are essential components, though their optimal concentrations have not been determined.

Additional studies are required for determining an optimal lung preservation solution.

Keywords

Euro-Collins solution · EP-TU solution · Low potassium dextran solution · Perfadex · University of Wisconsin solution · Celsior · ET-Kyoto solution

Although findings from numerous investigations of lung preservation solutions had been presented [1], a method that employed simple cold immersion without use of a preservation solution was applied for the first successful lung transplant in 1983, performed by the Toronto Lung Transplant Group [2]. Because a useful preservation solution was not created, for that initial procedure, they had to perform the donor operation at the same hospital where the recipient was receiving treatment, so as to minimize ischemic time. However, for cases with distant donor lung procurement,

S. Miyoshi (✉)
Koseikai Memorial Hospital, Suita, Japan

H. Matsuda et al. (eds.), *Heart and Lung Transplantation*,
https://doi.org/10.1007/978-981-96-8810-4_3

it was an important issue to develop a good lung preservation solution that is safe and reliable. This chapter presents a historical review of lung preservation methods, with focus on development of cold static preservation solutions.

3.1 Hypothermia

Successful cold static preservation is based on suppression of metabolism and catabolic enzymes in the targeted organ by use of hypothermia. However, cell swelling, acidosis, and production of radical oxygen species upon reperfusion are well-known side effects of hypothermia [3]. To overcome such undesirable consequences, several types of preservation solutions have been developed.

3.2 Preservation Solution

3.2.1 Euro-Collins Solution

Collins solution, a type of intracellular fluid (ICF) that includes phosphate buffer and glucose as the main composite materials, was developed by G.M. Collins for kidney preservation in 1969 [4]. Hypothermia impairs the activity of Na^+/K^+ ATPase, resulting in sodium being no longer extruded but passively entering affected cells. This creates a hyperosmolar intracellular environment, which subsequently leads to an influx of water, resulting in cell swelling. In the study by Collins [4], the authors speculated that elimination of concentration gradients for sodium and potassium ions between inside and outside of the cells would prevent ionic shifts and cell swelling. However, ionic shifts between inside and outside of cells were subsequently demonstrated to not cause cell swelling, which results in deterioration of renal function during preservation [5, 6]. Thereafter, glucose was thought to have an impermeant function and considered useful to prevent hypothermia-induced cell swelling. A modified mixture with magnesium eliminated, Euro-Collins (EC) solution, was presented by the Eurotransplant Foundation in 1976 [3, 7].

Haverich and colleagues presented experimental results in 1986 demonstrating that safe and reliable lung preservation for up to 24 h is possible using flush-perfusion with EC at 60 cc/kg over a period of 4 min with a pulmonary artery pressure of approximately 20 mmHg [8]. Since EC was already commercially available and widely used for abdominal organs, a pulmonary artery flushing technique with that solution followed by a simple topical hypothermia condition was rapidly adopted by most transplant centers for cases with distant procurement of donor lungs [9, 10]. Notably, a worldwide survey regarding pulmonary graft preservation solutions conducted in 1998 found that EC was used by 86 (77%) of 112 lung transplant centers, with a median maximum ischemic period accepted by those centers of 7 h. However, only 58 (67%) of 86 centers using EC expressed satisfaction with the quality of the preserved graft [11].

3.2.2 Low Potassium Dextran Solutions

3.2.2.1 EP-TU Solution

Applications of extracellular fluid (ECF)-type solutions for lung preservation have been experimentally investigated for a long period, as it became evident that ICF types have a disadvantage based on their use potentially causing K^+-induced pulmonary vasoconstriction. Kondo and his colleagues demonstrated that better lung preservation could be achieved with an ECF-type rather than an ICF-type solution in a canine model of lung transplantation [12]. Thereafter, during the mid-1980s, that group developed several different ECF-type phosphate-buffered solutions with high Na^+ and relatively low K^+, along with 2% dextran 40 and 1% glucose, which were termed extracellular phosphate-buffered solution type 1, 2, and 3 (Ep1, 2, and 3, respectively) [13]. Later, Ep4 was developed by adding K_2HPO_4 to Ep3 to strengthen its buffering capacity (Table 3.1), which was demonstrated to successfully maintain lung preservation for up to 96 h in a canine transplant model [14, 15]. Dextran 40 in each of those solutions functions as an oncotic agent and keeps water in the intravascular compartment, while it also reduces aggregation of erythrocytes and platelets, and may exert an antithrombotic effect, even following reperfusion, by coating the endothelial surface. These actions might prevent primary graft dysfunction (PGD), as platelet accumulation on the endothelial surface has been identified as a factor responsible for ischemia-reperfusion injury [15].

Recently, Ep4 has become commercially available as EP-TU (Cell Science & Technology Institute, Sendai, Japan) and applied to clinical lung transplantation cases in Japan. Okada and colleagues reported preliminary results of 10 cases of lung transplantation (3 single, 7 double lung transplants), for which EP-TU was utilized for organ preservation [16]. In those cases, the average graft ischemic times for the first and second grafts were 431 and 571 min, respectively, while average PGD grade ranged from 0.5 to 1.0 and average PaO2/FiO2 ratio from 350 to 400 Torr during the first 48 h following intensive care unit admission. The survival rates at 30 days and 5 years were 90% and 80%, respectively. EP-TU is now widely used by lung transplant centers in Japan for lung preservation.

3.2.2.2 LPD Solution

The Toronto Lung Transplant Team evaluated an extracellular fluid-type solution created by modifying Ep3, mentioned above, with primary factors included for maintaining pH at 7.4 and a K^+ level of 4 mmol/L [17]. As compared with the original Ep3, the Na^+ level was increased to 168 mmol/L, while the phosphate radical level was reduced to 36.7 mmol/L (Table 3.1). Additionally, glucose was not added. This modified solution was thus termed low-potassium dextran (LPD). Keshavjee and colleagues presented results obtained with a canine single lung transplant model demonstrating that LPD provided a significantly better immediate function for a preserved lung as compared to EC [17]. Furthermore, another of their studies demonstrated that both dextran 40 and a low concentration of potassium in LPD contributed significantly to uniformly excellent 12-h lung preservation noted in the same canine single lung transplant model [18]. In another study using a canine single lung

Table 3.1 Composition of various lung preservation solutions

	EC	Ep1	Ep2	Ep3	Ep4 EP-TU	LPD	Perfadex Plus	UW	Celsior	ET-Kyoto
Na^+	10	117	136	140	142	168	138	25	100	107
K^+	115	4.1	3.8	3.9	26.2	4	6	120	15	42
Cl^-	15	95	96	97	97	103	142	20	42	NA
Mg^{2+}	(−)	4	4	4	4	2	0.8	5	13	(−)
SO_4^{2-}	(−)	4	4	4	4	2	0.8	(−)	(−)	NA
Raffinose	(−)	(−)	(−)	(−)	(−)	(−)	(−)	30	(−)	(−)
Trehalose	(−)	(−)	(−)	(−)	(−)	(−)	(−)	(−)	(−)	117
Lactobionate	(−)	(−)	(−)	(−)	(−)	(−)	(−)	100	80	(−)
Mannitol	(−)	(−)	(−)	(−)	(−)	(−)	(−)	(−)	60	(−)
Glucose (g/L)	35.1	10	10	10	10	(−)	0.91	(−)	(−)	(−)
Dextran 40 (g/L)	(−)	20	20	20	20	20	50	(−)	(−)	(−)
HES(g/L)	(−)	(−)	(−)	(−)	(−)	(−)	(−)	50	(−)	29
HCO_3^-	10	(−)	(−)	(−)	(−)	(−)	(−)	(−)	(−)	NA
PR	57.5	7.8[a]	23.6[a]	50.1[a]	65	36.7	0.8	25	(−)	24
Histidine	(−)	(−)	(−)	(−)	(−)	(−)	(−)	(−)	30	(−)
THAM	(−)	(−)	(−)	(−)	(−)	(−)	2	(−)	(−)	(−)
Osmolarity (mOsm/L)	375	304	318	339	364	335	292	330	320	598
pH	7.4	6.4	6.7	7.2	7.5	7.4	7.35	7.4	7.3	NA

Abbreviations: *EC* Euro-Collins, *Ep* extracellular phosphate-buffered, *EP-TU* extracellular phosphate-buffered Tohoku University, *LPD* low potassium dextran, *UW* University of Wisconsin, *ET-Kyoto* extracellular trehalose-Kyoto, *HES* hydroxyethyl starch, *PR* phosphate radical, *THAM* tris hydroxymethyl aminomethane, *NA* not available. All units expressed in mmol/L unless otherwise indicated. PR is $H_2PO_4^-$ plus HPO_4^{2-}

[a]Data from Ref. [14]

transplant model, Date and colleagues found that addition of 1% glucose to LPD provided better preservation of inflated lungs stored for 24 h at 10 °C [19]. Thus, a series of experiments of LPD conducted by Keshavjee and Date and their colleagues reconfirmed that the original Ep3 is superior to EC and showed that a low concentration of potassium, dextran 40, and glucose are essential components. Also, Handa and colleagues demonstrated that Ep4 is better than Ep3, as it elevated the phosphate radical concentration from 50.1 to 65 mmol/L [14], thus indicating its superiority for lung preservation as compared to LPD, with a low phosphate radical level (36.7 mmol/L) and without glucose.

3.2.2.3 Perfadex

Based on findings obtained in extensive laboratory experiments suggesting that LPD is superior to EC for lung preservation, a Swedish company (Kabi Pharmacia AB, Uppsala, Sweden) developed Perfadex, which is LPD containing dextran 40 (50 g/L), Na^+ (138 mmol/L), K^+ (6 mmol/L), Mg^{2+} (0.8 mmol/L), Cl^- (142 mmol/L), SO_4^{2-} (0.8 mmol/L), $H_2PO_4^- + HPO_4^{2-}$ (0.8 mmol/L), and glucose (0.91 g/L), with a pH value of 6. Steen and associates used a pig single lung transplant model and demonstrated that use of Perfadex resulted in safe 12-h lung preservation [20]. Furthermore, in another of their experiments [21], prior to its use, the preservation solution was titrated to a pH level of 7.35 ± 0.05 with Addex tris hydroxymethyl aminomethane (THAM) at 0.24 ml/L, and the findings demonstrated excellent pulmonary function after pulmonary and bronchial artery perfusion with Perfadex at room temperature, followed by 24 h of cold atelectatic storage in Perfadex. Based on the results of these examinations, Perfadex has been used for clinical lung transplantation at many centers, though its efficacy in clinical settings remains controversial.

Aziz and colleagues presented results of a retrospective analysis of the outcome of 69 consecutive lung allografts retrieved and used for transplantation [22]. Donor lungs flushed with EC were used in 37 patients and those flushed with Perfadex in 32 patients, with no significant differences in mean chest roentgenogram score, arterial alveolar oxygen tension ratio, mean ventilation time, mean intensive therapy unit stay, or death caused by primary organ failure between the groups. In another study, Nath and colleagues also obtained results showing that lung preservation with Perfadex as compared with EC did not improve early gas exchange, or impact 90-day or 1-year mortality [23]. On the other hand, Rabanal and colleagues demonstrated that the PO2/FiO2 ratio was significantly better with use of Perfadex as compared to EC at the time of arrival to the intensive care unit (ICU), as well as 12 and 24 h later [24]. Furthermore, the duration of mechanical ventilatory support and ICU stay was also shorter in the Perfadex group. Additionally, Christian and colleagues [25] presented findings indicating that graft preservation using Perfadex leads to better immediate and intermediate graft function after pulmonary transplantation, and results in better long-term survival.

The rights to Perfadex were acquired by XVIVO Perfusion in 1999. Then in 2018 the company developed and marketed a new version named Perfadex Plus, which is pre-supplemented with calcium ions (0.5 mmol/L) and THAM (2 mmol/L), thus it can be used without prior addition, or mixing of the buffer and electrolytes [26]. Handa and colleagues presented findings showing that buffer capacity is an important factor for lung preservation and that Ep4 with phosphate radical at 65 mmol/L was better than Ep1, 2, or 3 with a lower concentration [14]. Thus, it is considered that 0.8 mmol/L of phosphate radical plus 2 mmol/L of THAM in Perfadex Plus might not be an adequate concentration. As compared to other solutions, glucose level, an important factor for lung preservation, is low in Perfadex Plus (Table 3.1). Steen and associates explained that the purpose of the high concentration of dextran 40 (50 g/L) in Perfadex is to counteract cell swelling induced by cold ischemic storage [20]. However, dextran 40 cannot penetrate capillary membrane pores, thus is not able to protect parenchymal cells of the lung from swelling. It is therefore considered that hypothermic-induced cell swelling may not be an important factor for lung preservation, different as compared to solid organs. This issue will be discussed later.

3.2.3 University of Wisconsin (UW) and Celsior Solutions

3.2.3.1 UW Solution

The UW group developed a preservation solution for solid organs in the mid-1980s [27]. The UW solution contains lactobionate and raffinose, which show impermeant characteristics for prevention of hypothermia-induced cell swelling [28]. This solution has been shown to provide effective preservation of pancreas [29], liver [30], and kidney [31] in experimental animals. Thus, we evaluated it for lung preservation using a previously reported rabbit lung preservation model [32, 33].

The UW solution is an ICF type that contains potassium (120 mmol/L) and sodium (25 mmol/l). However, an ECF-type solution was previously shown to be superior to an ICF-type (EC) for lung preservation [17, 18, 34]. Therefore, standard UW was compared with a modified UW (M-UW) solution containing a low level of potassium (K: 4 mmol/L), an LPD solution considered to be best in a previous study presented by our group (K: 4 mmol/L), and simple surface cooling using rabbit lungs [32]. For the three groups with use of a solution, the lungs were flushed in situ ($n = 5$ in each group), then the heart-lung block was harvested and stored at 10 °C for 30 h, while for the surface cooling group, the lungs were harvested without flushing, and simply immersed in saline and stored. For assessments, the stored lungs were ventilated with room air and perfused with fresh venous blood at a rate of 40 ml/min for 10 min. Oxygen tension of effluent blood after 10 min of perfusion in the M-UW (95 ± 6 mmHg) and LPD (99 ± 4 mmHg) groups was significantly higher as compared to that in the surface cooling (61 ± 7 mmHg) and UW (51 ± 7 mmHg) groups, while there was no significant difference between the M-UW and LPD groups, or between the surface cooling and UW groups.

The superiority of LPD and M-UW as compared to the original UW for lung preservation can be explained by their low potassium concentration. Perfadex, an LPD solution, and UW have become commercially available, with both applied for lung preservation in clinical settings. Arnaoutakis and colleagues retrospectively reviewed the UNOS dataset for adult primary lung transplant patients (2005–2008) who received donor lungs recovered with use of UW or Perfadex [35]. Of 4455 patients, 4161 (93.4%) received lungs preserved using Perfadex and 294 (6.6%) with UW. There was no significant difference for mortality between the flush solutions when all were examined together. However, patients in the upper two lung allocation score quartiles (Q3: 37.8–45.4, Q4: >45.4) that received lungs preserved using Perfadex had a greater 1-year survival rate (81.5% vs. 73.5%, $p = 0.02$). Multivariate analysis showed that use of UW resulted in an increased risk of 1-year mortality [Hz ratio 1.77 (1.21–2.58), $p = 0.003$] as compared to Perfadex. Thus, the superiority of Perfadex was clinically proven with the largest cohort examined in recent years.

M-UW and LPD both have a low potassium content, though M-UW also contains lactobionate and raffinose, which have impermeant qualities, shown to be extremely important for extending solid organ preservation. That leads to questions regarding why M-UW did not provide superior results as compared to LPD in those experiments. Since lung function was shown to be well preserved with the LPD solution as well as with M-UW, it was speculated that hypothermic-induced cell swelling may not occur or be reduced in lungs preserved with either of those solutions. In the experiment performed by our group, lungs were stored in an inflated condition at 10 °C indicating that oxygen in the alveoli may have been supplied by diffusion, not only to lung parenchymal cells but also to endothelial cells [32]. Thus, by using oxygen, ATP could be produced in those cells in a preserved lung. Additionally, Date and colleagues demonstrated that lung cells can maintain an aerobic metabolism during cold storage preservation by use of oxygen in alveoli [36]. For that study, lungs were also stored at 10 °C, a temperature at which the activity of Na^+/K^+ ATPase may be preserved [37]. Thus, by using ATP as an energy source, Na^+/K^+ ATPase may maintain Na^+/K^+ pumps in the cellular membrane, which can prevent or reduce hypothermia-induced cell swelling. In another study, Date and colleagues found that despite results showing that preservation at 10 °C provided significantly better lung function as compared to 4 °C, the ATP levels were not significantly different at the end of the 18-h preservation period [38]. It is thus speculated that when using preservation at 4 °C, Na^+/K^+ ATPase activity might be nearly stopped without ATP consumption and that hypothermic-induced cell swelling might be possibly occurring in such preserved lungs. Because LPD does not contain an impermeant factor, its use will likely not prevent hypothermia-induced cell swelling, which might occur in parenchymal cells at 4 °C. Therefore, maintenance of low-level cellular metabolism may be an important factor for lung preservation.

3.2.3.2 Celsior

A modified version of UW was introduced in 1994 for cardiac preservation and termed Celsior [39], after which it became commercially available. Remadi and colleagues demonstrated that use of Celsior was safe and highly effective for clinical cardiac transplantation cases [40].

Celsior is an ECF type, composed of the original UW, with raffinose (impermeant component), hydroxyethyl starch (HES) (colloid), and phosphate radical (buffer) eliminated, and mannitol (impermeant) and histidine (buffer) added (Table 3.1). Additionally, glutamic acid, which helps with production of energy in anaerobic conditions, is also included. Celsior provides antioxidant action for preservation of organs with permanently reduced glutathione, histidine, lactobionate, and/or mannitol.

Since it is an ECF-type solution, Celsior has been applied for lung preservation. Sommer and colleagues compared Perfadex with Celsior for amelioration of lung ischemia-reperfusion injury by using a single pig lung transplant model, with the results demonstrating that an increase in pulmonary vascular resistance index ($p = 0.01$) and sequestration of neutrophils ($p = 0.08$) were less pronounced in the Celsior group [41]. They concluded that while both solutions can provide safe pulmonary preservation for up to 24 h of cold ischemia and have effects on surfactant activity to the same extent, Celsior provides slightly superior endothelial preservation. After obtaining favorable experimental data, Gohrbandt and colleagues [42] compared lung preservation with Perfadex and Celsior in cases of clinical transplantation and noted a trend for better survival ($p = 0.09$) and increased freedom from bronchiolitis obliterans syndrome ($p = 0.03$) in the Celsior group, despite prolonged ischemic times. Since extirpated donor lungs are preserved at 4 °C, which may induce hypothermia-induced swelling, Celsior with an impermeant component could prevent cell swelling, resulting in better lung preservation as compared to Perfadex without such a component.

3.2.4 ET-Kyoto

ET-Kyoto, developed at the University of Kyoto, is an ECF-type solution that contains trehalose (disaccharide), phosphate, gluconate, HES, N-acetylcysteine, nitroglycerin, dibutyryl cAMP, ethanol, and propylene glycol. Experimental results showed that it is superior to both EC and UW for lung preservation [43, 44]. Thereafter, ET-Kyoto was used for 26 cases of lung transplantation performed from 2002 to 2012 [45]. The mean graft ischemic time for the recipients was 483.8 ± 19.0 min, though oxygenation capacity after reperfusion and recovery of respiratory function were both acceptable despite the long ischemic time, and survival rate at 5 years after transplantation was 85.1%. Presently, ET-Kyoto is commonly used for clinical lung transplantation in Japan.

The characteristics of these preservation solutions are summarized in Table 3.1.

3.3 Temperature for Donor Lung Preservation

The temperature used for donor lung preservation is another important factor with effects on graft function. Wang and colleagues performed a systematic evaluation to determine which temperature is optimal for rabbit lung preservation and their findings showed that 10 °C was superior to 38 °C, 34 °C, 15 °C, and 4 °C [33]. Using a canine model, Date and colleagues also demonstrated that lung preservation at 10 °C was superior to that at 4 °C [38]. Furthermore, recent clinical studies have also demonstrated superior graft preservation at 10 °C as compared with storage in an ice cooler, commonly considered the gold standard [46]. As noted above, it has been shown that Na^+/K^+ ATPase activity is preserved at 10 °C [37], which is speculated to result in maintaining Na^+/K^+ pumps in the cellular membrane, resulting in reduction or prevention of hypothermia-induced cell swelling. This indicates that when a donor lung is preserved at 10 °C, an impermeant factor would not be needed, though glucose is required as an energy source for ATP production. On the other hand, at 4 °C the activity of Na^+/K^+ ATPase may be nearly stopped, with Na^+/K^+ pumps then sequentially halted, resulting in hypothermic-induced cell swelling. Therefore, when a donor lung is preserved at 4 °C, it is considered that inclusion of an impermeant factor in the preservation solution is necessary.

3.4 Conclusion

This chapter presents a historical review of developments and testing of flushing and cold static preservation solutions for lungs obtained for transplantation. Findings have shown that important factors are a low level of potassium as well as dextran 40, buffer, and glucose. Nevertheless, the temperature of the solution may have greater effects on the various elements. Additional investigations are necessary for development of an optimal lung preservation solution.

References

1. Toledo-Pereyra LH, Hau T, Simmons RL, Najarian JS. Lung preservation techniques. Ann Thorac Surg. 1977;23:487–94.
2. Toronto Lung Transplant Group. Unilateral lung transplantation for pulmonary fibrosis. N Engl J Med. 1986;314:1140–5.
3. Maathuis MHJ, Leuvenink HGD, Ploeg RJ. Perspectives in organ preservation. Transplantation. 2007;83:1289–98.
4. Collins GM, Bravo-Shugarman M, Terasaki PI. Kidney preservation for transportation. Initial perfusion and 30 hours' ice storage. Lancet. 1969;2:1219–22.
5. Downes DL, Hoffmann RM, Huang J, Belzer OF. Mechanism of action of washout solution for kidney preservation. Transplantation. 1973;16:45–53.
6. Green CJ, Pegg DE. Mechanism of action of "intracellular" renal preservation solutions. World J Surg. 1979;3:115–20.
7. Annual Report Eurotransplant International Foundation. Leiden. Eurotransplant International Foundation; 1976.
8. Haverich A, Aziz S, Scott WC, et al. Improved lung preservation using Euro-Collins solution for flush-perfusion. Thorac Cardiovasc Surg. 1986;34:368–76.
9. Colquhoun IW, Kirk AJ, Au J, et al. Single-flush perfusion with modified Euro-Collins solution: experience in clinical lung preservation. J Heart Lung Transplant. 1992;11:S209–14.

10. Baldwin JC, Frist WH, Starkey TD, et al. Distant graft procurement for combined heart and lung transplantation using pulmonary artery flush and simple topical hypothermia for graft preservation. Ann Thorac Surg. 1987;43:670–3.
11. Hopkinson DN, Bhabra MS, Hooper TL. Pulmonary graft preservation: a worldwide survey of current clinical practice. J Heart Lung Transplant. 1998;17:525–31.
12. Kondo T, Fujimura S, Yamauchi A, et al. Successful preservation of canine lung for 24 hours by simple cooling method. Jpn J Transplant. 1984;19:295–9.
13. Fujimura S, Handa M, Kondo T, et al. Successful 48-hour simple hypothermic preservation of canine lung transplants. Transplant Proc. 1987;19:1334–6.
14. Handa M, Fujimura S, Kondo T, et al. A study of preservation solution for 48- and 96-hour simple hypothermic storage of canine lung transplants. Tohoku J Exp Med. 1989;159:205–14.
15. Okada Y, Kondo T. Preservation solution for lung transplantation. Gen Thorac Cardiovasc Surg. 2009;57:635–9.
16. Okada Y, Matsumura Y, Date H, et al. Clinical application of an extracellular phosphate-buffered solution (ET-TU) for lung preservation: preliminary results of a Japanese series. Surg Today. 2012;42:152–6.
17. Keshavjee SH, Yamazaki F, Cardoso P, et al. A method for safe twelve-hour pulmonary preservation. J Thorac Cardiovasc Surg. 1989;98:529–34.
18. Keshavjee SH, Yamazaki F, Yokomise H, et al. The role of dextran 40 and potassium in extended hypothermic lung preservation for transplantation. J Thorac Cardiovasc Surg. 1992;103:314–25.
19. Date H, Matsumura A, Manchester JK, et al. Evaluation of lung metabolism during successful twenty-four-hour canine lung preservation. J Thorac Cardiovasc Surg. 1993;105:480–91.
20. Steen S, Sjoberg T, Massa G, et al. Safe pulmonary preservation for 12 hours with low-potassium-dextran solution. Ann Thorac Surg. 1993;55:434–40.
21. Steen S, Kimblad PO, Sjoberg T, et al. Safe lung preservation for twenty-four hours with Perfadex. Ann Thorac Surg. 1994;57:450–7.
22. Aziz TM, Pillay TM, Corris PA, et al. Perfadex for clinical lung procurement: is it an advance? Ann Thorac Surg. 2003;75:990–5.
23. Nath DS, Walter AR, Johnson AC, et al. Does Perfadex affect outcomes in clinical lung transplantation? J Heart Lung Transplant. 2005;24:2243–8.
24. Rabanal JM, Ibanez AM, Mons R, et al. Influence of preservation solution on early lung function (Euro-Collins vs Perfadex). Transplant Proc. 2003;35:1938–9.
25. Christian M, Heinrich F, Hermann R, et al. Lung procurement by low-potassium dextran and the effect on preservation injury. Transplantation. 1999;68:1139–43.
26. Perfadex Plus (XVIVI, Gothenburg, Sweden); https://www.xvivogroup.com/products-services/perfadex-plus/. Accessed 10 Feb 2025.
27. Wahlberg JA, Southand JH, Belzer FO. Development of a cold storage solution for pancreas preservation. Cryobiology. 1986;23:477–82.
28. Beltzer OF, Southard JH. Principles of solid-organ preservation by cold storage. Transplantation. 1988;45:673–6.
29. Wahlberg JA, Love R, Landegaad L, et al. 72-hour preservation of the canine pancreas. Transplantation. 1987;43:5–8.
30. Jamieson NV, Sundberg R, Lindell S, et al. Preservation of the canine liver for 24-48 hours using simple cold storage with UW solution. Transplantation. 1988;46:517–22.
31. Ploeg RJ, Goossens D, McAnulty JF, et al. Successful 72-hour cold storage of the dog kidney with UW solution. Transplantation. 1988;46:191–6.
32. Miyoshi S, Shimokawa S, Schreinemakers H, et al. Comparison of the University of Wisconsin preservation solution and other crystalloid perfusates in a 30-hour rabbit lung preservation model. J Thorac Cardiovasc Surg. 1992;103:27–32.
33. Wang LS, Yoshikawa K, Miyoshi S, et al. The effect of ischemic time and temperature on lung preservation in a simple ex vivo rabbit model used for functional assessment. J Thorac Cardiovasc Surg. 1989;98:333–42.

34. Yamazaki F, Yokomise H, Keshavjee SH, et al. The superiority on an extracellular fluid solution over Euro-Collins' solution for pulmonary preservation. Transplantation. 1990;49:690–4.
35. Arnaoutakis GJ, Allen JG, Merlo CA, et al. Low potassium dextran is superior to University of Wisconsin solution in high risk lung transplant recipients. J Heart Lung Transplant. 2010;29:1380–7.
36. Date H, Matsumura A, Manchester JK, et al. Changes in alveolar oxygen and carbon dioxide concentration and oxygen consumption during lung preservation. Maintenance of aerobic metabolism during lung preservation. J Thorac Cardiovasc Surg. 1993;105:492–501.
37. Martin DR, Scott DF, Downes GL, Belzer FO. Primary cause of unsuccessful liver and heart preservation: cold sensitivity of the ATPase system. Ann Surg. 1972;175:111–7.
38. Date H, Lima O, Matsumura A, et al. In a canine model, lung preservation at 10 degrees C is superior to that at 4 degrees C. J Thorac Cardiovasc Surg. 1992;103:773–80.
39. Menasche P, Termignon JL, Pradier F, et al. Experimental evaluation of Celsior, a new heart preservation solution. Eur J Cardiothorac Surg. 1994;8:207–13.
40. Remadi JP, Baron O, Roussel JC, et al. Myocardial preservation using solution in cardiac transplantation: early results and 5-year follow-up of a multicenter prospective study of 70 cardiac transplantations. Ann Thorac Surg. 2002;73:1495–9.
41. Sommer SP, Warnecke G, Hohlfeld JM, et al. Pulmonary preservation with LPD and Celsior solution in porcine lung transplantation after 24h of cold ischemia. Eur J Cardiothorac Surg. 2004;26:151–7.
42. Gohrbandt B, Simon AR, Warnecke G, et al. Lung preservation with Perfadex or Celsior in clinical transplantation: a retrospective single-center analysis of outcomes. Transplantation. 2015;99:1933–9.
43. Fukuse T, Hirata T, Ueda M, et al. Effects of Euro-Collins, University of Wisconsin, and new extracellular-type trehalose-containing Kyoto solutions in an ex vivo rat lung preservation model. Transplantation. 1996;62:1212–7.
44. Wada H, Liu CJ, Hirata T, et al. Effective 30-hour preservation of canine lungs with modified ET-Kyoto solution. Ann Thorac Surg. 1996;61:1099–105.
45. Ikeda M, Bando T, Yamada T, et al. Clinical application of ET-Kyoto solution for lung transplantation. Surg Today. 2015;45:439–43.
46. Ali A, Hoetzenecker K, de la Cruz JLCC, et al. Extension of cold static donor lung preservation at 10°C. NEJM Evid. 2023;2(6):EVIDoa2300008. https://doi.org/10.1056/EVIDoa2300008.

Part III

Mechanical Circulatory Support

Mechanical Circulatory Support in Advanced Heart Failure: Acute Support, Ventricular Assist Device, Bridge to Transplantation, and Bridge to Recovery

4

Hikaru Matsuda, Goro Matsumiya, Motonobu Nishimura, Takafumi Masai, and Yuji Miyamoto

Abstract

Mechanical circulatory support (MCS) evolved with advances in cardiac surgery, where postcardiotomy shock was a problem. In the 1990s, percutaneous cardiopulmonary support (PCPS) was introduced as a less invasive system. Subsequently, direct left ventricular support with a ventricular assist device (VAD) was introduced for patients with severe heart failure, such as those eligible for heart transplantation (bridge to transplantation). This chapter presents a historical review of our efforts in such MCS and, in particular, the achievements of implantable VADs at Osaka University. In addition to the above-mentioned "bridge to transplantation" strategy, the "bridge to recovery" strategy has been developed and the current progress is presented.

H. Matsuda (✉)
Yoshiken-kai Shion Hospital, Osaka, Japan

The University of Osaka, Suita, Osaka, Japan
e-mail: hmatsudahuhs@gmail.com

G. Matsumiya
Department of Cardiovascular Surgery, Chiba University Graduate School of Medicine, Chiba, Japan
e-mail: matsumg@faculty.chiba-u.jp

M. Nishimura
Kawasaki Hospital, Kobe, Hyogo, Japan

T. Masai
Osaka Keisatsu Hospital, Osaka, Japan

Y. Miyamoto
Otemae Hospital, Osaka, Japan
e-mail: ymiyamoto@otemae.gr.jp

H. Matsuda et al. (eds.), *Heart and Lung Transplantation*,
https://doi.org/10.1007/978-981-96-8810-4_4

Keywords

PCPS · Heart transplantation · Mechanical circulatory support · Ventricular assist device · Bridge to transplantation · Bridge to recovery · Regenerative therapy · Destination therapy · Impella

4.1 Introduction

The history of mechanical circulatory support (MCS) for heart failure dates back to the introduction of a disposable centrifugal pump in the 1980s and its integration with a membrane oxygenator to provide percutaneous cardiopulmonary support (PCPS) in the early 1990s. This system was effective in emergencies, but limited efficacy and durability led to a shift to ventricular assist devices (VADs) for more direct support. The Toyobo VAD, an extracorporeal air-driven pulsatile VAD, was the main device used in the 1980s for patients with severe heart failure who were comparable to the candidates for heart transplantation. Then, in the 1990s, the choice shifted to implantable left ventricular VAD (LVAD) such as TCI-HM and Novacor to prepare for heart transplantation aiming bridge to transplantation (BTT). Continuous-flow VADs demonstrated further evolution in treatment strategies for end-stage heart failure, extending to destination therapy (DT). In reviewing the background of these historical steps of MCS, we look back at our efforts at Osaka University (OU), from the early 1990s to 2005 where heart transplantation started in 1999. And also the issue surrounding current practice of MCS is discussed.

4.2 Percutaneous Cardiopulmonary Support

In the early days, the heart-lung machine was used for cardiogenic shock after heart surgery, but it was highly invasive and of limited life-saving value. Subsequently, MCS entered a new era with the advent of the simple centrifugal pump, BioMedicus BP-80 (Medtronic Inc. USA). Especially in combination with a membrane artificial lung, a new system of percutaneous cardiopulmonary support was introduced in the 1980s [1]. We also developed such a system as PCPS collaborated with Terumo Corporation (Tokyo, Japan) for commercial use [2]. The indication was extended from heart failure after cardiac surgery to intensive care units and cardiology laboratories [3], but the salvage rate in cardiac surgery was limited. It was clear that such peripheral vascular approaches were less effective in directly unloading the failing left ventricle.

In addition, another circulatory assist system by transcutaneous-transatrial septal cannulation to the left atrium for direct left ventricular unloading has been developed [4]. This concept is used in sophisticated systems such as Tandem Heart®. PCPS is now widely used as ECMO (extracorporeal membrane oxygenation) and its role as temporary circulatory or respiratory support is widely accepted.

4.3 Ventricular Assist Devices

MCS, which can directly reduce the left ventricular load, made remarkable progress in Japan in the late 1980s with the development of pulsatile left ventricular VADs (LVADs). One such device was introduced in the early 1980s by Toyobo Inc. (Osaka, Japan) in collaboration with the National Cardiovascular Center (NCVC, Osaka, Japan) (Fig. 4.1a). The VAD was named as Toyobo-NCVC LVAD (Toyobo-LVAD), and a multicenter clinical trial was conducted involving 92 patients in 1989, many of whom had difficulty weaning from extracorporeal circulation [5]. A pediatric version of this device was also initially developed (stroke volume 20 ml) and used in two infants after Fontan surgery in 1988 [6].

The first model of Toyobo-LVAD was the left atrial drainage type, which caused the problems of intraventricular thrombus formation, and then changed to the left ventricular apical drainage type after 1999 with improved results even in the long-term supports [7, 8]. In July 1992, a 17-year-old high school student with dilated cardiomyopathy and severe heart failure was implanted with a Toyobo-LVAD. After implantation, the patient's ventilator was removed and his general condition improved, but his heart function did not recover. Because the chance of heart transplantation was not realistic at that time, we asked Dr. Frazier of Texas Heart Institute (Houston Texas, USA) about the possibility of heart transplantation there, and the patient was transported by charter jet to the USA with an extracorporeal VAD. He underwent a successful heart transplant as the first case of BTT in our situation [9] and has been doing well for more than 30 years.

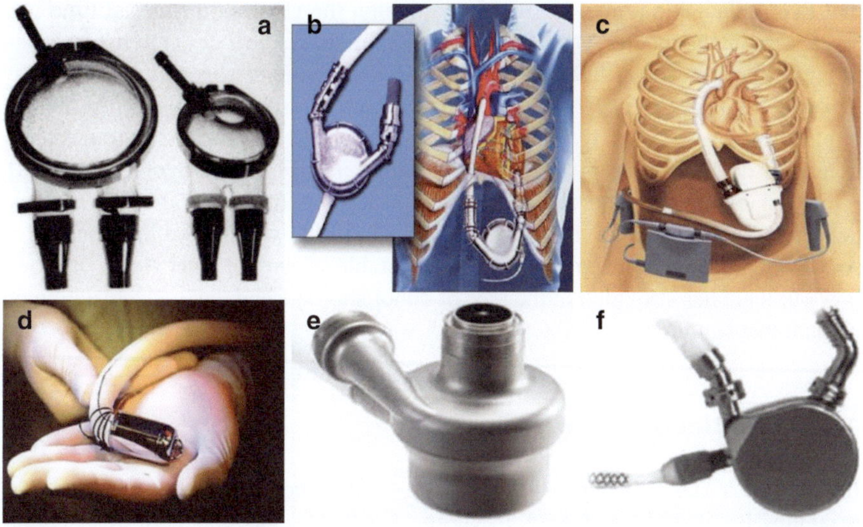

Fig. 4.1 Pictures of LVADs utilized in the early days for bridge to transplantation. Upper (left to right); (**a**) Toyobo, (**b**) TCI-HM(VE), (**c**) Novacor. Lower (left to right); (**d**) Jarvik 2000, (**e**) EVAHEART, and (**f**) DuraHeart

4.3.1 Implantable VADs

One of the pioneering implantable LVAD could be the pneumatically driven TCI-HeartMate IP (Thoratec Corp., CA, USA), and this VAD has been applied widely for BTT from 1986 to 1990s mainly in the USA [10]. As the next step, completely implantable device of electrically driven, vented VAD (HeartMateVE, Fig. 4.1b) was introduced in 1991 [11] and took over the HeartMateIP VAD. In 2001, the result of the REMATCH trial with the HeartMate VE was reported as the historic milestone of MCS for end-stage heart failure and marked the beginning of DT [12]. In addition, a prototype of Novacor LVAD (World Heart Com., Ottawa, Canada) was introduced to North America as a wearable, electrically powered VAD in 1984 and wide clinical application started in 1993(Fig. 4.1c) [13].

Influenced by the above advances in MCS, the introduction of implantable LVADs has been promoted in Japan because patients with advanced cardiomyopathy require long-term mechanical support aiming for possible heart transplantation. First, TCI's air-driven HeartMateIP was imported on a university initiative and implanted in two cases by 1996. Then the wearable electric type was promoted nationally, and HeartMateVE [14] and Novacor (Baxter, Novacor Division, Oakland, CA, USA) [15] were introduced through national multicenter clinical trials.

At OU, the clinical application of such VADs has continued and as of 1997, 16 myopathy patients with end-stage heart failure compatible with transplant candidates received VAD therapy by Toyobo LVAD, TCI-IP, and Novacor [7]. Later in 2003, a total of 55 cases of LVAD support were counted including 22 implantable types: Novacor 9, HeartMate-IP 11, and HeartMate-VE 2 [16]. In this series, comparison of survival rates between extracorporeal and implantable devices showed that the implantable type was superior, although the maximum survival time was 3 years. Actually, the first heart transplantation under the new organ transplantation law was done in Feb. 1999 to a 43-year-old male patient who was supported by Novacor for 4 months [17]. As this, Japanese heart transplantation was resumed by implantable LVAD as bridge use. The following second and third heart transplantations were done at NCVC by Dr. Kitamura, both were bridged by Toyobo LVAD [18].

Such a unique situation with a persistent need for extracorporeal VADs was due to the extraordinary delay in settling the legislation as well as the high barrier of social insurance reimbursement for the implantable system. In other words, it shows how our team has struggled in the face of donor shortage and delayed legislation on organ transplantation.

4.3.2 Continuous-Flow VADs

Implantable VADs have been shifted from pulsatile to continuous flow type, and the axial flow Jarvik 2000 (Fig. 4.1d, Jarvik Inc. NY, USA), the pioneer of this technology, was introduced in 2005 to OU supported by research funding. Dr. Frazier was invited from Houston, Texas, to assist in the implantation of the first two cases [19]. This model was finally approved for social reimbursement later in 2013. The number of cases for which this device was indicated increased due to its minimally invasive implantation procedure, low rate of pocket infection, and portable characteristics [20]. Among them, a female patient of 73 years of age with biventricular heart failure was supported in the context of destination therapy [21].

As for continuous-flow VADs, Sun Medical Technology Research Corp. (Nagano, Japan) and Terumo Corp. (Tokyo, Japan) subsequently developed EVAHEART(Fig. 4.1e) [22] and DuraHeart(Fig. 4.1f) [23], respectively. The actual steps involved in these device developments are reviewed in the Journal of Artificial Organ under the title "How people worked" in 2020 [24].

4.3.3 Achievements with VAD

Our experience of such VADs from 1992 to 2006, where organ transplantation law was settled in 1997, is summarized in Fig. 4.2 . As a note, after the organ transplantation law was revised in 2010, the number of heart transplants has increased to over 100 per year in 2023. As an additional data, out of the 15 heart transplants at OU up to 2007, 11 patients were BTT with VADs and 3 patients were also transplanted abroad on the devices. There was no mortality at the time of transplantation (Table 4.1). As shown here, the heart transplantation in Japan has taken the steps with VAD from the start providing remarkable outcomes by BTT strategy.

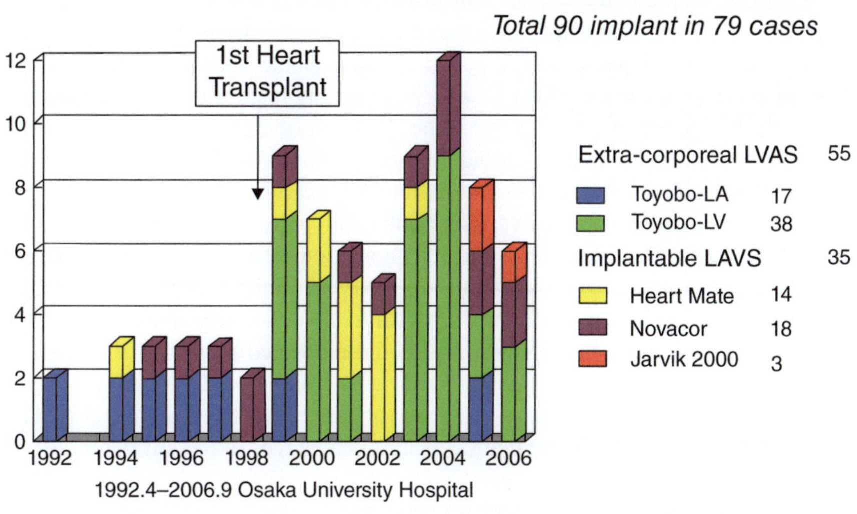

Fig. 4.2 Trends of the device selection in 90 LVAD implants from 1992 to 2006

Table 4.1 Summary of successful BTT patients; divided by the device used during the early phase of heart transplantation at Osaka University (including 3 patients transplanted abroad)

Device	N	Support period; days () average
Toyobo-LA	1	118
Toyobo-LV	3	21–954(388)
TCI-IP	3	515–1233(380)
Novacor	6	124–1090(690)
Jarvik 2000	1	359
Total	14	21–1233(590)

LA left atrium, *LV* left ventricle

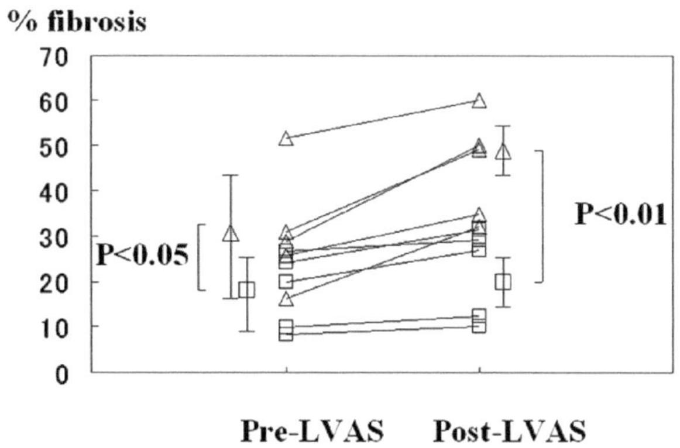

Fig. 4.3 Change of myocardial fibrosis during LVAD support in recovered (triangle) and non-recovered group (square). *LVAS* left ventricular assist system. (Source: Ref. [25] with permission)

4.3.4 Bridge to Recovery (BTR)

In the process of preparing a heart transplantation program in the 1990s, long-term support by VAD was mandatory because of the delay in legislation, and during that period some cases, 4 out of 22 supported by implantable VADs, could be weaned showing as bridge to recovery [16]. Due to the severe shortage of donors, we started to explore the bridge to recovery strategy in the 1990s, and even in dilated cardiomyopathy, it can be expected if the myocardial fibrosis was limited as described below [25].

From 2000 to 2004, 11 patients (mean age 27.9 years) with end-stage heart failure and dilated cardiomyopathy were supported with pulsatile LVADs for more than 6 months. Among them, 5 patients showed significant recovery of cardiac function and successfully underwent LVAD removal. Myocardial biopsies at the time of LVAD implantation and at the time of removal (recovery, transplantation, or death) showed that myocardial fibrosis was less in the recovered group (17.7% ± 8.2%) compared to the non-recovered group (30.5% ± 13.2%) before LVAD implantation. At the time of recovery, %fibrosis was also less in the recovered group [25] (Fig. 4.3). The results showed that a lower degree of fibrotic changes in the left ventricle was predictive of recovery.

In addition, adjunctive treatment by gene transfection and cell transplantation under LVAD support has been developed as the next step of bridge to recovery strategy [26]. One of the attempts is the application of autologous skeletal myoblast sheet, and there have been some patients responding to this therapy of regenerative approach combined with LVAD support [27, 28].

4.3.5 J-MACS

Since the resumption of heart transplantation in 1999, the role of the VAD as a BTT has become more important. In fact, since 2000, the introduction of implantable VADs in addition to conventional external VADs has led to a situation where most patients on the waiting list are supported by a VAD, as the priority of heart allocation in the system remains unchanged. The number of VADs has increased to more than 100 cases per year since 2013. This situation necessitated a national registry, and the J-MACS (Japanese Registry for Mechanically Assisted Circulatory Support) was established in 2009 [29]. In its 2017 report, among the annual registrations, the number of implantable types in particular has increased since 2011, with the total number of patients exceeding 300 in 2015. A comparison of survival rates between extracorporeal and implantable types shows that there is no significant difference up to 1000 days (Fig. 4.4). This indicates that although home care is not possible, the

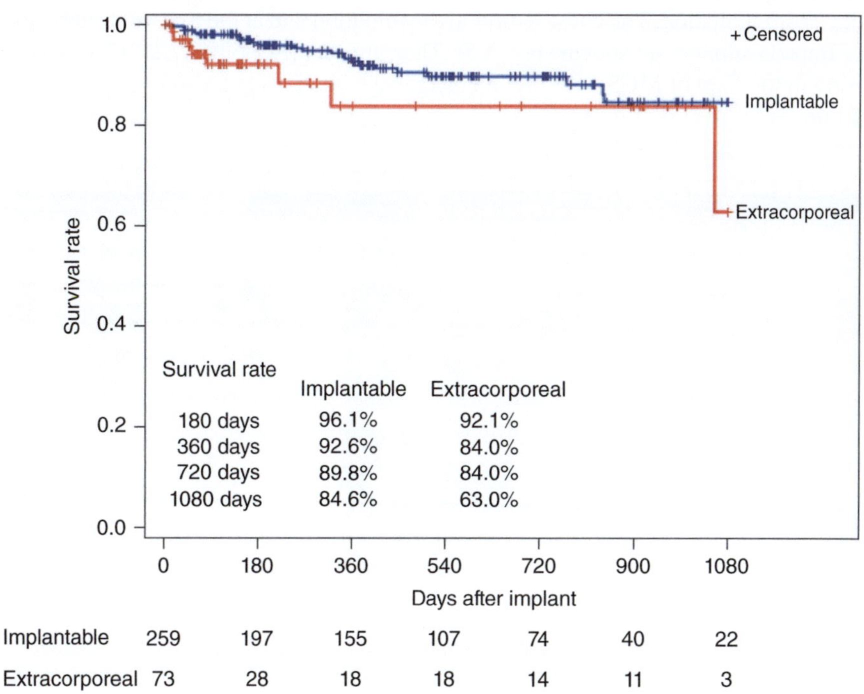

Fig. 4.4 Comparison of survival rates between extracorporeal (Toyobo LVAD) and implantable LVADs over 3 years. (Source: Ref. [29] with permission)

extracorporeal type provides long-term stable support with careful management by the transplant teams.

4.3.6 Update in Percutaneous VAD

One of the recent breakthroughs in MCS is the advent of the catheter-based flow device represented by Impella (ABIOMED, Danvers, MA, USA). The developmental history of intraarterial axial flow blood pump has been long since HemoPump™ (Medtronic, Inc., Minneapolis, MN) was introduced in around 2004. Currently, Impella 5.5 (SmartAsisst®) is demonstrating remarkable progress as the new style of less invasive catheter VAD [30]. In fact, under the new UNOS heart allocation policy, this new modality has been extended to BTT and recent data from UNOS showed favorable results in a cohort of 464 patients [31]. Here, we show a representative case supported by Impella 5.5 for post-myocardial infarction.

Case Presentation The patient is a 66-year-old male who suffered severe left ventricular dysfunction after acute myocardial infarction due to left main coronary artery obstruction. He required temporary PCPS for life saving after emergent percutaneous intervention under ImpellaCP. On the 7th day, switched to Impella 5.5, and finally, the device was removed on the 49th day, after active rehabilitation under device implantation. The chest X-rays at the initiation and at the time of termination of Impella support are shown (Fig. 4.5). Thus, this catheter-type VAD seems promising in the field of MCS not only in emergency situations but also in chronic heart failure.

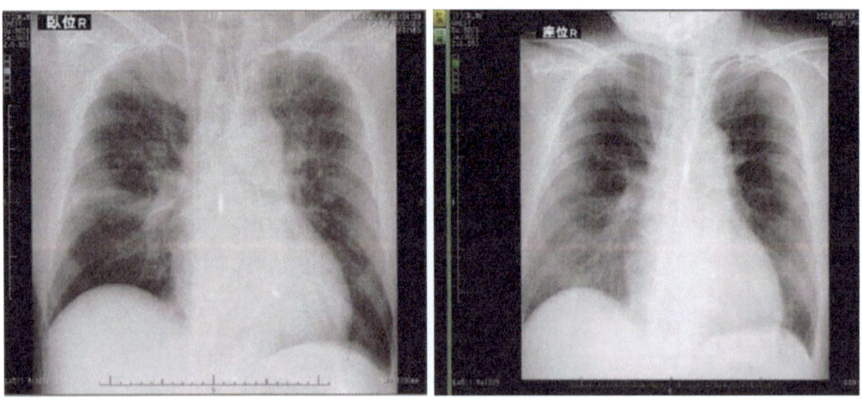

Fig. 4.5 Chest X-rays of a patient supported by Impella 5.5. Left: On the first day of Impella CP implantation under PCPS support. Right: after switched to Impella 5.5 (on the day of removal). Body of Impella is seen in place (ascending aorta). (Courtesy of Dr. Hisashi Satoh, Higashitakarazuka Satoh Hospital, Takarazuka, Hyogo, Japan)

4.4 Summary

Because of the severe donor shortage in Japan, heart transplantation is still in developing state with an average waiting time of nearly 5 years. On the other hand, implantable VADs are playing an increasingly central role in the treatment of end-stage heart failure, extending to BTT, DT, and BTR. As the shortage of donors is addressed at the national level, further refinements in the indications for VADs are expected, leading to an integrated end-stage heart failure category covering BTT and DT as one category of end-stage heart failure. Furthermore, the breakthrough strategy for BTR should be implemented in combination with a regenerative approach.

Addendum

DT is presented in Chap. 5 and pediatric VAD is presented in Chap. 15 in this book.

References

1. Philips SJ, Zeff RH, Kongtahworn C, et al. Percutaneous cardio-pulmonary bypass: application and indication for use. Ann Thorc Surg. 1989;47:121–3.
2. Sawa Y, Nishimura M, Hayashi Y, et al. Clinical evaluation of percutaneous cardiopulmonary support using a centrifugal pump for patients with postcardiotomy shock. In: Matsuda H, editor. Rotary blood pumps, new developments and current application. Tokyo: Springer; 2000. p. 97–106.
3. Matsuda H, Matsuwaka R, Kaneko M, et al. Analysis of clinical factors for survival after left and biventricular bypass using centrifugal pump following open heart surgery in infants and adults. Artif Organs. 1990;14:382–6.
4. Satoh H, Kobayashi T, Nakano S, et al. Clinical application of percutaneous left ventricular support with a centrifugal pump. ASAIO J. 1993;39:153–5.
5. Takano H, Taenaka Y, Noda H, et al. Multiinstitutional studies of the National Cardiovascular Center ventricular assist system: use in 92 patients. ASAIO Trans. 1989;35:541–4.
6. Matsuda H, Taenaka Y, Ohkubo N, et al. Use of a paracorporeal ventricular assist device for postoperative cardiogenic shock in two children with complex cardiac lesions. Artif Organs. 1988;12:423–30.
7. Nishimura M, Ohtake S, Sawa Y, et al. Left ventricular assist system as a bridge to heart transplantation: the role and the strategy in Japan. Transplant Proc. 1999;31:1997–9.
8. Masai T, Sawa Y, Ohtake S, et al. Hepatic dysfunction after left ventricular mechanical assist in patients with end-stage heart failure: role of inflammatory response and hepatic microcirculation. Ann Thorac Surg. 2002;73:549–55.
9. Matsuwaka R, Matsuda H, Kaneko M, et al. Overseas transport of a patient with an extracorporeal left ventricular assist device. Ann Thorac Surg. 1995;59:522–3.
10. Frazier OH, Duncan JM, Radovancevic B, et al. Successful bridge to heart transplantation with a new left ventricular assist device. J Heart Lung Transplant. 1992;11:530–7.
11. Frazier OH. First use of an untethered vented electric left ventricular assist device for long-term support. Circulation. 1994;89:2908–14.
12. Rose EA, Gelijns AC, Moskowitz AJ, et al. Long-term use of a left ventricular assist device for end-stage heart failure. N Engl J Med. 2001;345:1435–43.

13. Portner PM, Jansen PGM, et al. Improved outcomes with an implantable left ventricular assist system: a multicenter study. Ann Thorac Surg. 2001;71:205–9.
14. Omoto R, Kyo S, Nishimura M, et al. Japanese multicenter clinical evaluation of the HeartMate vented electric left ventricular assist system. Artif Organs. 1995;8:34–40.
15. Masai T, Kadoba K, Miyamoto Y, et al. Application of wearable Novacor left ventricular assist system patients with end-stage cardiomyopathy: Osaka experience. In: Akutsu T, Koyanagi H, editors. Heart replacement-artificial heart 6. Tokyo: Springer; 1998. p. 210–6.
16. Matsuda H, Matsumiya G. Current status of left ventricular assist devices: the role in bridge to transplantation and future perspectives. J Artif Organs. 2003;6:157–61.
17. Matsuda H, Fukushima N, Sawa Y, et al. First brain dead donor heart transplantation under new legislation in Japan. Jpn J Thorac Cardiovasc Surg. 1999;47:499–505.
18. Kitamura S, Nakatani T, Yagihara T, et al. Cardiac transplantation under new legislation for organ transplantation in Japan. Report of two cases. Circ J. 2000;64:333–9.
19. Yoshioka D, Matsumiya G, Toda K, et al. Clinical results with the Jarvik 2000 axial flow left ventricular assist device: the Osaka University Experience. Artif Organs. 2014;17:308–14.
20. Kohno H, Matsumiya G, Sawa Y, et al. The Jarvik 2000 left ventricular assist device as a bridge to transplantation: a Japanese registry for mechanically assisted circulatory support. J Heart Lung Transplant. 2018;37:71–8.
21. Kamata S, Sakaguchi T, Miyagawa S, et al. The first clinical case in Japan of destination therapy using the Jarvik 2000 left ventricular assist device. J Artif Organs. 2010;13:170–3.
22. Yamazaki K, Litwak P, Tagusari O, et al. An implantable centrifugal blood pump with recirculating purge system (cool-seal system). Artif Organs. 1998;22:466–74.
23. Nojiri C, Kijima T, Maekawa J, et al. Development status of the Terumo implantable left ventricular assist system. Artif Organs. 2001;25:411–3.
24. Matsuda H. Development of ventricular assist device and heart transplantation in Japan: how people worked. Artif Organs. 2020;44:544–60.
25. Matsumiya G, Monta O, Fukushima N, et al. Who would be a candidate for recovery during prolonged mechanical left ventricular support in idiopathic dilated cardiomyopathy? J Thorac Cardiovasc Surg. 2005;130:699–704.
26. Miyagawa S, Sawa Y, Taketani S, et al. Myocardial regenerative therapy for heart failure: hepatocyte growth factor enhances the effect of cellular cardiomyoplasty. Circulation. 2002;105:256–61.
27. Sawa Y, Yoshikawa Y, Toda K, et al. Safety and efficacy of autologous skeletal myoblast sheets (TCD-51073) for the treatment of severe chronic heart failure due to ischemic heart disease. Circ J. 2015;79:991–9.
28. Domae K, Miyagawa S, Toda K, et al. New treatment strategy for severe heart failure: combination of ventricular assist device and regenerative therapy. J Artif Organs. 2021;24:1–5.
29. Nakatani T, Sase K, Oshiyama H, et al. Japanese registry of mechanically assisted circulatory support; First report. J Heart Lung Transplant. 2017;36:1087–96.
30. Ramzy D, Soltesz EG, Silvestry S, et al. Improved clinical outcomes associated with the Impella 5.5 compared to the Impella 5.0 in contemporary cardiogenic shock and heart failure patients. J Heart Lung Transplant. 2023;42:553–7.
31. Cevasco M, Shin M, Cohen W, et al. Impella 5.5 as a bridge to heart transplantation: waitlist outcomes in the United States. Clin Transplant. 2023;37(10):e15066.

Role of Implantable Ventricular Assist Device in End-Stage Heart Failure: Bridge to Transplantation and Destination Therapy

5

Daisuke Yoshioka and Shigeru Miyagawa

Abstract

To date at Osaka University, six types of LVADs have been used clinically: Jarvik2000, EVAHEART, DuraHeart, HeartMate II, HeartMate 3, and HVAD. In a total of 281 patients, the 5-year survival rate was a satisfactory 71%. Currently, the total number of LVADs has reached over 300, and the long-term survival rate at 2 years was approximately 95% for HeartMate 3 implants.

In this report of long-term VAD therapy as bridge to transplantation (BTT), we have focused on the complications of the following: stroke, infection, aortic regurgitation, and right heart failure including tricuspid regurgitation. The characteristics of complications with long-term VAD support are analyzed to evaluate risk factors. In the neurological study, post-transplant MRI showed the presence of cerebral microbleeds very frequently. It was also found that underlying bacteremia significantly increased the risk of neurological complications in long-term VAD patients. Although the number of heart transplants is limited, our experience with long-term VAD as BTT may be helpful in further refining this treatment strategy. Also, the analysis of these patients from the view of complication at long-term support may give important information to the ongoing destination therapy (DT).

Keywords

Mechanically assisted circulatory support · Ventricular assist device · Continuous flow VAD · Heart transplantation · Bridge to transplantation · Right heart failure · Aortic regurgitation · Cerebral microbleeds · Destination therapy

D. Yoshioka (✉) · S. Miyagawa
Department of Cardiovascular Surgery, The University of Osaka Graduate School of Medicine, Suita, Osaka, Japan
e-mail: yoshioka@surg1.med.osaka-u.ac.jp; miyagawa.shigeru.med@osaka-u.ac.jp

H. Matsuda et al. (eds.), *Heart and Lung Transplantation*,
https://doi.org/10.1007/978-981-96-8810-4_5

5.1 Introduction

Worldwide, the number of patients with heart failure has been increasing as a result of the heart failure pandemic. Along with this trend, the number of heart transplants for end-stage heart failure has also increased. At the same time, the development of mechanically assisted circulatory support (MCS) has been remarkable with the introduction of implantable left ventricular assist devices (LVADs).

In Japan, instead of delaying heart transplantation, the application of VADs for severe heart failure has been organized since the early 1990s [1]. In our practice at Osaka University, the use of LVAD has started with pulsatile, extracorporeal, and implantable, considering bridge to heart transplantation (BTT) [2, 3]. The actual start of heart transplantation was in 1999 [4], but due to a marked shortage of donors and an average waiting time of about 3 years, the use of durable, implantable continuous-flow VADs began in 2011 [5]. After nearly 10 years of active management of heart transplant candidates, we have accumulated clinical experience with implantable LVADs in nearly 200 patients. Along with this approach, a bridge to recovery (BTR) strategy has also been conducted [6]. Since 2021, destination therapy (DT) has been initiated. This report discusses the current status of implantable LVADs in Japan from the perspective of our achievements at Osaka University.

5.2 Overview of Implantable LVAD

5.2.1 Current Status in Japan

According to a report by the J-MACS Committee of the Japanese Association for Thoracic Surgery in December 2023, 1458 patients had received LVAD implants in Japan since June 2011, with a mean age of 44 years and 1-year and 2-year survival rates of 93% and 90%, respectively [7]. The above cohort includes extracorporeal VADs, which were widely used prior to the official introduction of permanent implantable VADs. Since 2005, Osaka University has performed LVAD implantation for 281 patients with severe heart failure, achieving a 5-year survival rate of 71% (Fig. 5.1).

Currently, there has been a shift to continuous-flow implantable VADs, represented by HeartMateII and, more recently, HeartMate3. Data from HeartMate II alone, reported primarily by our members, showed a 3-year survival rate of 91% for patients younger than 59 years and 76% for patients 60 years and older [8]. The HeartMate 3 is now well accepted as the most commonly used device, and results continue to improve [9]. Although registry reports for HeartMate 3 are not yet available, a joint study by Osaka University and the National Cerebral and Cardiovascular Research Center (Suita, Japan) of 75 cases reported excellent survival rates of 94.7% at both 1 and 2 years [10] (Fig. 5.2). In this analysis, it should be noted that the HeartMate II cohort of 197 patients showed comparable results.

Regarding DT, the academic professionals related to MCS have published the guidelines [11] after the government approval as a new category of MCS in May

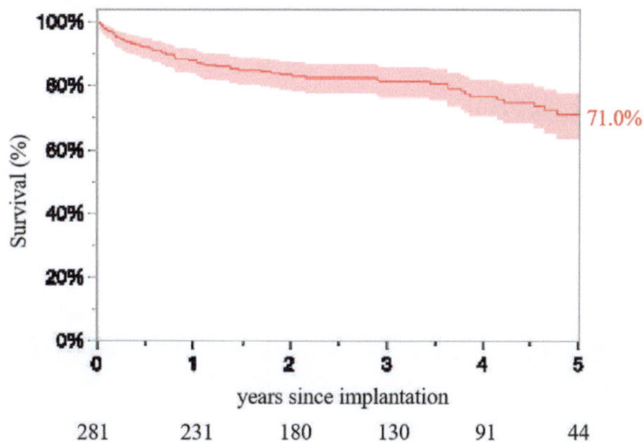

Fig. 5.1 Overall survival in 281 implantable LVAD patients (unpublished data)

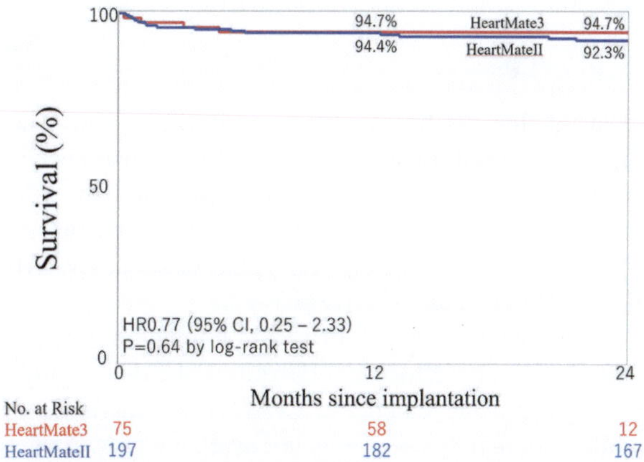

Fig. 5.2 Overall survivals after HeartMateII (*N* = 195) and HeartMate3 (*N* = 75) LVAD implantation Data are combined from two institutions; Osaka University Hospital and National Cerebral and Cardiovascular Center. (Source: Ref. [10] (open access))

2021. The number of patients enrolled in J-MACS has reached 98 so far, of which 90 were from HeartMate3 [7]. This group consisted of 73 male and 25 female patients, and the age at enrollment was 50–59 years in 22, 60–69 years in 46, and over 70 years in 10 patients, respectively. The outcome has not yet been reported.

As a social matter, the presence of a caregiver during home medical care is essential for VAD/transplant therapy. For BTT cases, 24-h support is mandatory during LVAD use until heart transplantation, while DT requires a minimum of 6 months of cohabitating caregiver support. Our experience suggested that approximately 10% of consultation cases could not proceed with VAD therapy due to a lack of caregivers [12]. Clinical research is being conducted to remove these obstacles and ensure patient safety.

5.2.2 Osaka Experience

Our first implantable VAD was made by introducing Jarvik 2000 continuous-flow implantable LVAD in 2005, the first case in Japan. By 2010 a total of 8 patients had

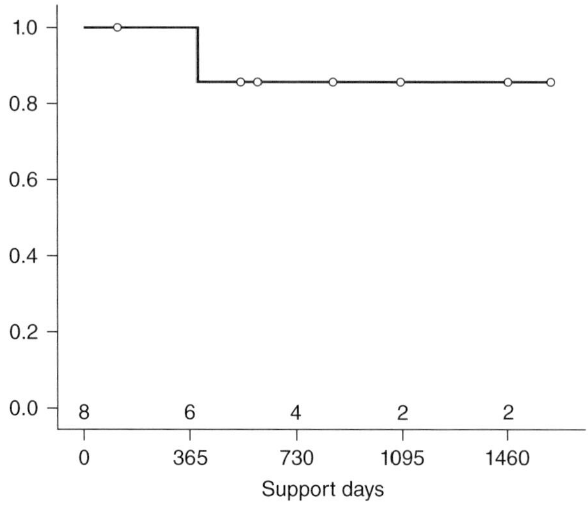

Fig. 5.3 Long-term survival rate after Jarvik2000 implantation. (Source: Ref. [13] with permission)

received this pin-bearing device for BTT [13]. Later, DuraHeart (Terumo Inc., Japan) was used for potential BTR before insurance reimbursement began [14]. In 2011, implantable LVADs were reimbursed by insurance in Japan as BTT for patients with severe heart failure awaiting heart transplantation. To date, six types of LVADs have been used clinically: Jarvik 2000, EVAHEART, DuraHeart, HeartMate II, HeartMate 3, and HVAD [13–17].

As shown in Fig. 5.1a of LVAD implantation for 281 patients, a 5-year survival rate was as satisfactory as 71% during the developing phase. In this chance of publishing our achievements in LVAD, our experience of Jarvik2000 may be worthwhile although this device is not available now. As described above, 8 patients had received this device, and the support period ranged from 388 to 1601 days because of the severe donor shortage, and 6 patients had reached transplantation with average support of 725 days. Overall survival rates at 1, 2, and 3 years were 100, 86, and 86%, respectively [13] (Fig. 5.3). Later in 2021, we attempted to implant Jarvik2000 to a 75-year-old woman as the first case of DT protocol [18].

5.3 VAD-Related Complications

5.3.1 Neurological Complications

Neurological complications have historically been the most frequent and fatal complications in LVAD patients. These complications are caused by thromboembolism within the artificial heart and bleeding associated with anticoagulation therapy. Thrombosis in the pump or around the cannulas in the left ventricle often leads to strokes. We have reported that approximately 10–20% of patients experienced severe neurological complications in early clinical studies involving devices like *DuraHeart* and *HVAD*, conducted before insurance reimbursement in Japan [14,

17]. Notably, Samura and his colleagues reported a significant relationship between acute postoperative LVAD flow rates and the occurrence of strokes in patients using *HeartMate II* [19].

In recent years, the availability of *HeartMate3* has dramatically reduced the incidence of neurological complications [9]. In that report, the 5-year stroke incidence for *HeartMate 3* is 0.05 events per patient-year, with a hazard ratio of 0.37 compared to *HeartMate II*. Specifically, pump thrombosis rates decreased to less than 10% of *HeartMate II* levels, at 0.05 events per patient-year. Japanese data obtained from two institutions, Osaka University and NCVC, show a 2-year stroke-free rate of 97% for *HeartMate 3*, a dramatic improvement compared to *HeartMate II*'s 80.4% [10].

In addition to thromboembolic-related neurological complications, infections frequently lead to neurological complications. Our study covering 164 LVAD patients demonstrated that bacteremia significantly increased the risk of neurological complications. Among 58 cases with bacteremia, 22% developed cerebral hemorrhage within 3 months, a significantly higher risk compared to 106 cases without bacteremia [20](Fig. 5.4). Since *HeartMate 3* requires a lower optimal INR than other devices, the 22% risk may be lower, but vigilance for infection-related neurological complications remains critical.

We also attempted the study of structural brain changes in LVAD patients using brain MRI after heart transplantation or VAD weaning, and 35 patients were analyzed [21](Fig. 5.5). Nearly all patients had cerebral microbleeds (CMBs), which

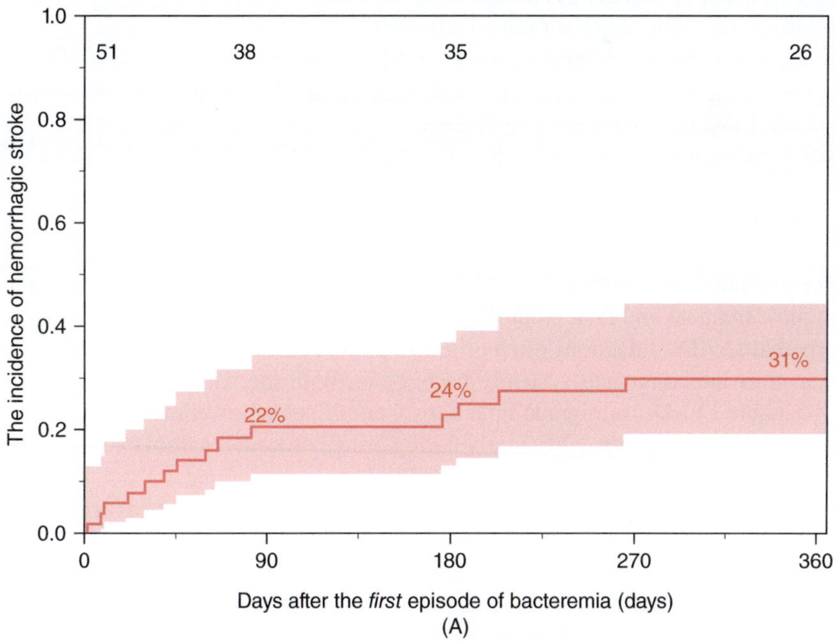

Fig. 5.4 The incidence of hemorrhagic strokes after the first episode of bacteremia. (Source: Ref. [20] (open access))

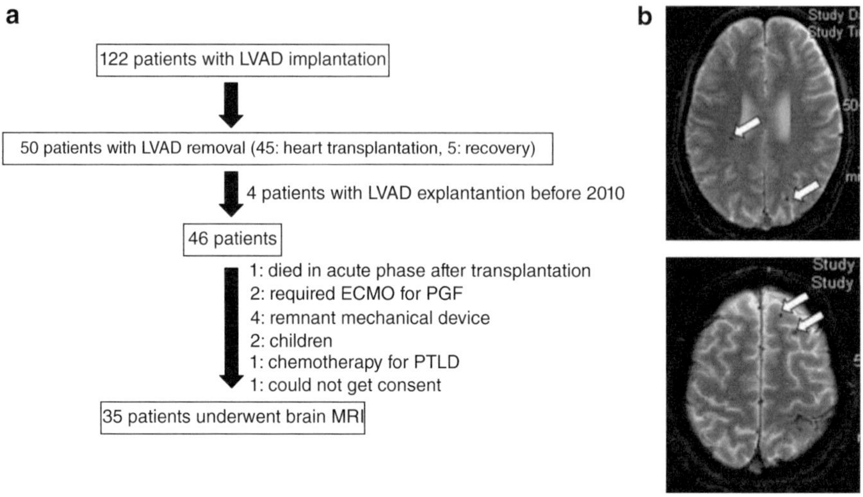

Fig. 5.5 Study of cerebral microbleeds after LVAD support. (**a**) Schema of patient selection for brain MRI examination. (**b**) Cerebral microbleeds were defined as homogeneous round foci <10 mm diameter with low signal intensity shown by T2-weighted MRI (white arrow). (Source: Ref. [21] with permission)

are typically seen only in the elderly in the general population, with a significantly higher number of lesions in patients with infections. In addition, a study from the Department of Neurology at Osaka University found that LVAD patients had more pronounced pathological brain atrophy on MRI compared to standard heart failure patients [22]. This study also provided interesting insights into the relationship between LVAD use and cognitive decline.

5.3.2 Infections

Like neurological complications, LVAD-related infections have long been among the most frequent and fatal complications associated with LVAD therapy. In extracorporeal LVADs, infections often originate at the cannula exit site, leading to vascular graft infections and systemic bacteremia. With the widespread adoption of implantable LVADs, retrograde infections from driveline insertion sites and infections of the LVAD pump, particularly during bridge procedures from extracorporeal to implantable LVADs, have been reported [23].

Regarding driveline infections, we identified diabetes as a risk factor for increased driveline infections using the J-MACS database [24](Fig. 5.6). We have used *DuraHeart* in clinical studies since 2009, observing frequent infections in cases involving bridge procedures from extracorporeal LVADs [5]. LVAD pump infections are particularly challenging to treat and associated with poor prognosis. Imaoka et al. proposed a treatment algorithm for pump infections, including debridement and pump replacement [25]. Domae and his colleagues reported a case

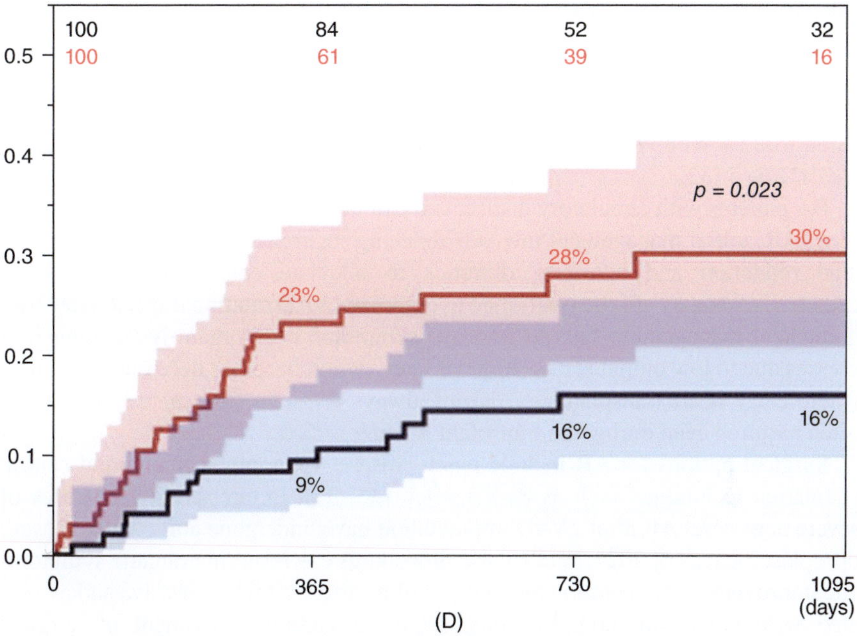

Fig. 5.6 Incidence of driveline infection in propensity-matched HeartMateII patients. Red line: patients with diabetes, black line: patients without diabetes. (Source: Ref. [24] (open access))

of successful treatment of pump infections in *HVAD*, an implantable LVAD without a pump pocket [26].

Preventing driveline infections is critical to avoiding retrograde pump infections. Recently, Imaoka et al. reported that driveline fixation methods can effectively reduce driveline infections [27].

5.3.3 Aortic Regurgitation (AR)

The development of new-onset aortic regurgitation (AR) during LVAD support is a relatively common complication, occurring in 20–25% of patients with *HeartMate II* within the first year post-implantation. This condition arises as LVAD support directs all blood flow from the left ventricle through the LVAD, leading to persistent closure of the aortic valve. This constant closure results in pathological fusion and degeneration, contributing to AR [28].

Progressive AR causes recirculation of blood flow through the regurgitant valve, which can lead to low cardiac output syndrome even when LVAD flow remains normal. Reports have indicated that the incidence of new-onset AR increased with the transition from pulsatile-flow devices like *HeartMate XVE* to continuous-flow devices like *HeartMate II* [29]. Continuous-flow LVADs are particularly associated with a higher incidence of new-onset AR in cases where the aortic valve remains persistently closed [30]. A recent report from Columbia University Irving Medical Center (NY) suggested that *HeartMate 3* has a similar incidence of new-onset AR compared to *HeartMateII* [31]. However, sub-analysis from the *Momentum Trial* indicated that the 2-year freedom from severe AR was 92% with *HeartMate3* compared to 82% with *HeartMateII*, suggesting a lower incidence of severe AR with *HeartMate 3* [32].

For patients with circulatory insufficiency or heart failure symptoms due to new-onset AR, initial management involves reducing regurgitant volume through afterload reduction and adjusting diuretics to alleviate congestion. Right heart catheterization may also be performed to optimize LVAD rotational speed. However, if medical management fails to improve symptoms or if organ dysfunction progresses due to low output status, surgical intervention becomes necessary. In Japan, where early heart transplantation is not always feasible, surgical intervention is often required even during the transplant waiting period.

Surgical options for AR include patch closure, valve replacement, and central coaptation techniques such as Park's stitch [33, 34]. In our activity, 17 cases of severe new-onset AR after LVAD implantation have undergone aortic valve closure or replacement as of 2024. While these procedures can result in dramatic symptomatic improvement, reoperation involving cardiac arrest is highly invasive and associated with significant complications, requiring careful assessment of surgical indications based on preoperative heart failure status and right heart dysfunction. In 5 out of the 17 cases, temporary right ventricular assist devices (RVADs) or ECMO were required postoperatively.

Treatment options for AR remain limited in our practice, with no available devices for addressing AR in LVAD patients. Internationally, transcatheter aortic valve replacement (TAVR) has been increasingly reported for managing new-onset AR in LVAD patients [35].

5.3.4 Right Heart Failure (RHF)

RHF in LVAD patients can be classified into acute-phase occurring shortly after LVAD implantation and chronic-phase developing later. RHF reduces pulmonary circulation, which subsequently decreases left ventricular preload and leads to reduced LVAD flow. This decline in LVAD flow can compromise organ perfusion, resulting in organ dysfunction. Additionally, increased venous pressure due to RHF contributes to organ congestion and decreased perfusion pressure (the difference between arterial and venous pressures), further exacerbating organ dysfunction.

From our experiences, it was suggested that patients with significant right ventricular diastolic dysfunction were more prone to postoperative RHF [36]. Elevated central venous pressure (CVP) due to RHF can impair renal function even in the absence of decreased renal artery blood flow [37]. Reduced urine output due to renal dysfunction can exacerbate CVP elevation and interstitial edema, creating a vicious cycle. RHF-induced CVP elevation also leads to hepatic congestion, which can progress to congestive hepatopathy and ultimately cirrhosis [38]. Similarly, venous pressure elevation causes intestinal congestion, leading to malabsorption and nutritional deficiencies. Intestinal mucosal dysfunction can increase the risk of bacterial translocation [39].

Patients with late-phase RHF have higher rates of rehospitalization, as well as increased incidence of strokes, gastrointestinal bleeding, and coagulation disorders due to reduced autoregulatory capacity and venous pressure elevation [40]. The incidence of RHF after LVAD implantation is approximately 10–15%, depending on severity, and late-phase RHF tends to persist longer [41]. Takeda and his colleagues identified risk factors for late-phase RHF, including reduced right ventricular contractility, elevated CVP, smaller left ventricular diameter, and higher BUN levels [42]. Conditions such as arrhythmogenic right ventricular cardiomyopathy, hypertrophic cardiomyopathy with significant diastolic dysfunction, and restrictive cardiomyopathy are particularly prone to both acute and late-phase RHF [43, 44]. Additionally, in dilated cardiomyopathy cases, mild right ventricular dysfunction at the time of LVAD implantation may progress to late-phase RHF due to disease progression during long-term support.

The incidence of late-phase RHF does not significantly differ between *HeartMateII* and *HeartMate3*. Randomized prospective trials comparing these devices over 5 years found no significant differences in RHF incidence [45]. However, some reports suggest higher rehospitalization rates for *HeartMate3*, though these studies often fail to distinguish between RHF and left heart failure [46]. Clinical studies from our group comparing the two devices over 2 years similarly found no significant differences in RHF incidence, though differences in patient backgrounds due to advancements in device technology must be considered [9]. Despite device improvements, RHF remains a major cause of rehospitalization, requiring meticulous management.

Tricuspid regurgitation (TR) can also contribute to RHF by causing circulatory insufficiency in the right heart. Patients with a tricuspid annular diameter ≥41 mm at the time of LVAD implantation are at higher risk of late-phase RHF, regardless of whether tricuspid annuloplasty was performed [47]. However, preventive tricuspid annuloplasty has been reported to have limited efficacy in reducing TR progression and preventing RHF [48], and this is confirmed by our experience [49] (Fig. 5.7). Complete prevention of late-phase worsening of TR may require tricuspid valve replacement with a prosthetic valve, but further studies are needed to confirm its effectiveness.

In cases of severe right ventricular dysfunction, simultaneous implantation of an RVAD may be necessary, resulting in a biventricular assist device (BiVAD) configuration. Since the era of extracorporeal VADs, we have reported poor outcomes for patients requiring BiVADs [50]. In Japan, where heart transplant waiting times can exceed several years, successful bridging to transplantation for BiVAD patients has relied almost exclusively on implantable BiVADs. We have exclusively performed the successful bridged patients to heart transplantation using implantable BiVADs, employing devices like *HVAD* and *Jarvik 2000* as RVADs [51–54].

The above-described major complications associated with long-term LVAD support are summarized in Table 5.1.

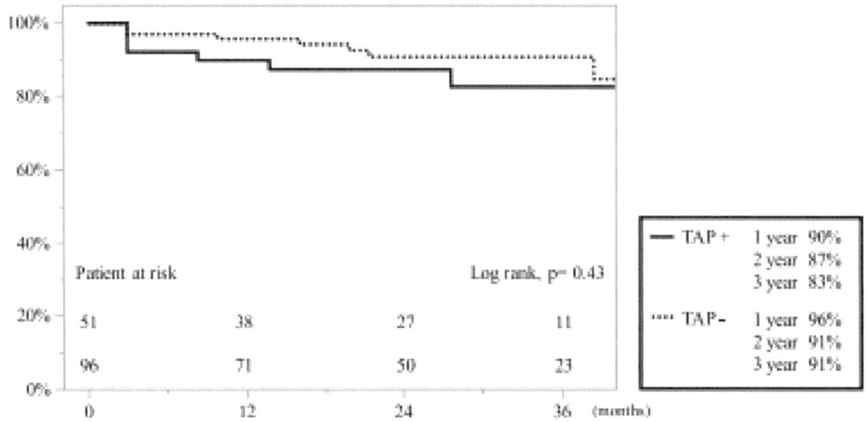

Fig. 5.7 The Kaplan-Meier analysis of late right ventricular failure-free rates according to concomitant tricuspid annuloplasty(TAP). Solid line: patients with TAP, dashed line: patients without TAP. (Source: Ref. [47] with permission)

Table 5.1 Characteristics of complications with long-term LVAD support

Type of complication	Frequency	Risk of mortality	Management	References
Drive-line infection	10–30%@2 years	NA	Debridement	[8, 22, 25]
Pocket infection	5–10%	26%@1 year 39%@2 years	Debridement, pump exchange	[23, 24]
AR	5–10%@2 years	NA	Aortic valve closure, heart transplantation	[29, 30]
RVF	10–20%@3 years	50–70%@3 years	Inotropes, RVAD, heart transplantation	[39, 40, 43]
Ischemic stroke	3–10%@2 years	10–20%@ 3 months	Thrombectomy, Anticoagulation	[8, 9, 17]
Hemorrhagic stroke	10–20%@2 years	>50% @ 3 months	Cease anticoagulation, craniotomy	[18]

5.4 Summary

Implantable VAD, especially the continuous-flow type, has established the role in the management of end-stage heart failure, including BTT and DT. In Japan, under the severe donor shortage and limited number of heart transplantation, the role of durable VADs has been recognized as crucial in the field of heart failure. Under long-term support, various VAD-related complications such as stroke, infection, aortic regurgitation, and right heart failure have been reported. Specific strategy including biventricular support. The mechanism and management for such complications are provided.

References

1. Matsuda H. Development of ventricular assist device and heart transplantation in Japan: how people worked. Artif Organs. 2020;44:544–60.
2. Nishimura M, Ohtake S, Sawa Y, et al. Left ventricular assist system as a bridge to heart transplantation: the role and the strategy in Japan. Transplant Proc. 1999;31:1997–9.
3. Masai T, Kadoba K, Miyamoto Y, et al. Application of wearable Novacor left ventricular assist system patients with end-stage cardiomyopathy: Osaka experience. In: Akutsu T, Koyanagi H, editors. Heart replacement-artificial heart 6. Tokyo: Springer; 1998. p. 210–6.
4. Matsuda H, Fukushima N, Sawa Y, et al. First brain dead donor heart transplantation under new legislation in Japan. Jpn J Thorac Cardiovasc Surg. 1999;47:499–505.
5. Yoshioka D, Sakaguchi T, Saito S, et al. Initial experience of conversion of Toyobo paracorporeal left ventricular assist device to DuraHeart left ventricular assist device. Circ J. 2012;76:372–6.
6. Matsumiya G, Monta O, Fukushima N, et al. Who would be a candidate for recovery during prolonged mechanical left ventricular support in idiopathic dilated cardiomyopathy? J Thorac Cardiovasc Surg. 2005;130:699–704.
7. J-MACS Statistical Report in 2024. https://j-vad.jp/document/J-MACS%20Statistical%20Report%20_20240204.pdf. https://j-vad.jp/jmacs-report/. Accessed 11 Feb 2025.
8. Yoshioka D, Toda K, Ono M, et al. Clinical results, adverse events, and change in end-organ function in elderly patients with HeartMateII left ventricular assist device – Japanese multicenter study. Circ J. 2018;82:409–18.
9. Mehra MR, Uriel N, Naka Y, et al. A fully magnetically levitated left ventricular assist device – final report. N Engl J Med. 2019;380:1618–27.
10. Inoue K, Fujita T, Yoshioka D, et al. Short-term outcomes of magnetically levitated left ventricular assist device in advanced heart failure – the Japanese cohort. Circ J. 2022;86:1961–7.
11. Ando M, Ono M. Current issues of destination therapy in Japan: to achieve 5-year or even more survival. J Art Organs. 2024;27:203–11.
12. Saito S, Yoshioka D, Kawamura T, et al. The foremost and greatest barrier to end-stage heart failure treatment: the impact of caregiver shortage. J Artif Organs. 2025;28:192. https://doi.org/10.1007/s10047-024-01463-x.
13. Yoshioka D, Matsumiya G, Toda K, et al. Clinical results with Jarvik 2000 axial flow left ventricular assist device: Osaka University experience. J Artif Organs. 2014;17:308–14.
14. Sakaguchi T, Matsumiya G, Yoshioka D, et al. DuraHeart magnetically levitated left ventricular assist device: Osaka University experience. Circ J. 2013;77:1736–41.
15. Saito S, Yamazaki K, Nishinaka T, et al. Post-approval study of a highly pulsed, low-shear-rate, continuous-flow, left ventricular assist device, EVAHEART: a Japanese multicenter study using J-MACS. J Heart Lung Transplant. 2014;33:599–608.
16. Ono M, Sawa Y, Nakatani T, et al. Japanese multicenter outcomes with the HeartMate II left ventricular assist device in patients with small body surface area. Circ J. 2016;80:1931–6.
17. Nishi H, Toda K, Miyagawa S, et al. Initial experience in Japan with HeartWare ventricular assist system. J Artif Organs. 2014;17:149–56.
18. Kamata S, Sakaguchi T, Miyagawa S, et al. The first clinical case in Japan of destination therapy using the Jarvik 2000 left ventricular assist device. J Artif Organs. 2010;13:170–3.
19. Samura T, Yoshioka D, Toda K, et al. Risk of stroke early after implantation of a left ventricular assist device. J Thorac Cardiovasc Surg. 2019;157:259–67.
20. Yoshioka D, Sakaniwa R, Toda K, et al. Relationship between bacteremia and hemorrhagic stroke in patients with continuous-flow left ventricular assist device. Circ J. 2018;82:448–56.
21. Yoshioka D, Okazaki S, Toda K, et al. Prevalence of cerebral microbleeds in patients with continuous-flow left ventricular assist devices. J Am Heart Assoc. 2017;6(9):e005955. https://doi.org/10.1161/JAHA.117.005955.

22. Murase S, Okazaki S, Yoshioka D, et al. Abnormalities of brain imaging in patients after left ventricular assist device support following explantation. J Heart Lung Transplant. 2020;39:220–7.
23. Imamura T, Kinugawa K, Ono M, et al. Bridge-to-bridge left ventricular assist device implantation strategy vs. primary left ventricular assist device implantation strategy. Circ J. 2020;84:2198–204.
24. Yoshioka D, Toda K, Ono M, et al. Effect of diabetes mellitus on outcomes in patients with left ventricular assist device – analysis of data from a Japanese National Database. Circ J. 2022;86:1950–8.
25. Imaoka S, Samura T, Yoshioka D, et al. Clinical outcomes of left ventricular assist device pump infection. ASAIO J. 2023;69:1056–64.
26. Domae K, Toda K, Yoshioka D, et al. Complex HeartWare left ventricular assist device infection treated with pump exchange: clinical alert for the driveline location. J Artif Organs. 2021;24:377–81.
27. Imaoka S, Kashiyama N, Yoshioka D, et al. Clinical outcomes of modified left ventricular assist device driveline management. J Artif Organs 2024. https://link.springer.com/article/10.1007/s10047-024-01482-8. Accessed Feb 15 2025.
28. Hata H, Fujita T, Ishibashi-Ueda H, et al. Pathological analysis of the aortic valve after long-term left ventricular assist device support. Eur J Cardiothorac Surg. 2014;46:193–7.
29. Cowger J, Pagani FD, Haft JW, et al. The development of aortic insufficiency in left ventricular assist device-supported patients. Circ Heart Fail. 2010;3:668–74.
30. Jorde UP, Uriel N, Nahumi N, et al. Prevalence, significance, and management of aortic insufficiency in continuous flow left ventricular assist device recipients. Circ Heart Fail. 2014;7:310–9.
31. Malick A, Ning Y, Kurlansky PA, et al. Development of de novo aortic insufficiency in patients with HeartMate3. Ann Thorac Surg. 2022;114:450–6.
32. Uriel N, Milano C, Agarwal R, et al. Incidence and clinical correlates of de-novo aortic regurgitation with a fully magnetically levitated left ventricular assist device: a MOMENTUM 3 trial portfolio analysis. Eur J Heart Fail. 2023;25:286–94.
33. Atkins BZ, Hashmi ZA, Ganapathi AM, et al. Surgical correction of aortic valve insufficiency after left ventricular assist device implantation. J Thorac Cardiovasc Surg. 2013;146:1247–52.
34. Gyoten T, Morshuis M, Fox H, et al. Secondary aortic valve replacement in continuous flow left ventricular assist device therapy. Artif Organs. 2021;45:736–41.
35. Rali AS, Taduru SS, Tran LE, et al. Transcatheter aortic valve replacement and surgical aortic valve replacement outcomes in left ventricular assist device patients with aortic insufficiency. Card Fail Rev. 2022;8:e30.
36. Samura T, Yoshioka D, Asanoi H, et al. Right atrial pressure waveform predicts right ventricular failure after left ventricular assist device implantation. Ann Thorac Surg. 2019;108:1361–8.
37. Damman K, van Deursen VM, Navis G, et al. Increased central venous pressure is associated with impaired renal function and mortality in a broad spectrum of patients with cardiovascular disease. J Am Coll Cardiol. 2009;53:582–8.
38. Verbrugge FH, Dupont M, Steels P, et al. Abdominal contributions to cardiorenal dysfunction in congestive heart failure. J Am Coll Cardiol. 2013;62:485–95.
39. Sandek A, Bauditz J, Swidsinski A, et al. Altered intestinal function in patients with chronic heart failure. J Am Coll Cardiol. 2007;50:1561–9.
40. Rame JE, Pagani FD, Kiernan MS, et al. Evolution of late right heart failure with left ventricular assist devices and association with outcomes. J Am Coll Cardiol. 2021;78:2294–308.
41. Kapelios CJ, Lund LH, Wever-Pinzon O, et al. Right heart failure following left ventricular device implantation: natural history, risk factors, and outcomes: an analysis of the STS INTERMACS database. Circ Heart Fail. 2022;15:e008706.
42. Takeda K, Takayama H, Colombo PC, Y et al. Incidence and clinical significance of late right heart failure during continuous-flow left ventricular assist device support. J Heart Lung Transplant 2015;34:1024–1032.

43. Grupper A, Park SJ, Pereira NL, et al. Role of ventricular assist therapy for patients with heart failure and restrictive physiology: improving outcomes for a lethal disease. J Heart Lung Transplant. 2015;34:1042–9.
44. Patel SR, Saeed O, Naftel D, et al. Outcomes of restrictive and hypertrophic cardiomyopathies after LVAD: an INTERMACS analysis. J Card Fail. 2017;23:859–67.
45. Mehra MR, Goldstein DJ, Cleveland JC, et al. Five-year outcomes in patients with fully magnetically levitated vs axial-flow left ventricular assist devices in the MOMENTUM 3 randomized trial. JAMA. 2022;328:1233–42.
46. Vidula H, Takeda K, Estep JD, et al. Hospitalization patterns and impact of a magnetically-levitated left ventricular assist device in the MOMENTUM 3 trial. JACC Heart Fail. 2022;10:470–81.
47. Nakanishi K, Homma S, Han J, et al. Usefulness of tricuspid annular diameter to predict late right sided heart failure in patients with left ventricular assist device. Am J Cardiol. 2018;122:115–20.
48. Fujino T, Imamura T, Nitta D, et al. Effect of concomitant tricuspid valve surgery with left ventricular assist device implantation. Ann Thorac Surg. 2020;110:918–24.
49. Nakazato T, Yoshioka D, Toda K, et al. Impact of tricuspid regurgitation on late right ventricular failure in left ventricular assist device patients can prophylactic tricuspid annuloplasty prevent late right ventricular failure? J Cardiothorac Surg. 2021;16(1):99. https://doi.org/10.1186/s13019-021-01492-0.
50. Saito S, Sakaguchi T, Miyagawa S, et al. Recovery of right heart function with temporary right ventricular assist using a centrifugal pump in patients with severe biventricular failure. J Heart Lung Transplant. 2012;31:858–64.
51. Saito S, Sakaguchi T, Miyagawa S, et al. Jarvik 2000 biventricular assist device conversion from old pin-shaped bearing pumps to new conical bearing pumps. J Artif Organs. 2013;16:105–9.
52. Saito S, Sakaguchi T, Miyagawa S, et al. Biventricular support using implantable continuous-flow ventricular assist devices. J Heart Lung Transplant. 2011;30:475–8.
53. Sakaguchi T, Saito S, Yoshioka D, et al. Long-term biventricular support with rotary blood pumps in a patient with a noncontractile heart. J Thorac Cardiovasc Surg. 2013;146:e29–30.
54. Yoshioka D, Toda K, Yoshikawa Y, et al. Over 1200-day support with dual Jarvik 2000 biventricular assist device. Interact Cardiovasc Thorac Surg. 2014;19:1083–4.

Destination Therapy: Background and Future Prospects

6

Yoshiki Sawa

Abstract

In the treatment of end-stage heart failure, the role of mechanical circulatory support represented by a durable ventricular assist device (VAD) has been accepted worldwide as a bridge to transplantation (BTT) or destination therapy (DT). In the United States, the priority of such VADs has shifted to DT from original BTT, and the number of DT cases is increasing year by year, exceeding the number of heart transplants. In Japan, the application of implantable VAD has started from bridge to candidacy in the early period before the start of heart transplantation, and the long-term survivals on VAD as BTT under the prolonged waiting period over 5 years have been demonstrated to be comparable to that of heart transplantation. Based on such results of VAD treatment, the introduction of DT has started in April 2021. This article outlines the Japanese version of DT and the future prospects.

Keywords

Destination therapy · Heart transplantation · LVAD · End of life care · Bridge to transplantation · Bridge to recovery · Cost-effectiveness · HeartMate 3

6.1 Introduction

Heart transplantation for end-stage heart failure has been performed for more than half a century, since the first case in 1967, and has now reached an annual number of more than 5000 cases worldwide, having established itself. On the other hand, in addition to the severe shortage of donors, there have also been significant advances

Y. Sawa (✉)
Osaka Keisatsu Hospital, Osaka, Japan

H. Matsuda et al. (eds.), *Heart and Lung Transplantation*,
https://doi.org/10.1007/978-981-96-8810-4_6

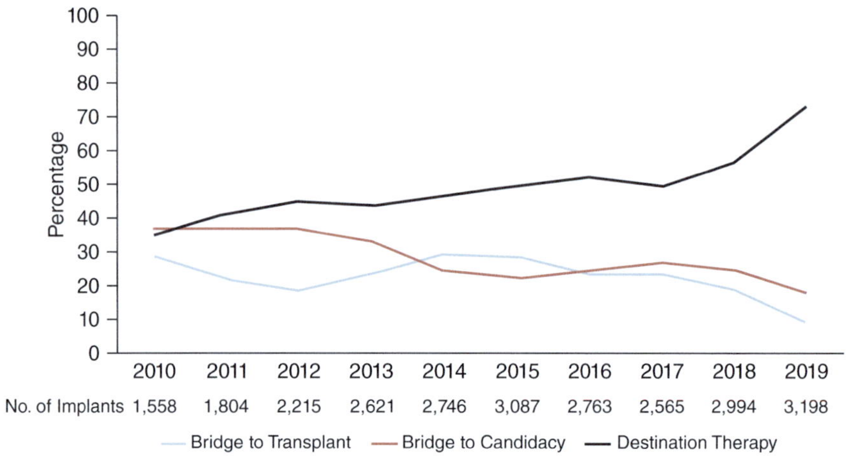

Fig. 6.1 Trends of LVAD application since 2010 to 2019 in the United States. After 2017, the number of DT (black-line) has been only increasing compared to the decline in bridge to transplant and bridge to candidacy. (Source: Ref. [1] with permission)

in the implantable left ventricular assist device (LVAD), and now destination therapy (DT), which considers this as the last line of treatment, works in conjunction with heart transplantation. In fact, the number of DT cases in the United States is increasing year by year exceeding the heart transplant numbers [1] (Fig. 6.1).

On the other hand, in Japan, although the start of heart transplantation was delayed, the treatment of advanced heart failure has been managed by VADs since the 1980s, most of which were extracorporeal devices. Consequently, there are many results in their use as a bridge to transplantation (BTT), and also active works to introduce implantable types since the early 1990s [2]. Based on such results of LVAD treatment, the steps toward the introduction of DT in Japan have progressed rapidly over the past 10 years reaching the actual start in April 2021 through the efforts of related academic professionals [3]. This article outlines the process of DT introduction in Japan and the future prospects.

6.2 History of LVAD Development and Introduction of DT in Europe and the United States

On August 8, 1966, DeBakey successfully fitted the world's first LVAD to a patient in shock after open-heart surgery following aortic valve replacement as a bridge to recovery (BTR) until cardiac function recovered. Since then, LVADs have been developed and clinically applied as a BTR or bridge to heart transplantation (BTT). As the safety of the device and its effectiveness in improving prognosis have gradually improved, interest has grown in the permanent use of LVADs as DT without the need for transplantation. To investigate the usefulness of long-term LVAD support, the REMATCH trial was conducted in 1998–2001, in which 129 patients with end-stage severe heart failure (EF < 25%, NYHA IV, ineligible for heart transplantation) were randomly divided into two groups: one group continued with maximum medical treatment, and the other group implanted with an implantable pulsatile-flow LVAD (HeartMate VE, Thoratec). The results showed that LVAD treatment not only improved heart failure symptoms compared with medical treatment, but also significantly improved the 1-year survival rate from 25% to 52% [4].

Since 2000, the development and clinical application of small, continuous-flow implantable LVADs with fewer device failures has progressed, and a randomized comparative trial was conducted on 200 patients with end-stage severe heart failure between the HeartMate II, a small continuous-flow implantable LVAD, and the HeartMate XVE (pulsatile-flow type), an improved version of the HeartMate VE, whose usefulness was shown in the REMATCH trial. As a result, the HeartMate II reduced the frequency of infections and strokes by half compared to the conventional HeartMate XVE, reduced the need for LVAD replacement surgery to one-eighth, and improved the 2-year survival rate from 24% to 58% [5].

Based on the above, the FDA approved HeartMate XVE as an LVAD for DT since 2003, and the HeartMate II since 2010, and Medicare (a government-run health insurance system for the elderly) has also been providing insurance reimbursement. The number of cases has increased rapidly since the HeartMate II came into use, and currently the number of DT-LVAD implants exceeds 1000 cases per year, surpassing the number of LVADs implanted for BTT purposes.

As for other models, a randomized comparative study of the use of HVAD (Medtronic) for DT with the HeartMate II was conducted in the United States (ENDURANCE trial). There was no difference between the two in the primary end point (2-year survival rate without serious cerebral complications or pump replacement), and the HVAD has been FDA-approved as a DT-LVAD since 2018 [5, 6]. On the other hand, in Japan, HeartMate III, which is covered by insurance as BTT, was conducted in clinical trials in the United States without being bound by the category of BTT or DT and was approved by the FDA.

In Europe, the approval (CE mark) of implantable LVADs does not currently distinguish between BTT and DT. In Europe and the United States, where DT has been introduced for more than 15 years, implantable LVAD treatment is started as DT (or bridge to candidacy: BTC), and if the patient is suitable for transplant, BTT is performed, but if the patient is not suitable for transplant, DT is performed. Conversely, even if LVAD implantation is performed as BTT, if the patient is no longer suitable for transplant (for example, cancer is discovered), treatment is continued as DT.

The difference between DT and BTT is the name of the classification based on whether the patient was able to achieve transplantation, and it seems that the idea of separating BTT and DT from the beginning and considering the suitability of each has not been done in Europe and the United States until recently.

As a consequence of above-described efforts in application of LVAD for heart failure introducing DT, the paradigm of heart failure management has been changed dramatically and further advances of device development and management protocol combined with refinements in medical therapy are demanding [1].

6.3 Controversial Issues

In contrast to the remarkable progress of LVAD and DT overseas, the following three concerns have been pointed out regarding the introduction of DT in Japan.

1. Given that the number of heart transplants is still only a tenth of that in other countries, there is concern that if the indications for implantable LVADs were expanded beyond BTT, the number of patients eligible for transplant would increase, leading to a further extension of the waiting period for transplants.
2. In Japan, where combined non-insured therapies (mixed medical treatments) are not permitted under the universal health insurance system, there is concern about the financial burden of relatively expensive implantable LVAD treatment (in our calculations, the cost of the initial hospitalization surgery for LVAD implantation at one's own expense in INTERMACS* 3 = 25–30 million yen + annual equipment maintenance costs: 1.5–2 million yen) if it were expanded beyond BTT. * [7].
3. There were concerns about the management of end-of-life care. In the event of DT, patients would end up with the device still implanted until the end of life, causing confusion in the medical field in Japan, where the Death with Dignity Bill has not yet been enacted. In order to resolve these issues, efforts have been made over the past 6 years by related academic societies, as described in the next section.

6.4 How Academic Professions Worked

Considering the above controversial issues, efforts by related academic societies have been made to introduce DT in Japan [3]. In detail, related academic societies started to introduce implantable LVAD-DT therapy with a working group discussion at the Council of Societies Related to Ventricular Assist Therapy (VAD Council) on April 12, 2013 (Working Group for the Discussion of Appropriate Indications for Implantable LVAD). Initially, the working group's discussions were based on the premise of corporate clinical trials, but on the other hand, there were opinions expressed by members of the VAD Council that the discussion on DT in Japan was insufficient and that it was premature to aim for drug approval straight from corporate clinical trials, and that including BTC in DT would lead to a further increase in the number of patients waiting for transplants and an extension of the waiting period for transplants, so they should be separated.

In order to gather opinions, the first meeting of the DT Study Group, which included experts in cardiology, cardiovascular surgery, medical economics, and medical ethics, was held on March 21, 2014, and it was proposed that guidelines for DT in Japan should be created from three perspectives:

1. The patient selection criteria.
2. The ethical appropriateness of end-of-life care, including palliative care.
3. Cost-effectiveness from the perspective of medical economics.

After that, four meetings of the Working Group, which included members of the seven societies and two research groups that make up the VAD Council, experts in medical ethics, palliative care, and medical economics, the Ministry of Health, Labor, and Welfare (observer), and the PMDA (observer), were held, and in December 2014, the VAD Council compiled the results in a document titled "Concepts for appropriate adaptation of implantable ventricular assist devices in Japan: Destination Therapy," which has been published on the websites of each society (http://www.jacvas.com/view_dt.html). Since 2016, a corporate clinical trial using HeartMate II has been conducted in accordance with this guideline.

6.5 Summary of the Guideline

6.5.1 Patient Selection

(a) The patient who is not expected to survive for more than 2 years by advanced heart failure (Stage D).
(b) The patient in whom the heart transplantation cannot be indicated, but can tolerate LVAD implantation surgery.
(c) The patient is expected to have a good prognosis by LVAD implantation.

The HeartMate risk score (HMRS) [8], which also considers age factors, has been proposed to predict "cases where the implantation surgery prognosis is considered to be good." For example, if a 70-year-old patient with alb = 3.5 g/dl, Crn = 1.0, and INR = 1.0 undergoes surgery at a facility with extensive experience in VAD, the patient's risk score is $0.0274 \times 70–0.723 \times 3.5 + 0.74 \times 1.0 + 1.136 \times 1.0 + 0.807 \times 0 = 1.2635$. This makes the patient a low-risk patient, and according to US data, the patient is expected to have a 1-year survival rate of over 80%.

Initially, the Working Group suggested that an upper age limit should be set for DT, but since there was no scientific evidence for an upper age limit, it was decided that no upper age limit should be set and that low-risk cases with guaranteed outcomes for so-called elderly patients aged 65 and over would be eligible for DT. Unlike BTT, cases will be selected by a multidisciplinary in-house review committee at each facility based on the guidelines, and the case will be reported to the VAD Council. In addition, each facility is obligated to register all DT cases in J-MACS (Japanese Registry for Mechanically Assisted Circulatory Support), just like BTT cases, and the results and case selection process are verified by the VAD Council to ensure the results.

Recently, Ando and Ono [9] have proposed six issues to be explored when starting DT and the flowchart for decision-making (Fig. 6.2). The issues to be explored are as follows: risk assessment, management ability of the device, improve the quality of life to prevent the complication, expand the number of facilities capable to support the DT patients, reduce the burden of caregivers, and establish the home palliative care system based on the advanced care planning. Their proposal should be formalized to obtain social acceptance widely.

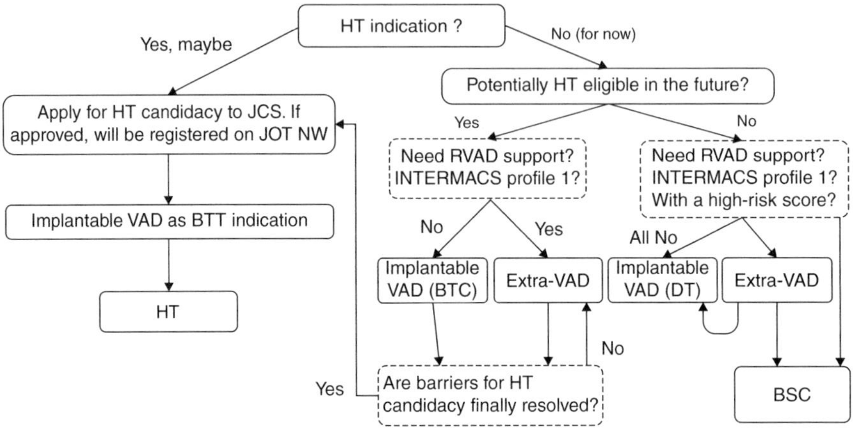

Fig. 6.2 The flow chart in the decision-making to apply LVAD in heart failure patients. *HT* heart transplantation, *RVAD* right VAD, *JCS* Japanese circulation society, *JOT NW* Japan organ transplant network, others see text. (Source: Ref. [9[(open access))

6.5.2 End-of-Life Care

End-of-life care is not unique to DT, but in DT, where the possibility of BTT is low, patients are forced to be aware of death, which is the end point of treatment, when starting treatment. It is considered important to explain end-of-life care in DT to the patient and family before treatment and to leave their wishes regarding end-of-life treatment in the form of an advance directive. When the patient reaches the end of life, it is important to provide palliative care to the patient and family, with an emphasis on the patient's wishes. At our hospital, when starting severe heart failure treatment, regardless of whether it is DT or BTT, the cardiovascular palliative care team (Kokorowa Care Team) explains end-of-life care and advance directives from an early stage and takes the time to explain and listen to the patient's wishes.

6.5.3 Cost-Effectiveness

Cost-effectiveness has been the major concern in VAD application to the end-stage heart failure, and DT is also a relatively new target of this issue. According to Gelijns and colleagues, the DT therapy has shown the cost-effectiveness of around $0.6 million per life year saving around $0.1 million compared to medical therapy [10]. Another report from the UK [11] provided evidence that HM3 LVAD therapy in advanced heart failure patients ineligible for heart transplantation may be cost-effective compared to medical therapy in the National Health Service UK-England context.

In the domestic matter, as national medical expenses increase, the cost-effectiveness of LVAD-DT, which is expensive per case, must be considered, where the national health insurance is universal, and it is necessary to make it a medical treatment that the public can accept. The cost of chronic maintenance dialysis (six million yen per year) is considered one indicator of the cost-effectiveness of medical expenses, but since the initial costs of LVAD treatment, such as the implanted device and surgery costs, are high, further improvement in the cost-effectiveness per year is expected by improving the life prognosis.

6.6 Domestic Issues

Since the government approval of the reimbursement of HM3 for DT in May 2021, a total of 98 patients have been registered to J-MACS [12]. The profile of this cohort is shown in Table 6.1. Actually, in 2 years from 2022 to 2023, 80 cases were enrolled indicating the rapid growth. In Japan, where long-term implantable LVAD treatment is the norm, whether DT or BTT, cooperation from doctors, medical staff, academic societies, companies, and government officials is essential. In this context, it will also be important to aim for the recovery of the patient's own heart by providing medical treatment, surgical treatment, regenerative treatment, cardiac rehabilitation, etc., in addition to long-term implantable LVAD treatment shown here as DT.

With the revision of insurance in 2016, even small hospitals can split the management fee (45,000 points per month) with the implantation facility by providing outpatient management at least once a month as an implantable LVAD management facility, as long as they have a certified artificial heart management technician or a certified extracorporeal circulation technician who has attended the designated educational seminar and artificial heart training course, a cardiovascular surgeon, or a cardiologist.

Therefore, it is expected that implantable LVAD patients will be managed more closely at local hospitals even if they are away from the implantation facility, and further expansion of certified artificial heart management technicians and the spread of implantable LVAD management facilities will be important in advancing heart failure treatment using implantable LVAD.

Table 6.1 Profile of the first 98 patients received LVAD as DT in Japan

Gender	Male 73, female 25
Age (year)	20–39:10, 40–49:10, 50–59:22, 60–69:46, 70–79:10
Disease	DCM:48, IHD:30, others:20
Intermacs profile	Level-1:1, Level 2: 49, Level 3: 42, Level 4–5: 10
Device	HM3: 90, others:8
Others (HM3) in average	Age 57.4 ± 10.8 year, BSA: 1.67 ± 0.21, BMI:22.1 ± 4.6

Data from J-MACS Report 2023, Ref. [12]

DCM dilated cardiomyopathy, *IHD* ischemic heart disease, *BSA* body mass index, *BMI* body mass index

6.7 Conclusion

LVAD therapy has been extensively expanded from the original BTT to non-transplant DT with well-acceptable outcomes providing better quality of life. However, DT has potentially controversial issues such as patient selection, cost-effectiveness, end-of-life care, major complications, and limited activities of daily living. For further refinement of DT strategy for end-stage heart failure, combined strategy with new pharmacological therapy and regenerative approach promoting BTR. Although the donor shortage is critical, we must make efforts to explore the more appropriate donor heart utilization system.

Finally, the current indication of LVAD has been separated to BTT or DT, and should be shifted to the US system, as seen after the heart allocation system revision, the priority of LVAD application may go to DT. However, in our situation of critical donor shortage, such a shift may not be realistic. Nevertheless, we need to consider the strategy of adopting the LVAD indication as a category for advanced heart failure, including BTT, DT, BTR, and BTC as an all-in-one category.

Acknowledgments In finishing this article, I would like to express my greatest respect to Dr. Shunei Kyo and Professor Koichiro Kinugawa, who have made great efforts to introduce DT in Japan.

References

1. Varshney AS, DeFilippis EM, Cowger JA, et al. Trends and outcomes of left ventricular assist device therapy. JACC Focus Semin JACC. 2022;79:1092–107.
2. Matsuda H. The development of ventricular assist device and heart transplantation in Japan: how people worked. Artif Organs. 2020;44:544–60.
3. Kinugawa K, Sakata Y, Ono M, et al. Consensus report on destination therapy in Japan: from the DT Committee of the Council for clinical use of ventricular assist device related societies. Circ J. 2021;84:1906–17.
4. Rose EA, Gelijns AC, Moskowitz AJ, et al. Long-term use of a left ventricular assist device for end-stage heart failure. N Engl J Med. 2001;345:1435–43.
5. Slaughter MS, Rogers JG, Milano CA, et al. Advanced heart failure treated with continuous-flow left ventricular assist device. N Engl J Med. 2009;361:2241–51.
6. Rogers JG, Francis D, Pagani FD, Tatooles AJ, et al. Intrapericardial left ventricular assist device for advanced heart failure. N Engl J Med. 2017;376:451–60.
7. Stevenson LW, Pagani FD, Young JB, et al. INTERMACS profile of advanced heart failure: the current picture. J Heart Lung Transplant. 2009;28:535–41.
8. Adamo L, Nassif M, Tibrewala A, et al. The Heartmate risk score predicts morbidity and mortality in unselected left ventricular assist device recipients and risk stratifies INTERMACS class 1 patients. JACC. 2015;3:283–90.
9. Ando M, Ono M. Current issues of destination therapy in Japan: to achieve 5-year or even more survival. J Artif Organs. 2024;27:203–11.
10. Gelijns AC, Russo MJ, Hong KN, et al. Dynamics of device innovation: implications for assessing value. Int J Technol Assess Health Care. 2013;29:365–73.
11. Lim HS, Shaw S, Carter AW, et al. A clinical and cost-effectiveness analysis of the HeartMate 3 left ventricular assist device for transplant-ineligible patients: a United Kingdom perspective. J Heart Lung Transplant. 2022;41:174–86.
12. J-MACS Report in 2023. https://j-vad.jp/document/J-MACS%20Statistical%20Report%20_20240204.pdf. Accessed 28 Dec 2024.

Part IV

Clinical Achievements in Heart and Lung Transplantation

7 Pioneering Heart Transplantation in Japan: A 25-Year Journey at Osaka University

Shunsuke Saito and Shigeru Miyagawa

Abstract

Over the past 25 years, Osaka University has played a pivotal role in advancing heart and heart-lung transplantation in Japan, contributing to improved survival outcomes and treatment options for end-stage heart failure patients. By the end of December 2023, a total of 184 patients had undergone heart or heart-lung transplantation: 181 heart transplants and 3 heart-lung transplants. Despite these advances, severe donor shortages persist, resulting in extended wait times, with the mean duration for Status 1 patients now approaching 5 years. To address this, the institution has maximized the use of marginal donors and developed an extensive bridge-to-transplant strategy using left ventricular assist devices (LVADs). Immunosuppression protocols have also evolved, improving long-term outcomes, with our 5- and 10-year survival rates reaching 93.8% and 89.0%, respectively. This review discusses ongoing challenges and potential avenues for addressing donor scarcity, including innovations in organ allocation, xenotransplantation, and alternative therapies such as regenerative medicine. Our findings underscore Osaka University's commitment to pioneering heart transplantation in Japan.

Keywords

Heart transplantation · Left ventricular assist device (LVAD) · Donor shortage · Immunosuppression · Heart-lung transplantation · Heart preservation · EXCOR

S. Saito (✉) · S. Miyagawa
Department of Cardiovascular Surgery, The University of Osaka Graduate School of Medicine, Suita, Osaka, Japan
e-mail: s.saito.cxb@osaka-u.ac.jp; miyagawa.shigeru.med@osaka-u.ac.jp

H. Matsuda et al. (eds.), *Heart and Lung Transplantation*,
https://doi.org/10.1007/978-981-96-8810-4_7

7.1 Introduction

It has been 25 years since the first heart transplant was performed in Japan under the Organ Transplantation Act in February 1999. Initially, organ donations across Japan were limited to approximately 10 cases per year. Following the enforcement of the Revised Organ Transplantation Act in July 2010, there was an increase in organ donations from brain-dead donors, leading to a rise in heart transplants, with 84 cases recorded in 2019. However, organ donations declined due to the impact of the COVID-19 pandemic, with only 54 and 59 heart transplants performed in 2020 and 2021, respectively. In 2022, as the severity and mortality rates associated with COVID-19 decreased, the number of organ donations began to increase, resulting in 79 heart transplants, followed by a notable rise to 115 cases in 2023. For the first time, the number of heart transplants exceeded 100 cases in a single year in Japan. However, in comparison with other countries, the number of heart transplants per capita remains extremely low, and the issue of organ scarcity remains unresolved.

This report offers a comprehensive review of the historical development and clinical outcomes of heart and heart-lung transplantation at Osaka University over the past 25 years.

7.2 Heart Transplant Cases at Osaka University

The number of heart and combined heart-lung transplants performed at Osaka University and the trends in Status 1 waiting days are shown in Fig. 7.1. Following the enactment of the Organ Transplantation Act in February 1999, the first heart

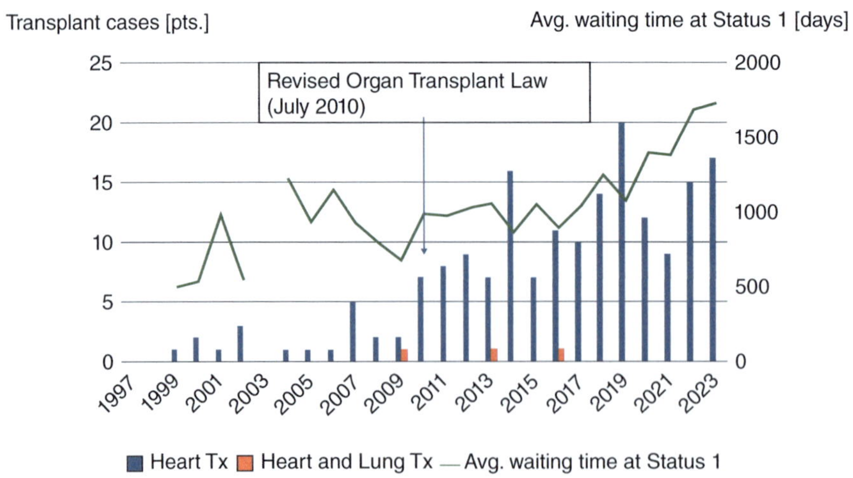

Fig. 7.1 Annual number of heart and heart-lung transplants performed at Osaka University, and trends in Status 1 waiting times. *Tx* transplantation

transplant in Japan was conducted at Osaka University [1]. For the subsequent decade, only about ten heart transplants were performed annually nationwide, with Osaka University conducting a few cases each year, reaching a maximum of five per year. In 2004, Japan's first heart transplant for an adult with congenital heart disease was performed [2], which was the university's eighth case. Additionally, in 2009, the institution conducted the country's first simultaneous heart-lung transplant [3]. To date, the only three heart-lung transplants performed in Japan have been carried out at Osaka University. After the revised Organ Transplantation Act took effect in July 2010, the increase in brain-dead donor organs also gradually led to an increase in heart transplants, with annual cases rising to around 10, occasionally exceeding 15.

However, the number of left ventricular assist device (LVAD) implants has consistently outpaced heart transplants, and the waiting period for Status-1 patients has notably lengthened (Fig. 7.2). Whereas the waiting time for heart transplants was previously about 3 years, the average now extends to nearly 5 years. Amid the severe shortage of cardiac donors, Osaka University has made various efforts to increase the number of heart transplants, including the effective use of marginal donors [4] and meticulous management of marginal recipients [5]. The story of VAD introdcution is also presented in Chaper 4 of this book.

By the end of December 2023, a total of 184 patients had undergone heart or heart-lung transplantation: 181 heart transplants and 3 heart-lung transplants; male: female = 117:67, with a mean recipient age of 35.5 ± 17.9 years. Following the 2010 revision to the Act, brain-dead organ donations from children under 15 became permissible, leading to the first heart transplant from a pediatric donor under 6 years old in 2012 [6]. Subsequently, in 2015, Berlin Heart EXCOR®(EXCOR) received

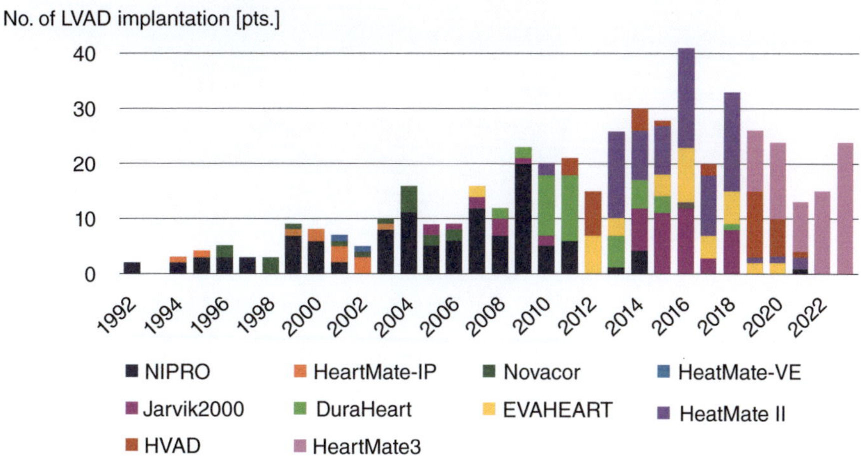

Fig. 7.2 Number of left ventricular assist devices (LVADs) implanted. *LVAD* left ventricular assist devices

insurance reimbursement [7], and a case report was published from Osaka University describing a 4-year-old child who developed failing Fontan 2 years after undergoing the Fontan procedure. The child received a heart transplant 465 days after the EXCOR was implanted [8]. In 2019, 17 pediatric heart transplants were performed nationwide in Japan. Reflecting these changes, heart transplants at Osaka University have been carried out across a broad age range (Fig. 7.3), with recipients aged 0–9 comprising 10% of cases and those aged 60–69 also comprising 10%, a noteworthy distribution.

The underlying diseases of heart transplant patients are shown in Fig. 7.4. Idiopathic dilated cardiomyopathy accounts for 52%, followed by dilated-phase hypertrophic cardiomyopathy at 14%. The high proportion of idiopathic cardiomyopathy cases is characteristic of Japan and consistent with the pattern at our institution. In contrast, ischemic cardiomyopathy, the most prevalent diagnosis in Western countries, represents only 10% of cases here. It is conceivable that ischemic cardiomyopathy cases may increase over time, approaching the proportions seen in Western countries.

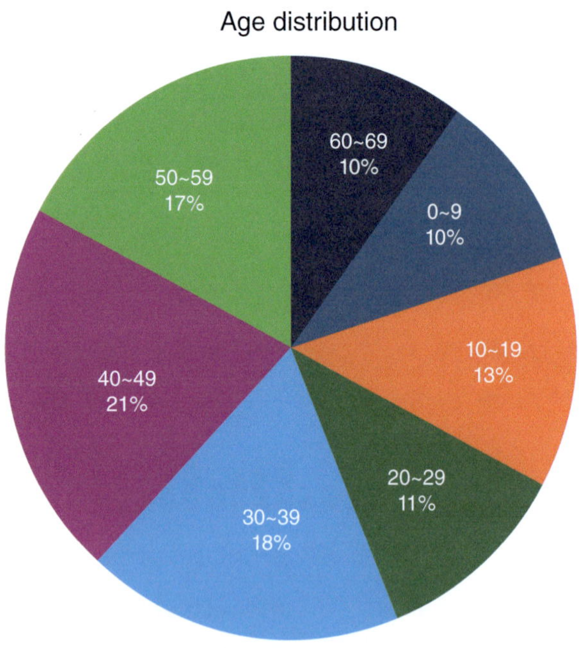

Fig. 7.3 Age distribution of heart transplant recipients

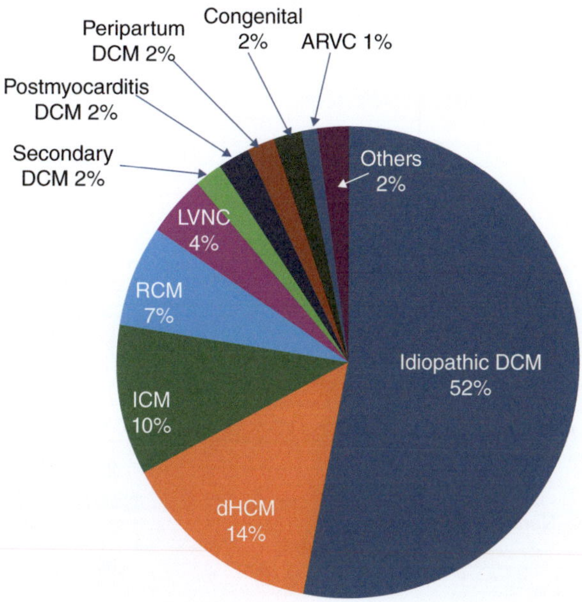

Fig. 7.4 Primary diseases of heart transplant recipients. *ARVC* arrhythmogenic right ventricular cardiomyopathy, *DCM* dilated cardiomyopathy, *dHCM* dilated phase hypertrophic cardiomyopathy, *ICM* ischemic cardiomyopathy, *LVNC* left ventricular noncompaction, *RCM* restrictive cardiomyopathy

7.3 Heart Transplant Waiting Status

The majority of heart transplant cases in Japan are patients who have been implanted with left ventricular assist devices (LVAD) as a bridge to transplant (BTT), with the external Toyobo LVAD (Nipro LVAD) previously being the primary device used [9]. At Osaka University, implantable LVADs were actively introduced even before they were approved for insurance coverage. Since the reimbursement for smaller continuous-flow implantable LVADs as BTT in April 2011, their use has significantly increased. Currently, continuous-flow implantable LVADs, such as HeartMate 3, HeartMate II, HVAD, EVAHEART, and Jarvik 2000, which support home-based treatment, are mainly used for patients awaiting transplants. Consequently, as of the end of December 2023, out of 178 heart transplant cases, only 20 patients had heart transplantation without an LVAD at our hospital, relying instead on continuous intravenous inotropic support, and there was only one pediatric Status-2 patient. The majority, 157 cases (88.2%), were BTT cases.

In recent years, most transplants have been for patients managed with continuous-flow implantable LVADs at home. Meanwhile, the number of pediatric transplants after EXCOR Pediatric support is gradually increasing, with 15 cases reaching heart transplantation.

Regarding the durable LVADs in recent practice, the high survival rates have been seen from the experience at Osaka University and National Cardiovascular Center [10], and the survival curve of HeartMate 3 at Osaka University is shown in Fig. 7.5. As the number of new registrations on the transplant waiting list continues

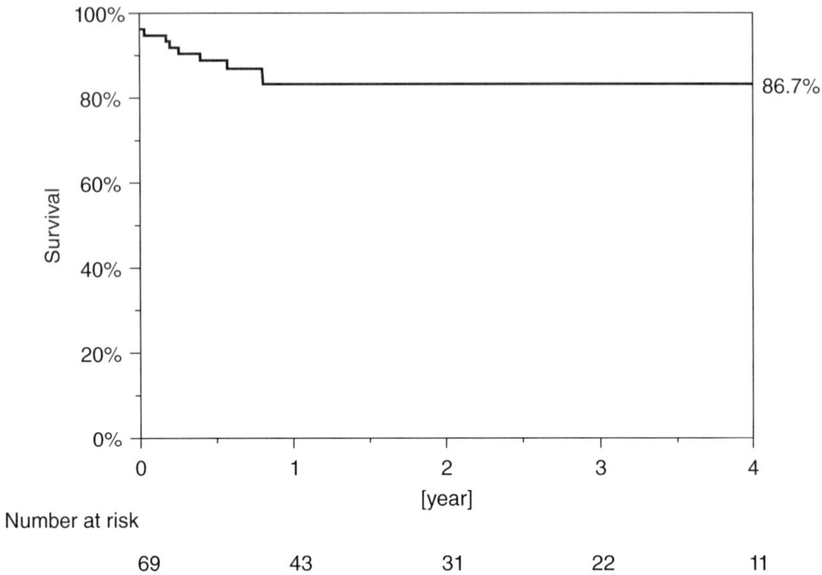

Fig. 7.5 Survival rate of patients implanted with HeartMate 3 ($n = 69$) at Osaka University

to exceed the number of transplants, there is currently no trend that the duration of LVAD support and the waiting time for transplantation will decrease.

7.4 Cardioplegia Solutions and Transplant Procedures

Initially, the cardioplegia solution used for the first few cases was Modified Collins solution, based on Euro-Collins solution. However, from around 2005, Celsior solution was adopted and used exclusively through 2023. Due to recent increases in the cost of Celsior solution and delays in the delivery time, it has been replaced by UW solution. There have been no observed differences in transplant outcomes or postoperative myocardial injury markers due to the change in cardioplegia solution (Fig. 7.6).

Regarding surgical technique, the Lower-Shumway method was employed for the first few cases, but since 2005, the bicaval or modified-bicaval method has been used. The modified-bicaval method is currently the standard approach; however, in anticipation of introducing domino transplantation for patients with severe biventricular failure, a reconsideration of the original bicaval method is also underway. No differences in transplant outcomes have been noted among the various surgical techniques.

Immunosuppressive Therapy For induction therapy, basiliximab is administered in cases with renal impairment or high-risk profiles. While some institutions use it extensively, basiliximab is currently not covered by insurance for heart

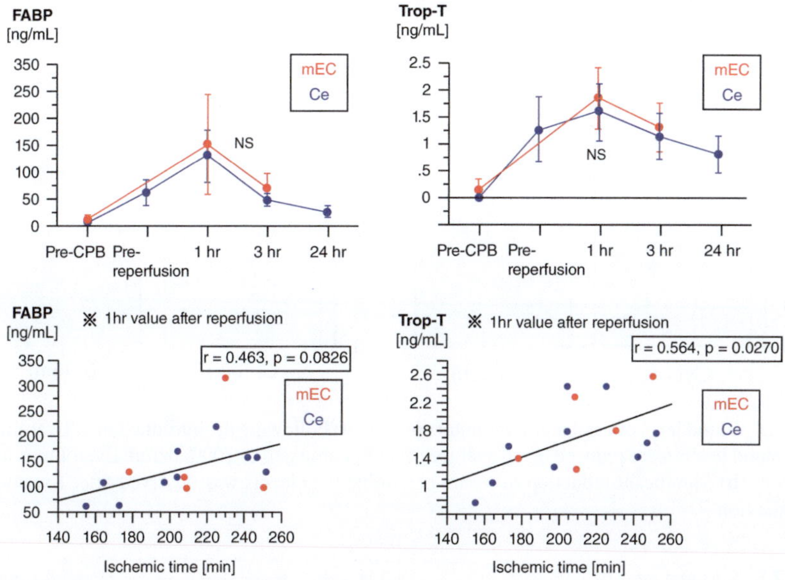

Fig. 7.6 Postoperative myocardial injury markers between myocardial preservation solutions by modified Collins solution (mEC) and Celsior solution (Ce). *FABP* fatty acid-binding protein, *Trop-T* Troponin T

transplantation in Japan, making its routine use challenging. A survey, led by the Japan Society for Transplantation, is currently underway to assess its utilization with the aim of securing insurance coverage. The advantage of delaying the introduction of calcineurin inhibitors (CNI) is substantial, and there is strong demand for expedited insurance approval.

For maintenance therapy, all patients receive a triple therapy regimen, including a CNI (either cyclosporine [CsA] or tacrolimus [Tac]), a metabolic antagonist (azathioprine or mycophenolate mofetil [MMF], with MMF now being used exclusively), and corticosteroids. In earlier cases, CsA was the CNI of choice; however, from around 2007–2008, Tac became the primary option, with CsA now reserved for patients with diabetes. Everolimus has not been used immediately after transplantation because of the risk of delayed wound healing side effects, and has been switched from MMF in patients with post-transplant coronary artery lesions, renal dysfunction, malignancy, and MMF intolerance. With the introduction of Everolimus, the CNI dosage can be reduced, resulting in lower blood CNI levels and consequent improvements in renal function (Fig. 7.7). For rejection treatment, steroid pulses are administered for cellular rejection, while plasmapheresis, intravenous immunoglobulin (IVIG), and rituximab are employed for antibody-mediated rejection (AMR) [11].

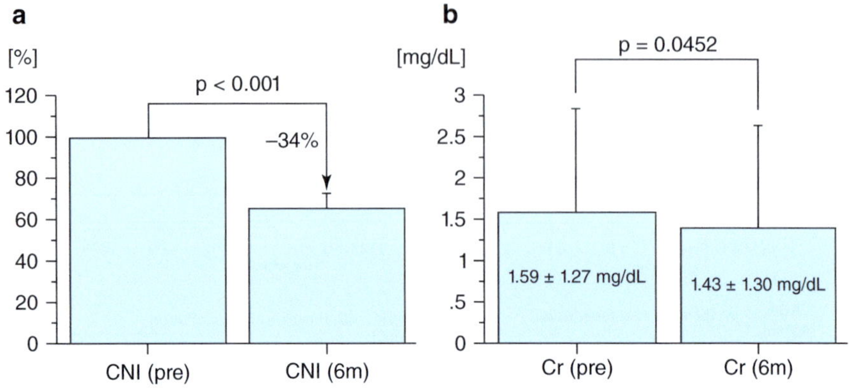

Fig. 7.7 Blood level of calcineurin inhibitors (CNI). (**a**) Following the introduction of Everolimus, CNI blood levels were reduced by an average of 34%, compared to 100% before Everolimus introduction. (**b**) Significant reduction in serum creatinine (Cr) levels was observed after Everolimus introduction

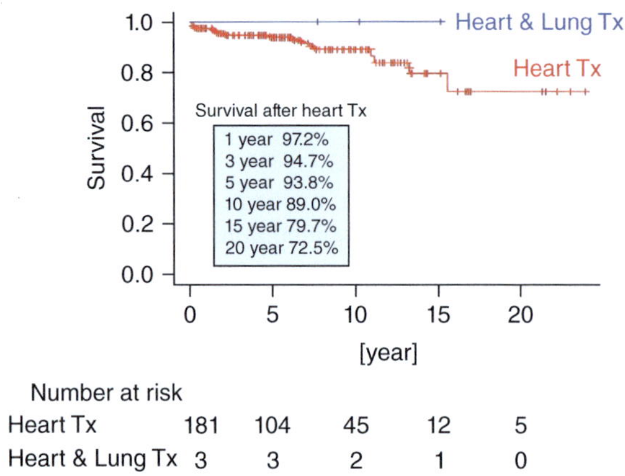

Fig. 7.8 Survival rates of heart and heart-lung transplant recipients at Osaka University. *Tx* transplantation

7.5 Post-transplant Survival Rate

The cumulative survival rates of patients who underwent heart and heart-lung transplantation as of December 2023 are shown in Fig. 7.8. All three cases of heart-lung transplantation have survived. The 5-, 10-, and 15-year survival rates for heart transplantation are 93.8%, 89.0%, and 79.7%, respectively, which are comparable to the result of Japan's heart transplant registry [12] and demonstrate higher postoperative survival than that of the International Society for Heart and Lung Transplantation (ISHLT) registry [13]. Among 20 cases of mortality observed over a maximum follow-up period of 23.9 years, causes of death included acute-phase infection and multi-organ failure (6 cases), late-phase infection (3 cases), malignancies, PTLD, sudden death (2 cases each), and others (Table 7.1).

Table 7.1 Cause of death in 20 patients after heart transplantation

	Cause of death	*N*
1	Post-operative acute phase infection/MOF	6
2	Remote phase infections	3
3	Malignancy	2
4	Post-transplant lymphoproliferative disorders	2
5	Sudden death	2
6	Primary graft dysfunction	1
7	Renal failure	1
8	Cardiac allograft vasculopathy	1
9	Stroke	1
10	Ruptured aortic aneurysm	1

MOF multiple organ failure

Table 7.2 Long-term survivors over 15 years after heart and heart/lung transplantation

Tx	Year of TX	Follow-up years	Age at Tx year-old	Current age year-old	Etiology	Bridging MCS	Status 1 days
Heart	2000	25	48	72	dHCM	Toyobo	356
Heart	2001	24	49	73	dHCM	Novacor	977
Heart	2002	23	22	45	dHCM	HeartMate IP	534
Heart	2002	22	37	59	PPCM	Toyobo	547
Heart	2002	22	39	61	DCM	(inotropes)	552
Heart	2007	18	34	52	DCM	Novacor	1051
Heart	2007	18	36	53	ICM	Toyobo	996
Heart	2007	18	45	62	DCM	Novacor	936
Heart	2007	17	40	58	DCM	Novacor	1166
Heart	2008	17	42	59	DCM	Jarvik2000	820
H/L	2009	16	35	51	DORV	(−)	0
Heart	2009	16	12	28	DCM	Toyobo	611
Heart	2009	15	50	65	DCM	EVAHEART	735
Heart	2010	15	54	69	DCM	Jarvik2000	525

DCM dilated cardiomyopathy, *dHCM* dilated phase hypertrophic cardiomyopathy, *PPCM* postpartum cardiomyopathy, *TX* transplantation, *DORV* double outlet right ventricle, *MCS* mechanical circulatory support

7.5.1 Long-Term Survivors

As another proof of our steps of heart and heart-lung transplantation, a list of patients alive beyond 15 years post-transplant is shown in Table 7.2. As of the end of 2024, a total of 16 patients have been followed up to 24 years as longest, and all except one among heart transplantation alone had bridged from VAD, nine patients supported by pulsatile VADs including extracorporeal Toyobo LVAD in 4. There were no retransplants nor major chronic rejection, and all had returned to non-restricted daily life.

7.6 Discussion

This report highlights the progress and challenges faced in heart and heart-lung transplantation at Osaka University over the past 25 years. The steady increase in transplant numbers, notably after the 2010 revision of the Organ Transplant Law, reflects improvements in Japan's organ donation system and heightened acceptance of heart transplantation as a treatment standard for end-stage heart failure. Yet, the persistent scarcity of donors in Japan has led to prolonged wait times, often exceeding 5 years, despite innovations such as the use of marginal donors. While the development of implantable LVADs has drastically reduced pre-transplant mortality, the extended wait times continue to impose a heavy burden on patients and caregivers.

The data suggest that, although survival rates among transplant recipients at Osaka University are comparable to or exceed national and international benchmarks, the unique distribution of primary heart conditions—most frequently idiopathic dilated cardiomyopathy—reflects both national demographic trends and unique aspects of the patient population in Japan. These results are critical as they underscore the need to optimize transplant candidacy criteria and further support for high-risk patients, such as those with advanced congenital heart diseases. There are also key operational challenges and considerations that remain. For instance, variations in myocardial preservation solutions and surgical techniques, while yielding equivalent outcomes thus far, suggest the potential for future optimization in surgical protocols.

The introduction of Everolimus in immunosuppressive therapy has shown potential benefits for long-term kidney function. However, limitations in the availability of certain induction agents, such as basiliximab, restrict widespread application and highlight the necessity for policy advancements in immunosuppressant coverage.

Looking forward, we are facing critical questions about alternative donor sources, such as donors after cardiac death and xenotransplantation, which are gaining traction internationally. These approaches, alongside advancing regenerative medicine and novel mechanical support options, represent promising avenues for reducing wait times and expanding treatment options for end-stage heart failure patients in Japan.

7.7 Conclusion

Heart transplantation has become an established standard treatment for end-stage severe heart failure in Japan, and the Department of Cardiovascular Surgery at Osaka University has consistently led the nation in advancing heart transplantation. However, the shortage of donors remains critically severe. Although advancements in implantable LVAD therapy have significantly reduced mortality among patients awaiting transplantation, the waiting period has markedly lengthened. To address these challenges, several issues must be addressed: Is the current organ allocation system adequate? Should Japan advance heart transplantation from donors following cardiac death, a practice becoming common in Western countries? What role will xenotransplantation play? Moreover, the development of novel therapies, including regenerative medicine as alternatives to transplantation, represents a critical area for the Department of Cardiovascular Surgery at Osaka University.

References

1. Matsuda H, Fukushima N, Sawa Y, et al. First brain dead donor heart transplantation under new legislation in Japan. Jpn J Thorac Cardiovasc Surg. 1999;47:499–505.
2. Matsuda H, Fukushima N, Ichikawa H, et al. Orthotopic heart transplantation for adult congenital heart disease: a case with heterotaxy and dextrocardia. Gen Thorac Cardiovasc Surg. 2017;65:47–51.
3. Sawa Y, Matsumiya G, Shigemura S, et al. First successful heart-lung transplantation in Japan: report of a case. Surg Today. 2013;43:1461–6.
4. Saito S, Matsumiya G, Ueno T, et al. Bench replacement of donor aortic valve before orthotopic heart transplantation. J Heart Lung Transplant. 2009;28:981–3.
5. Nakamura Y, Yoshioka D, Miyagawa S, et al. Successful heart transplantation after desensitization in a patient with extremely high panel-reactive antibody levels and pretransplant donor-specific antibody: a case report. Transplant Proc. 2018;50:4067–70.
6. Ueno T, Fukushima N, Sakaguchi T, et al. First pediatric heart transplantation from a pediatric donor heart in Japan. Circ J. 2012;76:752–4.
7. Kanaya T, Ueno T, Taira M, et al. Impact of long-term support with Berlin heart EXCOR® in pediatric patients with severe heart failure. Pediatric Cardiol. 2019;40:1126–33.
8. Hasegawa M, Tominaga Y, Watanabe T, et al. Successful bridge to transplantation with long-term support using Berlin heart EXCOR in a child with failing Fontan. General Thoracic Cardiovasc Surg. 2022;70:750–3.
9. Saito S, Matsumiya G, Sakaguchi T, et al. Fifteen-year experience with Toyobo paracorporeal left ventricular assist system. J Artif Organs. 2009;12:27–34.
10. Inoue K, Fujita T, Yoshioka D, et al. Short-term outcomes of magnetically levitated left ventricular assist device in advanced heart failure – the Japanese cohort. Circ J. 2022;86:1961–7.
11. Saito S, Matsumiya G, Fukushima N, et al. Successful treatment of cardiogenic shock caused by humoral cardiac allograft rejection. Circ J. 2009;73:970–3.
12. Japan Organ Transplantation Network. Heart Transplant Registry of Japan. http://www.jsht.jp/registry/japan/. Accessed 4 Mar 2025.
13. Singh TP, Cherikh WS, Hsich E, et al. Graft survival in primary thoracic organ transplant recipients: a special report from the international thoracic organ transplant registry of the International Society for Heart and Lung Transplantation. J Heart Lung Transplant. 2023;42:1321–33.

Lung Transplantation at Osaka University

8

Soichiro Funaki, Takashi Kanou, Chizu Kamon,
Masayoshi Inoue, Masato Minami, Meinoshin Okumura,
and Yasushi Shintani

Abstract

At Osaka University, we have performed 83 brain-dead donor (BDD) lung transplants, 11 bilateral living donor lobar lung transplants, and 3 combined heart-lung transplants. Survival rates in the BDD group for 5 and 10 years were 77.0% and 6.07% in single lung transplantation (*N* = 43), and 80.8% and 80.8% in bilateral lung transplantation (*N* = 35), respectively. There were 8 long-term sur-

S. Funaki (✉)
Department of Thoracic Surgery, Hyogo Medical University, Nishinomiya, Hyogo, Japan
e-mail: so-funaki@hyo-med.ac.jp

T. Kanou · Y. Shintani
Department of General Thoracic Surgery, The University of Osaka Graduate School of Medicine, Suita, Osaka, Japan
e-mail: yshintani@thoracic.med.osaka-u.ac.jp

C. Kamon
Department of Transplantation Medicine, The University of Osaka Hospital, Suita, Osaka, Japan
e-mail: kamon@hp-trpmed.med.osaka-u.ac.jp

M. Inoue
Division of Thoracic Surgery, Department of Surgery, Kyoto Prefectural University of Medicine, Kyoto, Japan
e-mail: mainoue@koto.kpu-m.ac.jp

M. Minami
Ashiya Municipal Hospital, Ashiya, Hyogo, Japan
e-mail: maminami1108@nifty.com

M. Okumura
National Hospital Organization Osaka Toneyama Medical Center, Toyonaka, Osaka, Japan
e-mail: okumura.meinoshin.hy@mail.hosp.go.jp

H. Matsuda et al. (eds.), *Heart and Lung Transplantation*,
https://doi.org/10.1007/978-981-96-8810-4_8

vivors of beyond 15 years, and late death in this group only developed in single lung transplantation. From these results, the superiority of bilateral lung transplantation has been confirmed. We have also done 3 combined heart and lung transplantation in 3 patients, and all are alive up to 16 years post-transplant. The characteristics of our practices in lung transplantation show a high frequency of combined repair of intracardiac lesions and also pulmonary artery hypertension. Here, we discuss chronic lung allograft dysfunction, role of surveillance bronchoscopy for acute rejection in relation to chronic lung allograft dysfunction (CLAD), and donor pool expansion by introducing transplantation from the donors after circulatory death.

Keywords

Lung transplantation · Living donor lobar lung transplantation · Ischemia/reperfusion injury · Chronic lung allograft dysfunction (CLAD) · Donor shortage · DCD · Heart-lung transplantation

8.1 Introduction

In 1983, Cooper and his colleagues at the University of Toronto successfully performed the world's first brain-dead donor (BDD) lung transplantation (LTx), and momentum for lung transplantation medicine increased [1]. In Japan, the start of clinical LTx was delayed for approximately 15 years as compared to North America and Europe due to the time required for the establishment of social consensus regarding the concept of brain death. LTx in Japan began with living donor lobar LTx (LDLLT) at Okayama University in 1998 [2], and Japan's first LTx from BDD was performed at Osaka University and Tohoku University in 2000 [3].

After LTx became reimbursed by social insurance in 2006 and the original organ transplantation law was revised in 2010, the number of BDD lung transplants has been steadily increasing and cumulative numbers have exceeded over 800 now [4] (Fig. 8.1). However, the average waiting time on the candidate list has been over 900 days, indicating that the number of donors is totally insufficient compared to that of desiring transplantation.

By the end of 2023, a total of 871 BDD lung transplantations, 293 LDLLT, and 3 combined heart and lung transplantation had been performed in Japan, and the outcomes of such cases have thus far been satisfactory with a five-year survival rate greater than 73% for both BDDLTx and LDLLT [5].

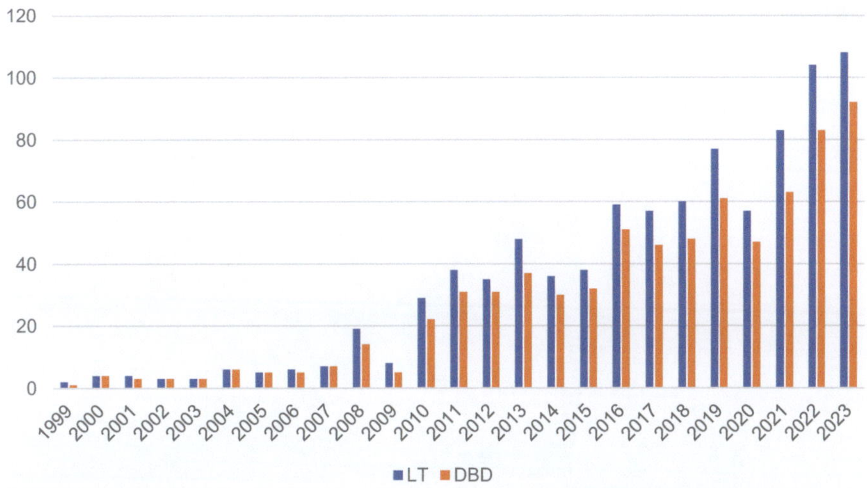

Fig. 8.1 Annual number of lung transplantation (LT) from brain-dead donor (BDD) in Japan. The number in each year is counted from April to next March. The number of BDDs is defined as the number of lung donations. (Data is reproduced from JOT Annual Report [4])

8.2 Basic Research on Lung Transplantation

Lung transplantation experiments were already being conducted on dogs by Professor Yoshio Ozawa (term from 1930 to 1959), and a newspaper article (1952) stated, "We aim to perform the procedure on humans" and "Since clots are likely to form if the lung veins are sutured, the sutures will be performed in the left atrium" (Fig. 8.2). Professor Kawashima (term from 1978 to 1998) began research into lung preservation and ischemia-reperfusion (I/R) injury. Professor Matsuda (term from 1991 to 2005) conducted active research using cell biochemical methods and animal experiments to elucidate the mechanism of ischemic damage that occurs during organ preservation. Notably, Akashi reported that the amount of intracellular ATP decreases rapidly as the disease progresses and that damage can be recovered by administering oxygen to the airway system of ischemic-preserved lungs [6].

Experimental LTx models that closely resemble clinical LTx are essential for the research for lung preservation and development of new transplant procedures. Mizuta developed a rat lung transplantation model using the cuff technique (Fig. 8.3). This method allows rat LTx without suturing the blood vessels and bronchi by attaching a cuff-like device to the blood vessels and bronchi of the transplanted lung [7]. This rat lung transplantation model "Mizuta's model" has greatly contributed to the following research topics [8–12].

Appropriate size matching between donor and recipient is critical for successful LTx. Chest size matching between the recipient's thoracic volume and the donor's

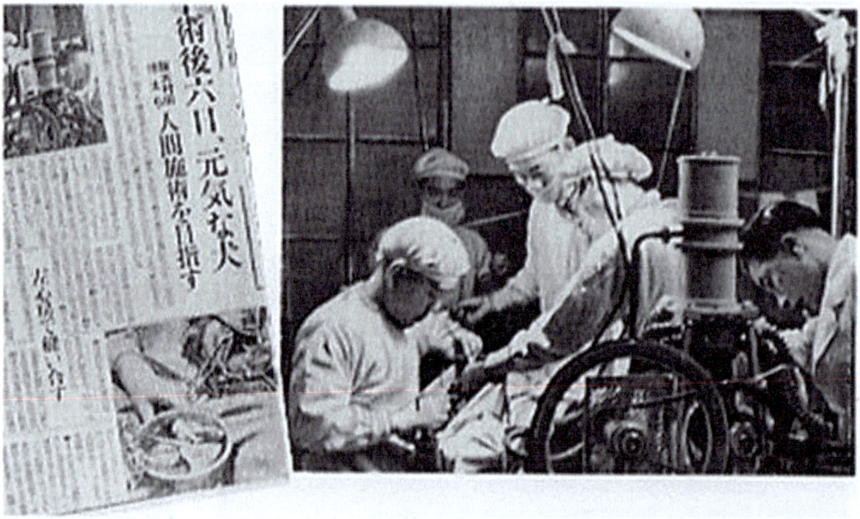

Fig. 8.2 A Japanese newspaper article (1952) stated "We aim to perform the procedure on humans"

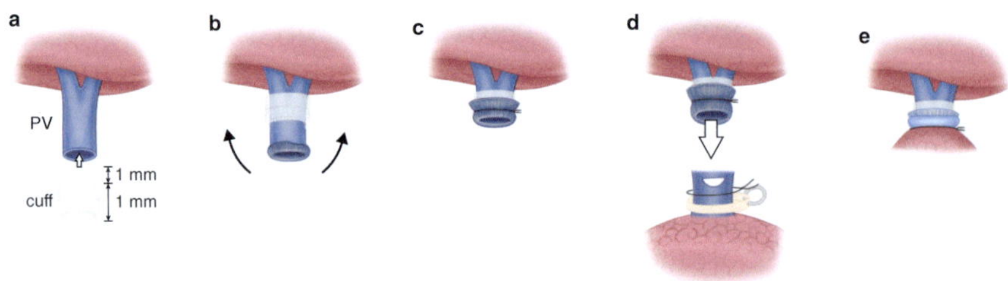

Fig. 8.3 Mizuta's cuff-technique in lung transplantation (Mizuta's model). The divided end of PV is passed through cuff (**a** and **b**) and everted over cuff. Circumferential suture secures cuff (**c**). Donor PV with cuff is inserted into recipient PV (**d**) and anastomosis is completed with circumferential suture (**e**). PA is also anastomosed in this way. (Courtesy of Dr. Takatoshi Mizuta)

lung volume was initially based on vertical and transverse radiologic dimensions of donor and recipient chests examined in heart-lung Tx [13]. Subsequently, Miyoshi and colleagues performed an exercise stress test on patients after LTx, and found a significant correlation between postoperative vital capacity (VC) and maximum oxygen uptake in patients with pulmonary fibrosis after single LTx [14]. Therefore, to obtain sufficient functional recovery after surgery, it is necessary to select a donor that has as large postoperative VC as possible. As the size of the thorax returns to its normal size, matching the size of the recipient's normal thorax to that of the donor will result in more accurate matching [15]. In current recipient selection criteria, pred-VC is used for size matching, with the donor's Pred-VC required to be between

70% and 130% of the recipient's Pred-VC for patients in cases over 18 years of age [16].

Research in the fields of immunology and biochemistry related to transplantation has also been actively conducted. In our department, the accumulated basic immunological knowledge developed from the research on thymus organized by Okumura has been transferred to transplant immunity, and experimentally demonstrated that Th17 is induced by IL6 at the site of rejection, and that suppressing Th17 alleviates the rejection reaction [17].

Primary graft dysfunction (PGD) is also one factor leading to poor LTx outcome and can be considered as a severe form of I/R acute lung injury. Kawamura conducted joint research with the University of Pittsburgh, and found that when LTx recipient rats and donor rats were inhaled with hydrogen gas, post-transplantation I/R injury was reduced, and transplanted lung showed that the gas exchange ability of hydrogen gas was improved through blocking the production of several proinflammatory mediators and reducing apoptosis [18, 19]. Kanou has also conducted research in collaboration with the University of Toronto using a rat LTx model for research on I/R lung injury, and reported a new treatment method by the inhibition of regulated necrosis, necroptosis [20]. Matsui demonstrated in a rat LTx model that Calpain, which can be used in clinical practice, reduces I/R lung injury by inhibiting necroptosis, and future clinical applications are expected [21].

8.3 Clinical Challenges in Lung Transplantation at Osaka University

8.3.1 Preparation for Lung Transplantation from a Brain-Dead Donor

Since 1987, many members of the First Department of Surgery have studied abroad at the University of Toronto and the University of Washington in St. Louis to learn about clinical LTx. Looking back to the domestic steps in preparation to start LTx from BDD, Dr. Nakahara, Associate Professor, established the Kinki Lung Transplant Study Group in 1991, aiming to establish the system for the management philosophy of fairness, objectivity, and transparency in LTx medical care. By this effort, we have built a system to strictly evaluate patients eligible for LTx. In September 1991, the LTx from BDD was officially approved by the Ethics Committee of Osaka University Medical School.

8.3.2 Actual Start of Lung Transplantation

The first case of LTx was a LDLLT from identical twin brothers performed on a 30-year-old man with multiple emphysematous bullae and bronchiectasis [22]. This case was the second LDLLT conducted in Japan in January 2000. He is still alive without restrictions in daily life for 24 years after transplantation.

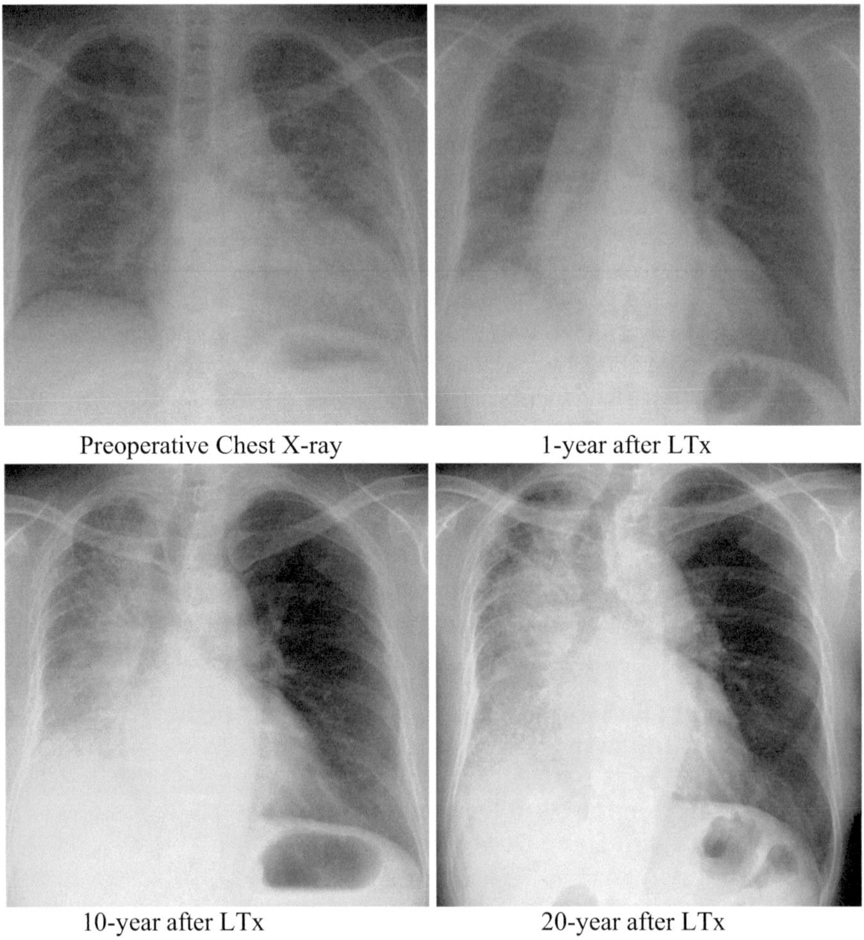

Fig. 8.4 Follow-up chest x-rays of patients received BDD LTx in 2000. From upper left to lower right; preoperative, at 1-year, at 10-year, and at 20-year post-transplantation

Actual start of LTx from BDD in Japan was in March 2000 with two single lung transplants from a single BDD successfully conducted at two institutions [3]. Our patient was a 48-year-old woman with idiopathic pulmonary fibrosis who underwent left single-LTx. Total ischemic time was 5 h and 37 min. The postoperative course was uneventful, and her progress was very satisfactory. She had a stable course for more than 20 years, mainly dependent on the transplanted left lung with progressive shrinkage of the contralateral native right lung (Fig. 8.4). Recently, she suffered from repeated pulmonary infections and died 23 years after the transplantation.

Second single LTx from a BDD was performed in 2001 for a patient with lymphangioleiomyomatosis. This patient experienced graft failure due to bronchial anastomotic stenosis and subsequently underwent single LTx on the contralateral side 6 years after the first surgery. This patient is alive while undergoing dialysis. Third LTx case was a patient with idiopathic pulmonary hypertension, which was the first bilateral LTx from BDD performed in Japan in the same year. The patient experienced no rejection and lived a normal life for more than 20 years.

8.4 Achievements

To date (as of September 2024), we have performed 83 BDD lung transplants, 11 LDLLT, and 3 combined heart-lung transplants from BDD. The demographics of these patients are shown in Table 8.1. In the BDD group, idiopathic interstitial lung disease and lymphangioleiomyomatosis account for more than half, followed by pulmonary arterial hypertension. In 78 patients of LTx from BDD operated before September 2023 (age: 2–64 years, 43 in average), the transplant procedures were 35 bilateral and 43 single LTx and the period on the waiting list until transplantation was 1249 days on average.

Including LDLLT, there were a total of 28 deaths (33.7%), and the causes were chronic lung allograft dysfunction (CLAD) in 8, including 2 with antibody-mediated rejection, malignancy in 6, PGD in 4, infection in 4, and other causes in 6. There were 5 hospital deaths in all, but not seen in recent practice.

The outcome of LTx from BDD is analyzed for patients who received LTx before the end of 2023 and presented by the 5-year and 10-year survival rates by the Kaplan-Meier method (Table 8.2 and Figs. 8.5 and 8.6). The bilateral LTx is obviously superior to the single LTx and there were no late deaths after 5 years of survival. Regarding the long-term survivors, we have 8 patients who survived more than 15 years after transplantation (Table 8.3). The longest survivor is the patient described above as the first LTx patient for BDD, who died 23 years after

Table 8.1 Demographics of patients who received BDD (brain-dead donor) and LDL (living donor lobal) lung transplantation at Osaka University

BDD	**86 cases**
Interstitial lung disease	26
Lymphangioleiomyomatosis	19
Pulmonary arterial hypertension	13
Chronic obstructive pulmonary disease	7
Eisenmenger syndrome	6
Bronchiolitis obliterans syndrome	4
Restrictive cardiomyopathy	2*
Double-outlet right ventricle	1*
Others	8
LDL	**11 cases**
Pulmonary hypertension	5
Bronchiectasis	2
Bronchiolitis obliterans syndrome	2
Interstitial lung disease	1
Others	1

*Heart-lung transplantation

Table 8.2 Comparison of the survival rates in lung transplantation (LTx) from BDD

Type of LTx	*N*	5-year survival rate %	10-year survival rate %
Single LTx	43	77.0	67.0
BL-LTx	35	80.8	80.8
Heart/lung Tx	3	100	100 (*N* = 2)

BL bilateral

Fig. 8.5 Overall survival curve of lung transplant recipients (*N* = 92)

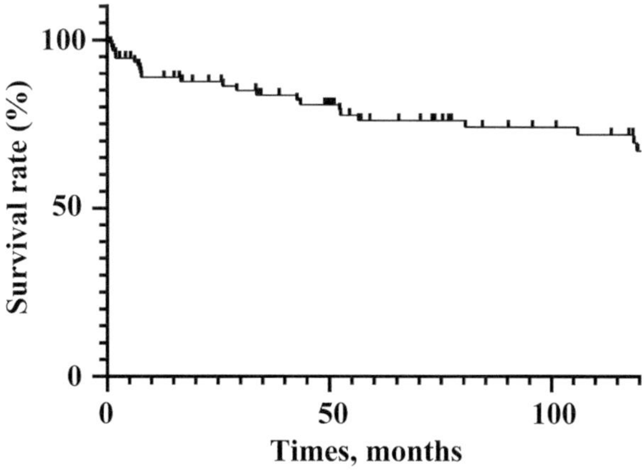

Fig. 8.6 Survival curves of lung transplant recipients; divided by transplantation procedures (*N* = 92). *SLL* single lung transplantation, *BLT* bilateral lung transplantation, *LDLLT* living-related lobar lung transplantation, *HLT*: heart and lung transplantation

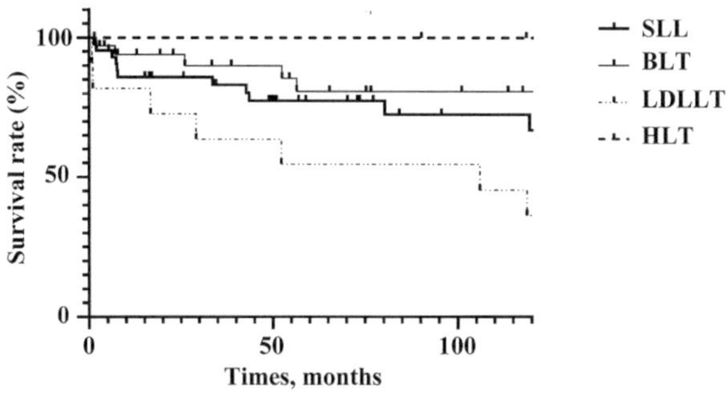

Table 8.3 Long-term survivors of BDD lung transplantation for more than 15 years

Type of LTx		Surviving period (year)	Mortality
Single LTx	(*N* = 3)	17 18[a] 23[a]	2
BL-LTx	(*N* = 4)	16 16 18 23	0
Heart/lung	(*N* = 1)	16	0

[a]Dead
BL bilateral

transplantation. Late death ($N = 2$) in this group occurred only in single LTx patients and none so far in bilateral LTx including three heart and lung transplant patients. The benefit of bilateral LTx is also shown here.

The characteristic of our LTx indicates the frequent association of cardiovascular diseases, including idiopathic pulmonary arterial hypertension (iPAH). In fact, 13 patients with iPAH have undergone bilateral LTx, and 2 patients received combined tricuspid valve repair for severe tricuspid regurgitation associated with right ventricular dysfunction. We have also actively performed bilateral LTx with intracardiac shunt closure for patients with Eisenmenger syndrome. Such an attempt was made in another case by bilateral LTx with ventricular septal defect (VSD) closure [23], and this strategy seems to be an alternative to heart-lung transplantation, especially in Japan where donor organ shortage is critical. This patient has been alive for more than 15 years. So far, bilateral LTx has been performed in 2 patients with VSD closure, 4 patients with atrial septal defect closure, and 1 with patent foramen ovale closure. In the contest of simultaneous repair of intracardiac lesions, an 11-year-old boy with an atrial septal defect and oversystemic pulmonary hypertension received LDLLT from his parents in 2002 [24]. He has returned to social activities well 16 years after LTx.

The first combined heart-lung transplant in Japan was performed at Osaka University in 2009 [25]. To date, only three combined heart-lung transplants have been performed in Japan, all of which have been performed in our department and are still alive (the details of the cases are described in Chap. 9). It has been carried out with keen cooperation from the cardiac surgery group, and it is thought that the environment in which thoracic surgery and cardiovascular surgery are in the same department at the former First Department of Surgery, Osaka University has led to these satisfactory lung transplant results [26].

8.5 Discussion

The Japanese National Lung Transplantation System was established immediately after the enactment of the Transplantation Law in 1997 based on the following three philosophies: (I) an institutional certification system based on strict standards, (II) a rigorous central monitoring system for transplant outcomes, and (III) a third-party review system to determine eligibility for patient registration [27]. The selection criteria were very stringent regarding the clinical, surgical, and ethical competence of the LTx teams, and for this reason, the designation of institution for LTx from BDD was limited to four university hospitals in the initial phase.

Of the 1167 patients who underwent LTx in Japan, 335 patients (228 LTx from BDD and 107 LDLLT) died, with 113 (33.7%) of the deaths due to infectious diseases [5]. In addition, in the acute period after transplantation, transplant lung dysfunction is a common cause of death, and the current situation is that organ preservation and I/R lung injury have not yet been overcome. Current research topics include the development of a new strategy using mesenchymal stem cells therapy for I/R lung injury and the development of lung preservation methods for cardiac arrest donor lungs by ex vivo machine perfusion [28].

CLAD is also the leading cause of death 1 year after LTx. The causes of CLAD are known to be acute transplant lung dysfunction, acute rejection (AR), infection, and gastroesophageal reflux disease, but the only progressive and effective treatment is re-transplantation, thus prevention of CLAD is important. In this context, Inoue reported that post-transplant surveillance bronchoscopy (SB) plays an important role in early detection of acute rejection and infection [29]. As the basic consideration, severe AR and human leukocyte antigen (HLA) mismatch has been reported to be potent risk factors of CLAD. The timely and accurate diagnosis of AR is required in order to optimize immunosuppressive therapy and preserve the pulmonary function of transplanted lungs. A single-center surveillance of SB after LTx in 45 patients at our institution was conducted and increased perioperative neutrophil to leukocyte ratio (NLR) was found as significantly associated with a higher odds ratio of AR [30] (Fig. 8.7).

Recently, the donor pool has been expanded overseas through the active introduction of donation after circulatory death (DCD). In particular, DCD after withdrawal of the life support system, controlled DCD, is the method of choice for LT when comparable reusable to those with BDD are expected. In the DCD Lung Transplant Registry of the International Society for Heart and Lung Transplantation, DCD accounts for approximately 10% of all lung transplants and the number has been increasing [30]. To safely use lungs for DCD, it is necessary to objectively evaluate the quality of donor lungs prior to transplantation. Reconditioning of donor lungs has attracted attention and is clinically applied mainly in North America. Various issues need to be resolved from an ethical and legal perspective [31], as well as the creation of systems such as methods for controlled DCD using extracorporeal lung perfusion [32]. We are currently conducting clinical research to explore the potential of DCD hoping that this will help in future efforts toward DCD [33].

In the field of oncology, the immune checkpoint pathway discovered by Drs. Tasuku Honjo and James P. Allison has been linked to innovative cancer immunotherapy and has produced significant results [34, 35]. Research on transplantation immunity based on this pathway is gradually progressing, and some transplants of other organs have been clinically applied [36]. In Japan, where there is a shortage of donors, even if a transplanted lung becomes dysfunctional, the chances of retransplantation are extremely low. We should contribute to transplantation medicine by actively conducting basic research on rejection and developing innovative methods to prolong the life of transplanted lungs.

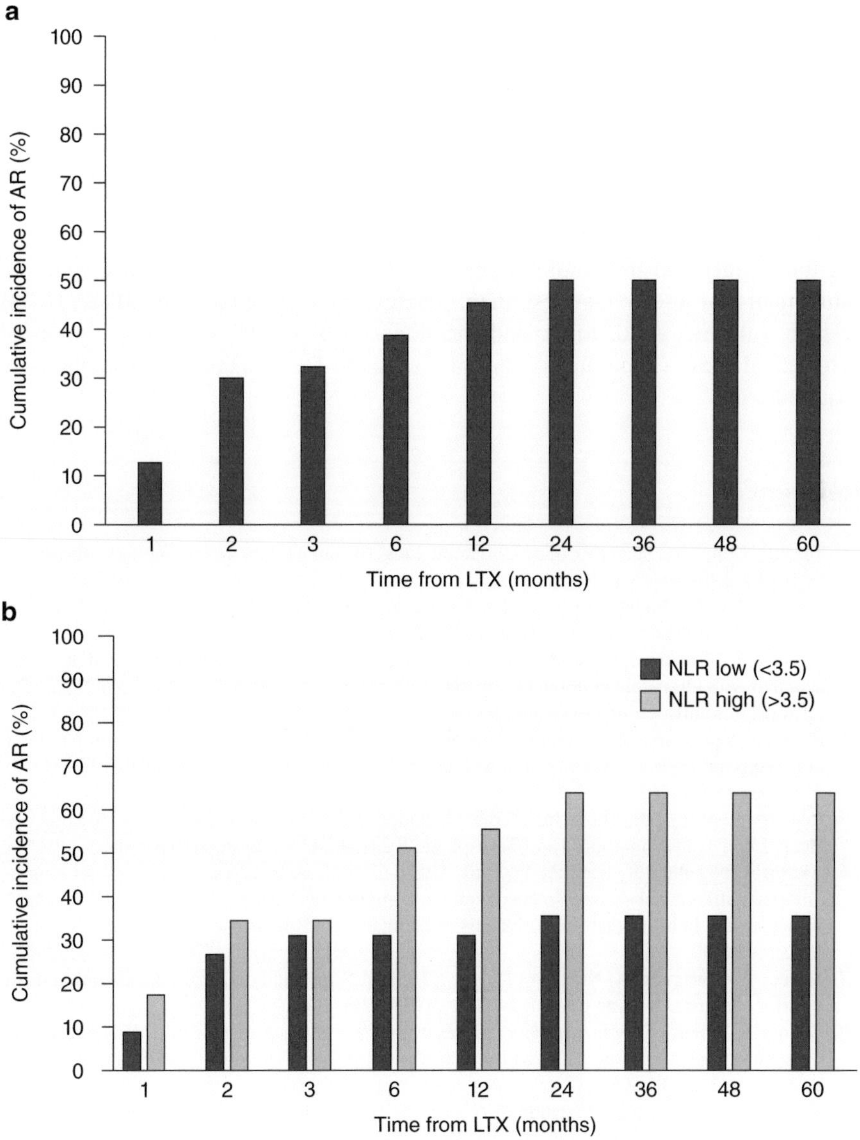

Fig. 8.7 Cumulative incidence of AR in post-transplant surveillance by broncho scope examination. In the entire cohort, 23 patients (52%) experienced AR during the 5-year follow-up period (**a**). The patients with higher NLR scores showed a higher cumulative incidence rate of AR in the 5-year follow-up period (**b**). *AR* acute rejection, *NLR* neutrophile to leukocyte ratio. (Source: Ref. 30 (open access))

8.6 Summary

LTx from BDD has been established as the gold standard for end-stage lung disease. In Japan, the start of BDD organ transplantation has been delayed until the actual start in 1999 for heart and 2000 for LTx. As shown in the national data and our analyses, the results of LTx especially of BDD has remained as 77% at 5 years in survival rate. Bilateral double LTx, in contrast, survival rate was as high as 80% at 5 and 10 years in our practice. Among the causes of mortality, infection, AR from I/R lung injury and immunologic rejection represented by CLAD have been the future matter of research interest. In this context, post-transplant surveillance by SB seemed valuable. Also, to expand the donor pool for LTx, the exploration of mechanical preservation and system of controlled DCD organ transplantation are required.

References

1. Toronto Lung Transplant Group. Unilateral lung transplantation for pulmonary fibrosis. N Engl J Med. 1986;314:1140–5.
2. Date H, Aoe M, Nagahiro I, et al. Living-donor lobar lung transplantation for various lung diseases. J Thoracic Cardiovasc Surg. 2003;126:476–81.
3. Miyoshi S, Minami M, Ohta M, et al. Single lung transplantation from a brain-dead donor for a patient with idiopathic pulmonary fibrosis. A breakthrough after new legislation in Japan. Jpn J Thorac Cardiovasc Surg. 2001;49:398–403.
4. Registry Report from Japan Organ Transplant Network: cummulative number of organ donation from brain-dead donor and transplantation: https://www.jotnw.or.jp/data/offer03.php. Accessed 15 Feb 2025.
5. Registry Report of Japanese lung Transplantation-2024: the Japanese Society of Lung and Heart-Lung Transplantation. Jpn J Transplant. 2024;59:243–9. (abstract in English).
6. Akashi A, Nakahara K, Kamiike W, et al. Attenuation of warm ischemic injury of rat lung by inflation with room air—assessment of cellular components and the surfactant in the bronchoalveolar lavage fluid in relation to changes in cellular adenosine triphosphate. Transplantation. 1993;55:24–30.
7. Mizuta T, Kawaguchi A, Nakahara K, Kawashima Y. Simplified rat lung transplantation using a cuff technique. J Thorac Cardiovasc Surg. 1989;97:578–81.
8. Yoon HE, Mizuta T, Minami M, et al. Exercise performance of rats after isogenic left or right lung transplantation followed by contralateral pulmonary artery ligation. J Heart Lung Transplant. 1996;15:605–11.
9. Minami M, Nakahara K, Matsumura A, et al. Histamine release from pulmonary mast cells after lung transplantation in rats. J Heart Lung Transplant. 1995;14:505–11.
10. Mizuta T, Fujii Y, Minami M, et al. Increased nitric oxide levels in exhaled air of rat lung allografts. J Thorac Cardiovasc Surg. 1997;113:830–5.
11. Utsumi T, Mizuta T, Fujii Y, et al. Nitric oxide production by bronchoalveolar cells during allograft rejection in the rat. Transplantation. 1999;67:1622–6.
12. Ohmori K, Takeda S, Miyoshi S, et al. Attenuation of lung injury in allograft rejection using NF-kappaB decoy transfection-novel strategy for use in lung transplantation. Eur J Cardiothorac Surg. 2005;27:23–7.
13. Otulana BA, Mist BA, Scott JP, et al. The effect of recipient lung size on lung physiology after heart-lung transplantation. Transplantation. 1989;48:625–9.

14. Miyoshi S, Trulock EP, Schaefers HJ, et al. Cardiopulmonary exercise testing after single and double lung transplantation. Chest. 1990;97:1130–6.
15. Miyoshi S, Schaefers HJ, Trulock EP, et al. Donor selection for single and double lung transplantation. Chest size matching and other factors influencing posttransplantation vital capacity. Chest. 1990;98:308–13.
16. Ministry of Health, Labor and Welfare: Selection Criteria for Lung Transplant Applicants (Recipients): https://www.mhlw.go.jp/content/10900000/001319473.pdf. Accessed 15 Feb 2025.
17. Nakagiri T, Inoue M, Morii E, et al. Local IL-17 production and a decrease in peripheral blood regulatory T cells in an animal model of bronchiolitis obliterans. Transplantation. 2010;89:1312–9.
18. Kawamura T, Huang CS, Peng X, et al. The effect of donor treatment with hydrogen on lung allograft function in rats. Surgery. 2011;150:240–9.
19. Kawamura T, Huang CS, Tochigi N, et al. Inhaled hydrogen gas therapy for prevention of lung transplant-induced ischemia/reperfusion injury in rats. Transplantation. 2010;90:1344–51.
20. Kanou T, Ohsumi A, Kim H, et al. Inhibition of regulated necrosis attenuates receptor-interacting protein kinase 1-mediated ischemia-reperfusion injury after lung transplantation. J Heart Lung Transplant. 2018;37:1261–70.
21. Matsui Y, Kanou T, Matsui T, et al. Protective effect of calpain inhibition during cold ischemia on ischemia-reperfusion injury after lung transplantation. Transplantation. 2023;107:1945–54.
22. Miwa T, Maruyama M, Matui S, et al. A case of multiple emphysematous bullae treated with living-donor lung transplantation from identical twin brothers. Nihon Kokyuki Gakkai Zasshi. 2001;39:877–81. (Abstract in English)
23. Inoue M, Minami M, Fukushima N, et al. Bilateral lung transplantation with closure of ventricular septal defect in a patient with Eisenmenger syndrome. Gen Thorac Cardiovasc Surg. 2010;58:25–8; discussion 29
24. Matsuda H, Minami M, Ichikawa H, et al. Living-related lobar transplantation and simultaneous atrial septal defect closure in a young patient with irreversible pulmonary hypertension: a case report. Heart Vessel. 2004;19:203–7.
25. Sawa Y, Matsumiya G, Shigemura S, et al. First successful heart-lung transplantation in Japan: report of a case. Surg Today. 2013;43:1461–6.
26. Shintani Y, Funaki S, Kanou T, et al. Integrated cardiothoracic team approach for complex lung transplantation procedures in Japan-current status and future direction. J Thorac Dis. 2023;15:5195–203.
27. Shiraishi T, Midorikawa K, Miyahara S, et al. The history of Japanese lung transplantation: the unique pathway to establishing the program and its initial success. J Thorac Dis. 2023;15:5204–12.
28. Kanou T, Nakahira K, Choi AM, et al. Cell-free DNA in human ex vivo lung perfusate as a potential biomarker to predict the risk of primary graft dysfunction in lung transplantation. J Thorac Cardiovasc Surg. 2021;162:490–9.
29. Inoue M, Minami M, Wada N, et al. Results of surveillance bronchoscopy after cadaveric lung transplantation: a Japanese single-institution study. Transplant Proc. 2014;46:944–7.
30. Kanou T, Minami M, Wada N, et al. Usefulness of a preoperative inflammatory marker as a predictor of asymptomatic acute rejection after lung transplantation: a Japanese single-institution study. J Thoracic Dis. 2020;12:4754–61.
31. Van Raemdonck DE, Keshavjee S, Levvey B, et al. 5-year results from the ISHLT DCD lung transplant registry confirm excellent recipient survival from donation after circulatory death donors. J Heart Lung Transplant. 2019;38:S103.
32. Matsuda H. Why is organ transplantation from cardiac death donors necessary in Japan? J Artif Organs. https://doi.org/10.1007/s10047-025-01493-z.

33. Matsuda H, Shintani Y, Miyagawa S. Current international status of organ donation after circulatory death viewed from heart and lung transplantation: expanding the donor pool by cross-sectional action among transplant organs. Jpn J Transplant. 2022;57:163–8. (Abstract in English)
34. Iwai Y, Terawaki S, Honjo T. PD-1 blockade inhibits hematogenous spread of poorly immunogenic tumor cells by enhanced recruitment of effector T cells. Int Immunol. 2005;17:133–44.
35. Kwon ED, Hurwitz AA, Foster BA, et al. Manipulation of T cell costimulatory and inhibitory signals for immunotherapy of prostate cancer. Proc Natl Acad Sci USA. 1997;94:8099–103.
36. Huang HJ, Schechtman K, Askar M, et al. A pilot randomized control trial of de novo belatacept-based immunosuppression after lung transplantation. Transplantation. 2024;108:777–86.

Combined Heart and Lung Transplantation: Report of Three Cases

9

Koichi Toda, Yoshiki Sawa, Meinoshin Okumura, and Yasushi Shintani

Abstract

While the early mortality rate after combined heart and lung transplantation (HLTx) is reported to be as high as 25%, three cases of HLTx have been performed at Osaka University with satisfactory long survival of 8.5–16 years. Although UNOS data indicated the risk of surgery is high in low-volume centers, HLTx could be safely performed in selected patients based on a surgical strategy that is meticulously discussed in a multidisciplinary transplant team. This review illustrates the details of three cases from the standpoint of surgical strategy in the very complex transplant procedure.

Keywords

Multi-organ transplant · Combined heart and lung transplantation · Eisenmenger syndrome · Restrictive cardiomyopathy · Secondary pulmonary hypertension · Donor shortage

K. Toda (✉)
Department of Cardiovascular Surgery, Dokkyo Medical University Saitama Medical Center, Koshigaya, Saitama, Japan

Y. Sawa
Osaka Keisatsu Hospital, Osaka, Japan

M. Okumura
National Hospital Organization Osaka Toneyama Medical Center, Toyonaka, Osaka, Japan
e-mail: okumura.meinoshin.hy@mail.hosp.go.jp

Y. Shintani
Department of General Thoracic Surgery, The University of Osaka Graduate School of Medicine, Suita, Osaka, Japan
e-mail: yshintani@thoracic.med.osaka-u.ac.jp

H. Matsuda et al. (eds.), *Heart and Lung Transplantation*,
https://doi.org/10.1007/978-981-96-8810-4_9

9.1 Introduction

According to reports from Europe and the United States, the early mortality rate after combined heart and lung transplantation (HLTx) is as high as 25%. To date, three cases of HLTx have been performed in Japan, all done at Osaka University. In this article, we reviewed the trends of HLTx in the world, looked back on our three cases discussing the specific surgical strategies in this complex transplant procedure.

9.2 History of Combined Heart and Lung Transplantation (HLTx)

HLTx is a surgical procedure in which the donor's heart and both lungs are removed as an en block from donor and anastomosed in four locations: the recipient's trachea, aorta, superior vena cava, and inferior vena cava. It was first performed successfully at Stanford University in 1982 [1] and has since been used to treat more than 3200 patients with end-stage heart and lung disease worldwide [2].

Until unilateral or bilateral lung transplantation was established, there was a time when HLTx was indicated for diseases that cause chronic respiratory failure including idiopathic pulmonary hemosiderosis, idiopathic pulmonary fibrosis, α1 antitrypsin deficiency, emphysema, and chronic obstructive pulmonary disease in addition to congenital heart disease with Eisenmenger syndrome, primary pulmonary hypertension, and cardiomyopathy with pulmonary hypertension. With the success of unilateral [3] and bilateral lung transplantation [4], the indications for lung transplantation for lung diseases such as emphysema and primary pulmonary hypertension are being established. In addition, among congenital heart diseases associated with Eisenmenger syndrome, intracardiac repair and bilateral lung transplantation have been shown to be treatment options for cases of repairable cardiac malformations such as atrial septal defect and ventricular septal defect (VSD), and we have succeeded in simultaneous surgery of VSD closure and bilateral lung transplantation for a case of Eisenmenger syndrome associated with VSD [5].

According to the International Thoracic Organ Transplant (TTX) registry of the International Society for Heart and Lung Transplantation, the annual reported number of HLTx surgeries performed worldwide peaked at 225 transplants in 1989 and 1990 and has progressively declined to only 38 total cases reported in 2015 [6].

9.3 Report on Three Cases of HLTx

In Japan, only three HLTx have been performed by January 2025, all done at Osaka University with long-term survivals. These three cases are summarized in Tables 9.1 and 9.2, and their clinical courses are described.

Table 9.1 Background of recipients and donors in three combined heart and lung transplantations

	Case 1	Case 2	Case 3
Recipient age (years)	35	26	22
Recipient sex	Male	Female	Male
Recipient height (cm)	155	152	166.5
Recipient weight (kg)	36.5	53	72.8
Predicted vital capacity of recipient (L)	3.921	3.218	4.729
Etiology	DORV/VSD/PDA Eisenmenger	RCM/PH	RCM/PH
Waiting time (years)	5.5 years	9 years	3 years
PAP (mmHg)	106/61(82)	142/68(101)	132/70(93)
PVR (wood units)	19.5	26.8	19.9
PCWP (mmHg)	7	31	33
Donor age (years)	30–40	30–40	40–50
Donor sex	Male	Female	Male
Donor height (cm)	165	151	170
Donor weight (kg)	50	48	70
Predicted vital capacity of donor (L)	4.362	3.024	4.357

DORV double outlet right ventricle, *PDA* patent ductus arteriosus, *RCM* restrictive cardiomyopathy, *PH* pulmonary hypertension, *PAP* pulmonary artery pressure, *PVR* pulmonary vascular resistance, *PCWP* pulmonary capillary wedge pressure

Table 9.2 Operative data and clinical outcomes in three patients who underwent combined heart and lung transplantation

	Case 1	Case 2	Case 3
Time for transportation	51 min	80 min	120 min
Time for explantation of recipient organs and hemostasis	2 h 38 min	2 h 17 min	1 h 8 min
Time for anastomosis	1 h 19 min	1 h 21 min	51 min
Donor organs ischemic time	4 h 7 min	3 h 49 min	4 h 27 min
LVEF at 5 years after HLTx	83%	80%	71%
PAP at 5 years after HLTx	16/7 (10) mmHg	18/5 (10) mmHg	25/9 (14) mmHg
FEV 1 at 5 years after HLTx	2.91 L	2.52 L	2.57 L
Survival	16 years Alive	11 years Alive	8.5 years Alive
NYHA class	I	I	I
Activity	He works 3 days in a week	She works 3 days in a week	He works 5 days in a week

FEV 1 forced expiratory volume in 1 s, *HLTx* combined heart and lung transplantation, *LVEF* left ventricular ejection fraction, *PAP* pulmonary artery pressure, *TR-PG* tricuspid regurgitation pressure gradient

Case 1 The first case was a 35-year-old male, born with double outlet right ventricle (DORV) with doubly committed VSD, patent ductus arteriosus, and coarctation of the aorta and he was diagnosed as Eisenmenger syndrome at the age of 5 years. Details of this case have already been reported [7]. Because of irreversible pulmonary hypertension and the impossibility of concomitant lung transplantation and intracardiac repair due to the expected prolonged cardiac and pulmonary ischemic time. He was registered as a candidate for HLTx in the Japan Organ Transplant Network in August 2003.

He underwent the HLTx in January 2009. The donor was a man in his 30 s. The size matching was good at heart (body weight) and lungs (predicted vital capacity) as shown in Table 1. Expected organ transport time was 1 h. We started the recipient operation, placing him on cardiopulmonary bypass after cross-clamping the donor aorta. The donor heart was perfused with 3 L of Celsior solution and the donor lung was perfused with 6 L of extracellular type trehalose-containing Kyoto solution, followed by the procurement of both organs in an en bloc procedure. After confirming successful procurement, recipient's ascending aorta was cross clamped and we divided the ascending aorta, superior vena cava, and inferior vena cava, and then closed the patent ductus arteriosus from inside of the pulmonary artery after division of the main trunk of the pulmonary artery. After dividing the bilateral main bronchus with a stapler, both sides of the pericardium were cut longitudinally at the dorsal position of phrenic nerves, followed by division of the left atrium and pulmonary artery. After extracting the left and right lungs, we dissected around the main trunk of the trachea up to above the bifurcation, with meticulous hemostasis of the many collateral vessels which was evident in preoperative CT scan (Fig. 9.1).

The en block graft was placed in the thoracic cavity so that the bilateral phrenic nerves were located on the ventral side of the hilum of the donor lung. First, tracheal

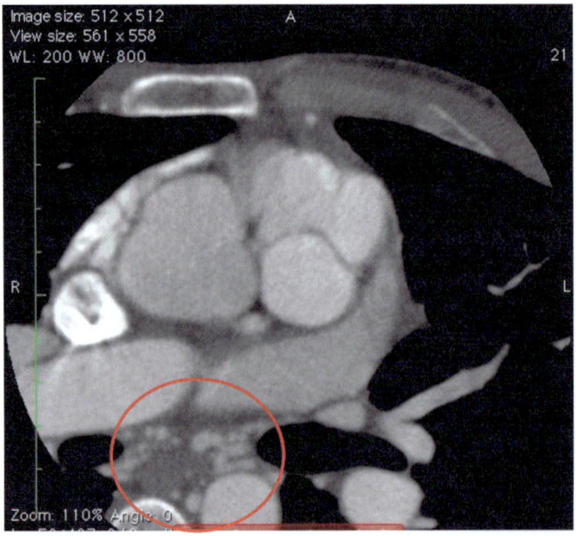

Fig. 9.1 Preoperative enhanced CT scan of the patient who underwent the first combined heart and lung transplantation. Red circle indicated collateral circulation from the bronchial artery, which required meticulous hemostasis before anastomosing trachea and large vessels

anastomosis was performed with continuous suturing of 3–0 monofilament. Subsequently, anastomosis of the ascending aorta and inferior vena cava was performed with continuous sutures. While anastomosing the superior vena cava, retrograde terminal warm cardioplegia was given through the coronary sinus with de-airing from aortic root. After the anastomosis was completed, the aortic cross clamp was removed, and the heart immediately resumed beating in sinus rhythm. He was easily weaned from cardiopulmonary bypass and chest was closed uneventfully. The operation time was 8 h 15 min, the cardiopulmonary bypass time was 4 h 38 min, the organ ischemic time was 4 h 7 min, and organ transport time was 51 min (Table 9.1). His postoperative course was uneventful, with scant bleeding and good organ functions. He was transferred out of the intensive care unit on postoperative day (POD) 13 and discharged to home on POD 66 without oxygen, infection, or rejection. He has been followed in the outpatient's clinic and has been doing well with good cardiopulmonary functions and no significant complications for more than 16 years (Table 9.2).

Case 2 The second case was a 26-year-old woman. She was diagnosed with restrictive cardiomyopathy and secondary pulmonary hypertension. Her LVEF and RVEF were reduced to 42% and 28%, respectively and pulmonary artery pressure exceeded systemic blood pressure (Table 9.1). She was registered as a candidate for HLTx in 2004, and a HLTx was performed in December 2013. Operation was performed as we did in the first case. Compared with the first case we encountered fewer collateral vessels around tracheal bifurcation and found vessel sealing devices useful for hemostasis. The time for explantation of recipient organs and hemostasis, time for anastomosis, the time for organ transport, and the organ ischemic time was 2 h 17 min, 1 h 21 min, 80 min, and 4 h 7 min, respectively (Table 9.2). Her postoperative course was also uneventful without infection or rejection and discharged to home without oxygen, infection, or rejection. She has been followed in the outpatient's clinic and has been doing well without significant complications for more than 11 years.

Case 3 The third case was a 22-year-old male patient with restrictive cardiomyopathy and secondary pulmonary hypertension (Table 9.1). He was registered as a candidate for HLTx at the age of 19, and after a three-year wait, he underwent a HLTx in June 2016. The surgery was performed in the same way as in previous cases. Although his postoperative cardio-pulmonary function was good, he suffered from mediastinitis due to tracheal anastomosis leakage. After the mediastinum and chest cavity required lavage and drainage, the omentum was transferred around the tracheal anastomosis. There was no recurrence of the infection and he was discharged to home at 4 months after surgery. Although hemostasis of the tracheal bifurcation is important, it was suggested that excessive hemostasis maneuvers may cause poor healing of the tracheal anastomosis. He has been followed in the outpatient clinic without significant complications for more than 8 years (Table 9.2).

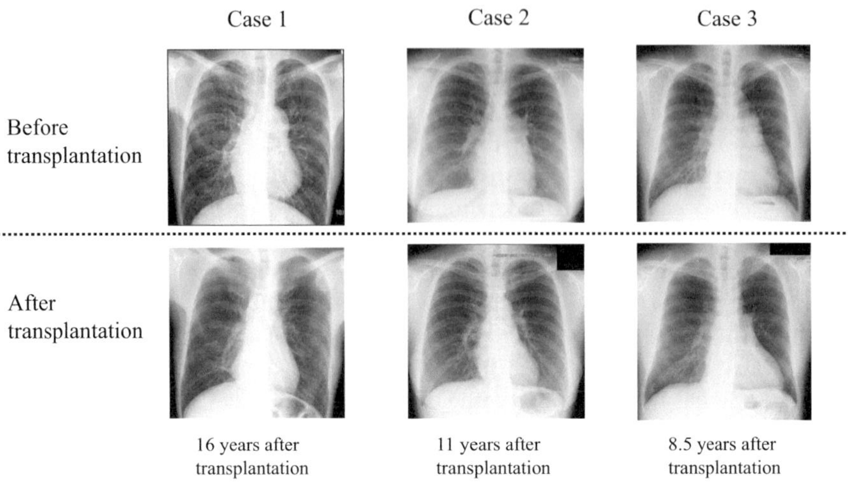

Fig. 9.2 Pre- and post-transplant chest X-rays of three patients who underwent combined heart and lung transplantation

Preoperative and follow-up chest-x-rays at 16, 11, and 8.5 years after transplant are shown in Fig. 9.2.

9.4 Outcomes of HLTx

The postoperative survival curve for all 3276 patients after HLTx in the ISHLT registry showed that the estimated time point at which 50% of the recipients have died was 4.5 years in adult and 3.6 years in pediatric [2]. The high mortality rate in the early postoperative period (25%) may also have an impact on long-term outcomes. Most perioperative deaths are related to hemorrhage or graft dysfunction, which is also associated with bleeding-related hemodynamic deterioration [8]. Because bleeding around the tracheal anastomosis is difficult to control after tracheal and large vessel anastomosis, complete hemostasis before anastomosis is important, especially in Eisenmenger syndrome, where collateral circulation is developed, and if there is a history of open-heart surgery, it is even more difficult to control the bleeding, and preoperative evaluation is important.

Dr. Shudo, who is originally from our group and currently working on cardiothoracic transplantation at Stanford University, analyzed the surgical results of HLTx in 997 patients using the UNOS database between 1987 and 2017 [9]. According to this, the one-year graft survival is 66.6%. The age of the donor was a significant risk factor and the donor age of non-survivor was 29.4 ± 13.0 years which was significantly higher than that of survivors (27.6 ± 12.1 years old). The transplant center volume was an important factor on the recipient side, and the top 1/4 of the centers with the highest number of cases performed better than other centers. Although the exact cause of the difference in outcomes among centers has not been analyzed, not only surgical technique, but also the multidisciplinary approach for preoperative and postoperative management is thought to be important.

In our experience of three HLTx cases, we learned the importance of multidisciplinary collaboration including collaboration between donor and recipient teams, and collaboration between cardiovascular surgeons and thoracic surgeons. Even in surgical techniques including hemostasis, the way of thinking differs depending on their specialties and hemostasis around the tracheal anastomosis needs to be carefully and meticulously done. Based on the experience of three cases, we predicted 1–2 h is necessary for explantation of recipient organs with complete hemostasis and 1 h for tracheal and large vessel anastomosis, and we performed the simulation of operative time course so that each of multidisciplinary team understands the time course of surgery in a donor side as well as in a recipient side (Fig. 9.3).

If there is a local donor and the preoperative CT scan of the recipient does not show abundant collateral circulation around the tracheal bifurcation, we estimate transport time is 1 h and that it takes 1 h for explantation of recipient's organs with complete hemostasis and 1 h for anastomosis of trachea and large vessels. In this case we can start explantation of the recipient's organs, after confirmation of donor organ arrival in the recipient hospital and the donor cardiopulmonary ischemia time can be within 4 h (Fig. 9.3a).

On the other hand, even if the expected transport time is 1 h, if abundant collateral circulations around the tracheal bifurcation are observed on preoperative CT scan of the recipient, as in Case 1, it is necessary to start the recipient organ removal as soon as it is confirmed that the procurement of donor's organs has been successfully performed. The donor organ arrives during recipient organ harvesting and hemostasis at tracheal bifurcation, and after confirming sufficient hemostasis, we can move on to anastomosis of the trachea and large blood vessels. Even if it takes 2 h for removal of heart and lungs from the recipient and 1 h for anastomosis, the donor cardiopulmonary ischemia time can be less than 4 h (Fig. 9.3b).

In patients with pulmonary hypertension and abundant collateral circulation around the tracheal bifurcation who is supported by bi-ventricular assist device (VAD), it may take more than 1 h to establish a cardiopulmonary bypass, and it is necessary to proceed with re-sternotomy before the donor organ is harvested (Fig. 9.3c). Regarding the transport time, even in cases where organ transportation takes 2 h and explantation of recipient's organs with complete hemostasis takes 2 h, it can be performed within 4 h of the donor cardiopulmonary ischemia time (Fig. 9.3d). On the other hand, if the transport time is 3 h, it is necessary to complete the hemostasis of the posterior mediastinum before donor organ arrival so that tracheal anastomosis can be started as soon as the donor organ arrives (Fig. 9.3e).

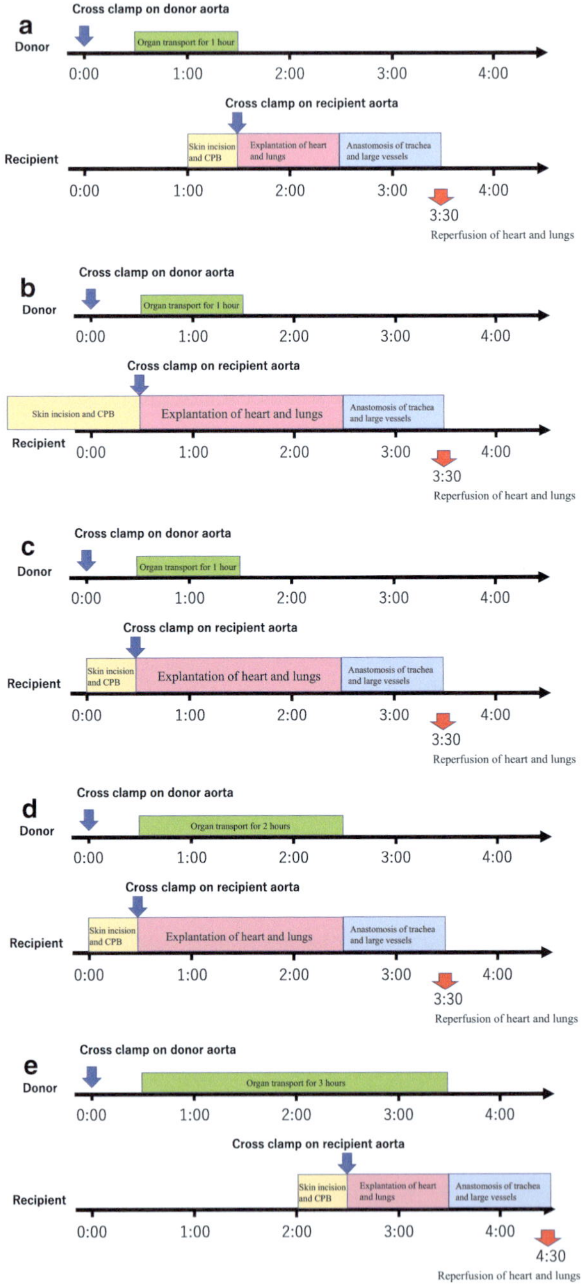

Fig. 9.3 Simulation of time course in donor and recipient operation in combined heart and lung transplantation. (**a**) Simulation in the case who required 1 h each for transport of donor heart, explantation of recipient's heart, and anastomosis of trachea and large vessels. (**b**) Simulation in the case who required 2 h for explantation of recipient's heart and 1 h each for transport of donor heart and anastomosis of trachea and large vessels. (**c**) Simulation in the case who required 1 h for re-sternotomy, 2 h for explantation of recipient's heart and 1 h each for transport of donor heart and anastomosis of trachea and large vessels. (**d**) Simulation in the case who required 2 h each for explantation of recipient's heart and transport of donor heart, and 1 h for anastomosis of trachea and large vessels. (**e**) Simulation in the case who required 3 h for transport of donor heart, and 1 h each for explantation of recipient's heart, and anastomosis of trachea and large vessels

9.5 Summary

Considering the fact that three organs are required to save one person's life, and the risk of surgery is high in facilities with less experience, HLTx may be indicated in limited cases. However, there are patients like ours who cannot be saved without HLTx and it is necessary to perform this combined transplantation in selected patients. Based on our experience, the surgical strategy is discussed in a multidisciplinary transplant team.

References

1. Reitz BA, Wallwork JL, Hunt SA, et al. Heart-lung transplantation: successful therapy for patients with pulmonary vascular disease. N Engl J Med. 1982;306:557–64.
2. Khush KK, Cherikh WS, Chambers DC, et al. The international thoracic organ transplant registry of the International Society for Heart and Lung Transplantation: thirty-sixth adult heart transplantation report – 2019; focus theme: donor and recipient size match. J Heart Lung Transplant. 2019;38:1056–66.
3. Toronto lung transplantation group unilateral lung transplantation for pulmonary fibrosis. N Engl J Med. 1986;314:1140–5.
4. Patterson GA, Cooper JD, Dark JH, et al. Experimental and clinical double lung transplantation. J Thorac Cardiovasc Surg. 1988;95:70–4.
5. Inoue M, Minami M, Fukushima N, et al. Bilateral lung transplantation with closure of ventricular septal defect in a patient with Eisenmenger syndrome. Gen Thorac Cardiovasc Surg. 2010;58:25–9.
6. Chambers DC, Yusen RD, Cherikh WS, et al. The registry of the International Society for Heart and Lung Transplantation: thirty-fourth adult lung and heart-lung transplantation report-2017; focus theme: allograft ischemic time. J Heart Lung Transplant. 2017;36:1047–59.
7. Sawa Y, Matsumiya G, Shigemura S, et al. First successful heart-lung transplantation in Japan: report of a case. Surg Today. 2013;43:1461–6.
8. Stoica SC, McNeil KD, Perreas K, et al. Heart-lung transplantation for Eisenmenger syndrome: early and long-term results. Ann Thorac Surg. 2001;72:1887–91.
9. Shudo Y, Wang H, Lingala B, et al. Evaluation of risk factors for heart-lung transplant recipient outcome: an analysis of the united network for organ sharing database. Circulation. 2019;140:1261–72.

Heart Transplantation in National Cerebral and Cardiovascular Center

10

Satsuki Fukushima, Kota Suzuki, Yuji Tominaga, Motoki Komori, Satoshi Kainuma, Yasumasa Tsukamoto, and Shigemitsu Iwai

Abstract

Since performing our first heart transplant in May 1999, the National Cerebral and Cardiovascular Center (NCVC) has been actively involved in left ventricular assist device (LVAD) therapy and heart transplantation for patients with severe heart failure. This report presents the clinical outcomes of heart transplantation at NCVC and our current activities.

The overall survival rates for heart transplantation at NCVC are 95%, 95%, and 87% at 5, 10, and 15 years, respectively, which are favorable compared to the International Society for Heart and Lung Transplantation (ISHLT) registry. While the number of heart transplants performed has been gradually increasing, the severe shortage of donors in Japan remains an ongoing issue, leading to prolonged waiting times for heart transplantation.

Key challenges in managing prolonged wait times include strategies for bridging patients in cardiogenic shock to durable LVAD therapy, approaches to man-

S. Fukushima (✉) · K. Suzuki · S. Kainuma
Division of Adult Cardiac Surgery, National Cerebral and Cardiovascular Center, Suita, Osaka, Japan
e-mail: s.fukushima@ncvc.go.jp; suzuki.kota@ncvc.go.jp; kainuma.satoshi@ncvc.go.jp

Y. Tominaga · M. Komori · S. Iwai
Department of Pediatric Cardiovascular Surgery, National Cerebral and Cardiovascular Center, Suita, Osaka, Japan
e-mail: tominaga.yuji@ncvc.go.jp; motokikomori0101@ncvc.go.jp; iwais@ncvc.go.jp

Y. Tsukamoto
Department of Transplant Medicine, National Cerebral and Cardiovascular Center, Suita, Osaka, Japan
e-mail: ytsuka@ncvc.go.jp

H. Matsuda et al. (eds.), *Heart and Lung Transplantation*,
https://doi.org/10.1007/978-981-96-8810-4_10

aging primary graft dysfunction, which is one of the leading causes of perioperative mortality, and aggressive utilization of marginal donors. We briefly discuss our current initiatives regarding these matters.

Keywords

Heart transplantation · Left ventricular assist device (LVAD) · Donor shortage · Marginal donor · Organ preservation solution · Modified bicaval method · EXCOR · Pediatric heart transplantation · Celsior solution · UW solution

10.1 Heart Transplant Cases at National Cerebral and Cardiovascular Center

The first heart transplantation at the National Cerebral and Cardiovascular Center (NCVC) was performed in May 1999. By May 2024, 210 transplants (143 male and 67 female recipients) had been performed. Until 2010, only a few transplants were performed annually. However, following the enactment of the revised Organ Transplantation Law in July 2010, the number of heart transplants gradually increased, reaching a record high of 32 transplants in 2023. The annual number of transplants is illustrated in Fig. 10.1. The average age of recipients at the time of transplantation was 39.7 ± 15.5 years. Recipients aged 0–9 years accounted for 7 cases (3.3%), while 22 cases (10.5%) involved elderly recipients aged 60 years or older. The age distribution of recipients is shown in Fig. 10.2. Of note, Kitamura et al. developed "the modified bicaval anastomosis technique" in the initial few cases, which is now the standard technique of heart transplantation in Japan.

Regarding the primary underlying diseases, dilated cardiomyopathy accounted for the highest proportion at 63%, followed by hypertrophic cardiomyopathy (10%) and ischemic cardiomyopathy (9%). The distribution of underlying diseases is presented in Fig. 10.3. Regarding pediatric heart transplants, the first heart transplantation under the age of 18 at NCVC was performed in January 2001. Then, 21 patients under the age of 18 underwent heart transplantation at NCVC between January

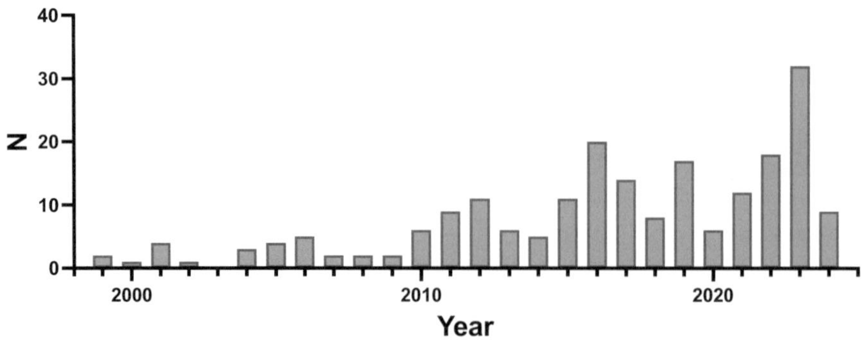

Fig. 10.1 Annual number of heart transplants (1999–May 2024)

Fig. 10.2 Recipient age at the time of transplantation

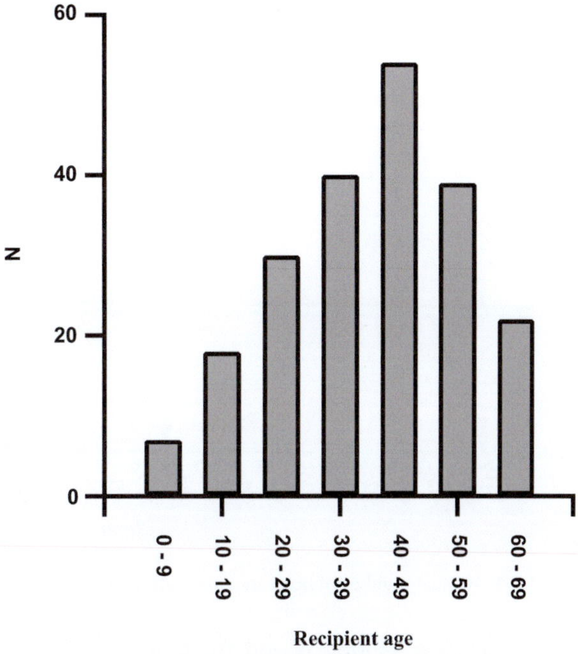

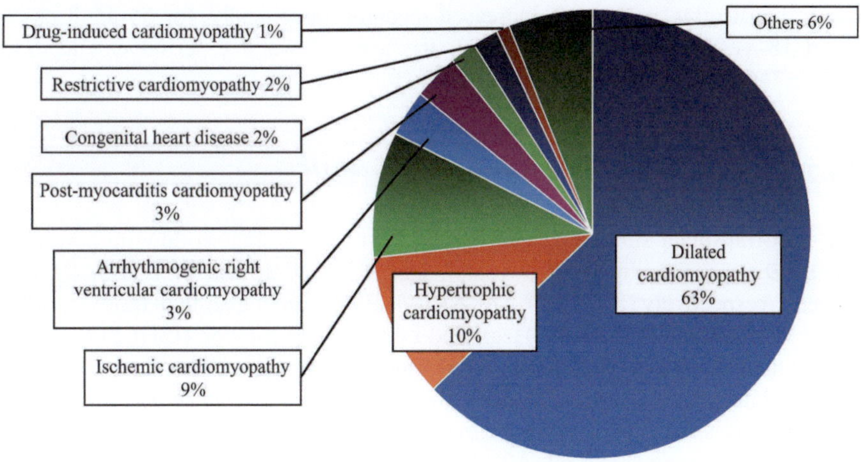

Fig. 10.3 Underlying cardiac disease

2001 and 2024. Regarding the annual trend in the number of transplant surgeries, almost all of the cases were performed after the revision of the Organ Transplant Act came into effect, and 11 cases (more than half of the total) were performed after 2023 after COVID-19 had subsided (Fig. 10.4). Of these, 7 cases (33%) were under 10 years old. The primary disease was dilated cardiomyopathy in 16 cases and other diseases in 5 cases.

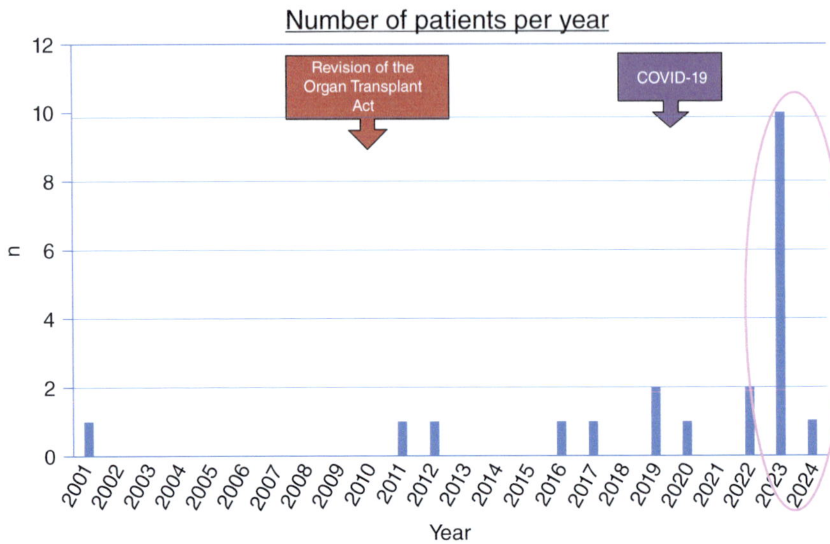

Fig. 10.4 Annual number of heart transplantation under the age of 18 (2001 to January 2024)

The average waiting period for transplantation across the entire period was 1424 ± 814 days (approximately 4 years). However, according to Japan's national trend, this waiting period has increased recently. Specifically, for 55 adult cases (aged 18 years or older) since 2020, the average waiting period extended to 1927 ± 716 days, exceeding 5 years.

10.2 Heart Transplant Outcomes at NCVC

The post-transplant survival rates at NCVC, with an average follow-up period of 7.0 ± 5.9 years (maximum 24.9 years), were 95%, 95%, and 87% at 5, 10, and 15 years, respectively (Fig. 10.5). These survival rates are higher than those reported in the International Society for Heart and Lung Transplantation (ISHLT) Registry. During the follow-up period, there were 15 mortality cases (4 in the acute phase and 11 in the late phase). Causes of death in the acute phase included cerebral complications in 2 cases and infections in 2 cases. The causes of death during the follow-up period are summarized in Table 10.1.

Several factors may contribute to the favorable post-transplant outcomes observed in Japan compared to reports from other countries. These include a lower proportion of ischemic cardiomyopathy cases (approximately 40% in ISHLT reports), a relatively younger recipient age (median 54 years, range 26–67 years in ISHLT reports), and a lower incidence of cardiac allograft vasculopathy [1]. On the other hand, a notable characteristic of heart transplantation in Japan is the high

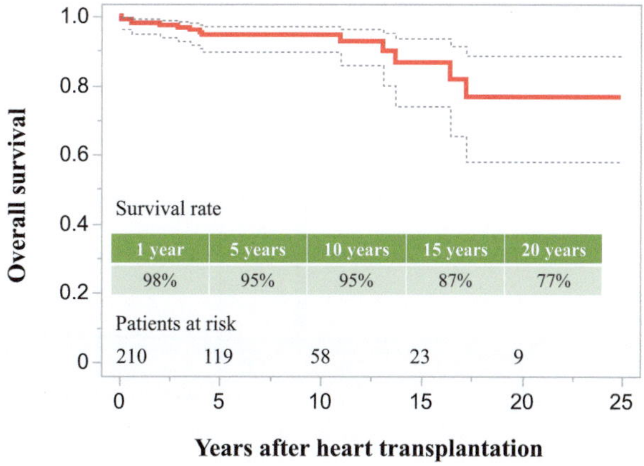

Fig. 10.5 Overall survival after heart transplantation

Table 10.1 Cause of death after heart transplantation

Cause of death	Number
Perioperative infection or MOF	2
Perioperative cerebral complication	2
Malignancy	3
Infection	3
Heart failure	1
PTLD	1
Unknown	4

MOF multiple organ failure, *PTLD* post-transplant lymphoproliferative disorders

proportion of elderly donors. At NCVC, 43% of adult heart transplant cases involved donors aged 50 years or older. The median ischemic time was 186 minutes (range 159–210 min), comparable to the ISHLT-reported data.

Regarding pediatric heart transplants, the median follow-up period after heart transplantation was 1.3 years, and the maximum was 12 years. The post-transplant survival rate at NCVC was 100% (Fig. 10.6). Conditions before heart transplantation included inotropes in 3 cases, implantable ventricular assist device (VAD) in 6 cases, and extracorporeal VAD in 12 cases. The Status 1 waiting period was 848 days, and the VAD support period was 710 days (maximum 4.0 years). Body weight differences at the time of transplant ranged from −24% to 157%, and the median donor cardiac ischemic time was 195 min (maximum 242 min). There was no severe acute rejection, and although two cases developed post-transplant lymphoproliferative disorders, both achieved complete remission. In conclusion, the outcomes of pediatric heart transplantation were considered as satisfactory. In the future, further improvements will be needed to manage long-term waiting periods, such as measures to prevent right heart failure, cerebrovascular disorders, and device infections after VAD placement.

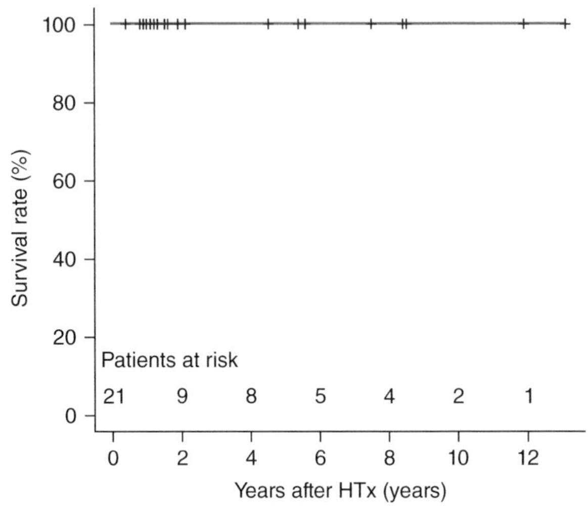

Fig. 10.6 Overall survival after heart transplantation in patients younger than 18 years

10.3 Heart Transplant Waiting Status/Left Ventricular Assist Device

Most heart transplant candidates at NCVC are patients with a left ventricular assist device (LVAD), similar to other institutions in Japan. Figure 10.7 illustrates the trends in LVAD use at NCVC up to 2024. In the 2000s, extracorporeal VADs were predominantly used. However, since the approval of implantable VADs for bridge-to-transplant (BTT) in 2011, their use has increased. Approximately 30 implantations are performed annually, including those for destination therapy. The overall survival rate of HeartMate3, the only implantable VAD currently available in Japan, is favorable, with 95.2% at 1 year and 93.3% at 2 years. This has contributed to the recent increase in heart transplant procedures.

To facilitate the conversion of patients with refractory cardiogenic shock to implantable VAD support or heart transplantation, we actively implement mechanical circulatory support, including Impella and extracorporeal VADs. In particular, for patients with elevated pulmonary vascular resistance, we have established a unique RALV-AOPA ECMO (Fig. 10.8), enabling biventricular support while adjusting pulmonary blood flow [2]. This approach aims to improve survival outcomes.

Regarding the treatment of LVAD therapy in pediatric patients, the first Berlin Heart EXCOR (BHE) pediatric implantation at NCVC was performed in April 2015 when EXCOR was insurance-reimbursed in Japan. Then, 26 patients under 18 underwent BHE implantation at NCVC between April 2015 and 2024. Median age and body weight at the time of BHE implantation was 12.4 months (interquartile range 9.0–57.3) and 7.5 kg (4.9–15.3). The post-BHE implantation survival rates were 92%, 76%, and 63% at 1, 2, and 3 years, respectively (Fig. 10.9).

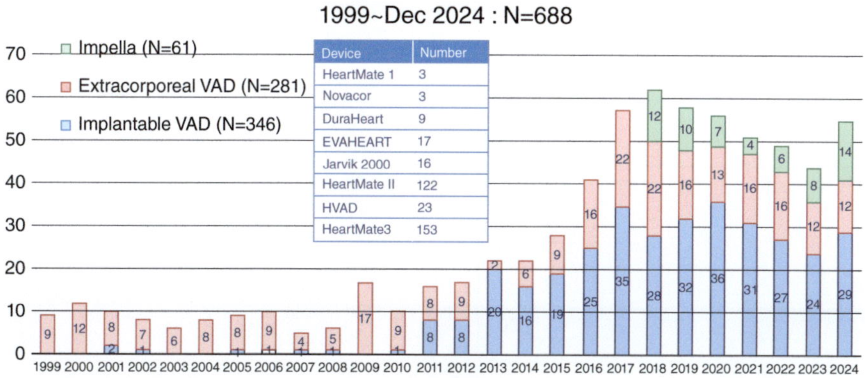

Fig. 10.7 Trends in the use of left ventricular assist device (LVAD)

Fig. 10.8 Schema of central RALV-AOPA ECMO. Central RALV-AOPA ECMO in which central cannulations were performed and then two inflows and two outflows were connected by two Y-connectors, which were in turn connected to one ECMO circuit. ECMO, extracorporeal membrane oxygenation. (Source; Ref. 2 with permission)

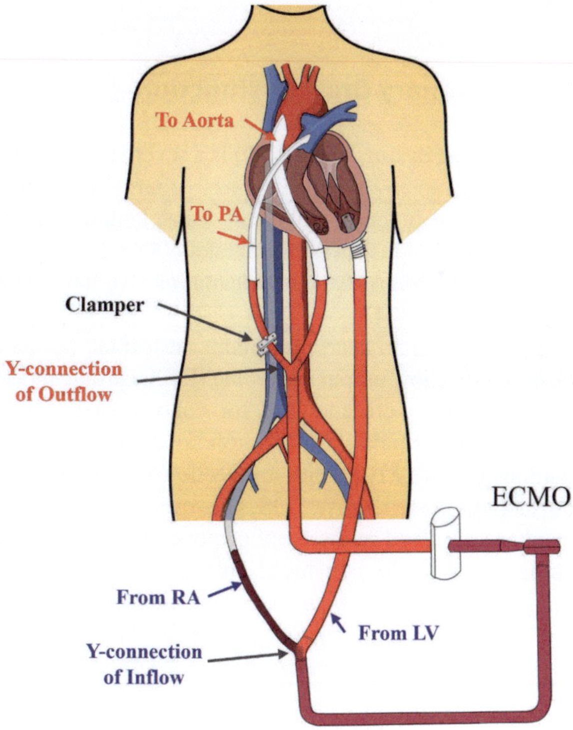

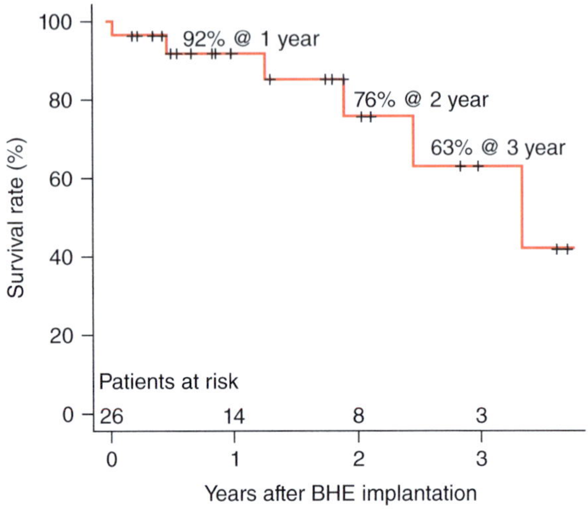

Fig. 10.9 Survival rate after Berlin Heart EXCOR (BHE) implantation

10.4 Primary Graft Dysfunction

Primary graft dysfunction (PGD) is a severe complication in the early postoperative period, characterized by impaired contractility and hemodynamic instability. Although the outcomes of heart transplantation in Japan are favorable, with a 10-year survival rate of approximately 90%, PGD remains a leading cause of early mortality following heart transplantation. We have published two papers analyzing risk factors for PGD.

First, among 36 heart transplants performed between 1999 and 2011, 7 cases of postoperative low output syndrome (LOS, cardiac index <2.2 L/min/m^2 or requiring IABP/ECMO) were analyzed for donor-related factors [3]. The study identified small left ventricular size (diastolic diameter <36 mm), high-dose catecholamine administration (≥10γ), and an ejection fraction (EF) of ≤55% as risk factors for developing postoperative LOS. However, all cases of LOS were successfully managed and resolved in the early postoperative period, with favorable long-term outcomes. The study concluded that expanding the acceptance of well-managed marginal donors may be a reasonable approach.

After the International Society for Heart and Lung Transplantation (ISHLT) published the definition of primary graft dysfunction (PGD) in 2013, we analyzed the risk factors and prognosis of PGD in 48 heart transplants performed between 1999 and 2014 [4]. Over 70% of the donors had at least one marginal factor, but only 6 cases (9.8%) developed PGD. Identified risk factors included high-dose catecholamine use in donors and a history of stroke in recipients. Although cases with PGD demonstrated significantly lower cardiac output at 6 months postoperatively during right heart catheterization (4.6 ± 0.8 vs. 5.8 ± 1.2 L/min, $p = 0.02$), no significant difference in 5-year survival rates was observed (83.3% vs. 93.3%, $p = 0.23$). More mechanical circulatory support (MCS) options are available now than in the previous era. Overcoming severe perioperative PGD with MCS may help to further improve heart transplant outcomes in Japan, indicating the need for further research.

10.5 Marginal Donor

It is well known that the number of organ donors in Japan is significantly lower than in Western countries, and the waiting period is substantially longer. Therefore, it is necessary to carefully evaluate and actively utilize marginal donors, including elderly donors and those with size mismatches. In 2024, we reported outcomes for heart transplants using donors aged 65 years or older [5]. Among 152 adult heart transplant cases, we compared 12 cases using donors aged 65 or older with 140 cases using younger donors in terms of background, perioperative factors, and mid-term outcomes. In the elderly donor group, higher E/e' and lower CI were observed 1 month post-operatively. By 1 year post-transplant, E/e' remained elevated, but CI was comparable between groups. The 3-year survival rate was significantly lower in the elderly donor group (81.5% vs. 97.8%, $p = 0.006$). However, since recipients in this group were also older (median age: 60 years), the study concluded that thoroughly evaluated heart transplants from elderly donors yielded acceptable results. In one case involving a 69-year-old donor, significant coronary artery disease was detected during planned coronary angiography on postoperative day 12, requiring CABG on day 17. This suggests that pre-procurement coronary angiography may be considered in selected cases.

We also have reported an analysis of the impact of donor-to-recipient size mismatch on heart transplantation outcomes. Among 111 heart transplantations performed by May 2018, 106 cases using the modified bicaval anastomosis technique [6] were categorized into three groups based on the donor-to-recipient weight ratio: the undersized group (<0.8, $N = 17$), the size-matched group (0.8–1.3, $N = 68$), and the oversized group (>1.3, $N = 21$). Survival rates and post-operative hemodynamic parameters were compared among the three groups. No significant differences in survival rates were observed among the groups. Regarding hemodynamics, while the cardiac index (CI) in the undersized group was lower 1 month post-operatively, no significant differences were observed at 6 months or 1 year post-transplant [7]. As noted, the shortage of donors in Japan remains a critical issue. Based on these findings, we have utilized the marginal donors, ensuring thorough evaluation and management.

10.6 Organ Preservation Solution

The Celsior solution has long been used as an organ preservation solution in Japan. However, in recent years, its supply has been discontinued, necessitating an alternative preservation solution selection. Since February 2023, NCVC has been using the University of Wisconsin (UW) solution. This section describes the initial impressions and safety of its use. One hundred sixty-six heart transplants at NCVC from 2014 to 2024 were included in the analysis, comparing perioperative data between the Celsior group (C group, $N = 114$) and the University of Wisconsin solution group (U group, $N = 52$). There were no significant differences in perioperative survival rates (C group vs. U group: 99.1% vs. 100%, $p = 0.79$) or peak postoperative CK-MB levels (58 [IQR: 43–84] vs. 51 [40–69], $p = 0.16$). The one-year survival rates were also comparable (98.2% vs. 98.1%, $p = 0.87$).

Additionally, there was no significant difference in the number of cases requiring postoperative MCS. However, the incidence of patients requiring three or more intraoperative defibrillation was significantly higher in the C group. In contrast, the number of patients requiring high-dose catecholamines postoperatively was significantly higher in the U group. These data suggest that the UW solution, which is widely used in various organ transplants, may be as safe as the Celsior solution for heart transplantation. Further case accumulation and detailed investigations are needed in the future.

10.7 Discussion

This report provides an overview of the clinical outcomes of heart transplantation at NCVC and the current challenges in this field. With improvements in the organ donation system, the number of transplants has been steadily increasing, reaching a record high of 32 cases in 2023. This trend is likely influenced by both the advancement of transplant medicine in Japan and an increase in organ donation. However, since 2020, the waiting period for adult cases has exceeded 5 years, highlighting the need for further measures to advance transplant medicine.

In summary, Japan's heart transplantation program has maintained favorable outcomes by making appropriate use of marginal donors, including elderly donors, despite the persistent challenge of donor shortages. Additionally, innovative systems such as RALV-AOPA ECMO have been utilized for cardiogenic shock cases to stabilize patients and facilitate the transition to durable LVAD therapy. However, the prolonged waiting period remains a significant issue, necessitating further expansion of donor availability, appropriate donor evaluation, and optimization of transplant eligibility criteria.

10.8 Conclusion

Heart transplantation has been established as the standard treatment for end-stage severe heart failure in Japan, and NCVC has contributed to the treatment of severe heart failure in the country. However, many challenges remain in transplant medicine, including a shortage of donors.

Acknowledgments Many surgeons, physicians, co-medical, and administration staff have contributed to heart transplantation at the National Cerebral and Cardiovascular Center. Special thanks go to the late Dr. Hisao Manabe, the late Dr. Tsuyoshi Fujita, Dr. Yasunaru Kawashima, Dr. Soichiro Kitamura, Dr. Toshikatsu Yagihara, Dr. Takeshi Nakatani, Dr. Yoshikado Sasako, Dr. Junjiro Kobayashi, Dr. Norihide Fukushima, Dr. Hajime Ichikawa, and Dr. Tomoyuki Fujita.

References

1. Kitamura S. Heart transplantation in Japan: a critical appraisal for the results and prospects. Gen Thorac Cardiovasc Surg. 2012;60:639–44.
2. Tadokoro N, Kainuma S, Tonai K, et al. Useful central mechanical circulatory support system for critical biventricular heart failure associated with high pulmonary vascular resistance. Artif Organs. 2024. https://doi.org/10.1111/aor.14906.
3. Fujita T, Toda K, Yanase M, et al. Risk factors for post-transplant low output syndrome. Eur J Cardiothorac Surg. 2012;42:551–6.
4. Seguchi O, Fujita T, Murata Y, et al. Incidence, etiology, and outcome of primary graft dysfunction in adult heart transplant recipients: a single-center experience in Japan. Heart Vessel. 2016;31:555–62.
5. Hada T, Seguchi O, Kitahata N, et al. Heart transplantation with super-aged donors older than 65 years. J Heart Lung Transplant Open. 2024;4:100083.
6. Kitamura S, Nakatani S, Bando K, et al. Modification of bicaval anastomosis technique for orthotopic heart transplantation. Ann Thorac Surg. 2001;72:1405–6.
7. Kakuta T, Fukushima S, Shimahara Y, et al. Benefits of the modified bicaval anastomosis technique for orthotopic heart transplantation from a size-mismatched marginal donor. Circ J. 2020;64:61–8.

Surgical Considerations in Heart Transplantation: Technical Viewpoint

11

Taichi Sakaguchi

Abstract

Heart transplantation has advanced significantly since Lower and Shumway introduced the biatrial anastomosis technique in the 1960s. Although this method is simple and reproducible, it can cause atrial enlargement and associated complications such as sinus node dysfunction and tricuspid regurgitation. The bicaval anastomosis technique addressed these problems by preserving the morphology of the right atrium through individual anastomoses of the superior and inferior vena cava. Further refinements with anastomotic modification have improved anastomotic ease and reduced complications such as anastomotic stenosis. Technically, complex congenital heart disease, including heterotaxy syndrome and failed Fontan, is challenging. In particular, partial heart transplantation for truncus arteriosus is one of the most exciting procedures recently introduced, changing the concept of heart transplantation and the management of complex congenital heart disease. The combination of 3D printing and virtual reality seems promising for the planning of transplantation procedures in various complex situations. Further technical refinements and the introduction of new techniques in heart transplantation are expected to provide more confident status as advanced medicine for end-stage heart failure.

Keywords

Heart transplantation · Biatrial anastomosis · Bicaval anastomosis · Modified bicaval anastomosis · Congenital heart disease · Partial heart transplantation · Heterotaxy syndrome · Failed Fontan · VAD

T. Sakaguchi (✉)
Department of Cardiovascular Surgery, Hyogo Medical University, Nishinomiya, Hyogo, Japan
e-mail: t-sakaguchi@hyo-med.ac.jp

H. Matsuda et al. (eds.), *Heart and Lung Transplantation*,
https://doi.org/10.1007/978-981-96-8810-4_11

11.1 Introduction

The history of heart transplantation began with the pioneering experimental studies of Lower and Shumway in the early 1960s [1]. They introduced the biatrial anastomosis technique, which became the standard method for orthotopic heart transplantation following the first transplant performed by Barnard in 1967. In the 1990s, the bicaval anastomosis technique was developed, preserving the donor's right atrium and utilizing separate anastomoses at the superior and inferior vena cava. By maintaining the morphology and function of the right atrium, this technique reduces complications such as late atrial enlargement, supraventricular arrhythmias, permanent pacemaker implantation, and tricuspid regurgitation. Today, it is the preferred method. This review outlines these techniques and their modifications.

11.2 Biatrial Anastomosis Technique (Fig. 11.1a)

1. *Recipient Heart Excision*

A median sternotomy is performed, and the aorta, superior vena cava (SVC), and inferior vena cava (IVC) are taped. After administering heparin, cannulation is performed on the ascending aorta near the origin of the brachiocephalic artery. SVC and IVC cannulation are done laterally to ensure a sufficient atrial cuff. Once the donor's heart is confirmed suitable, the aorta is clamped, and heart excision begins. Right atrial excision proceeds cranially to caudally along the atrioventricular groove, with the incision extending toward the coronary sinus while avoiding the IVC cannula. The aorta and pulmonary artery are transected above their respective valves. The left atrial dome is exposed by retracting the aorta and pulmonary artery,

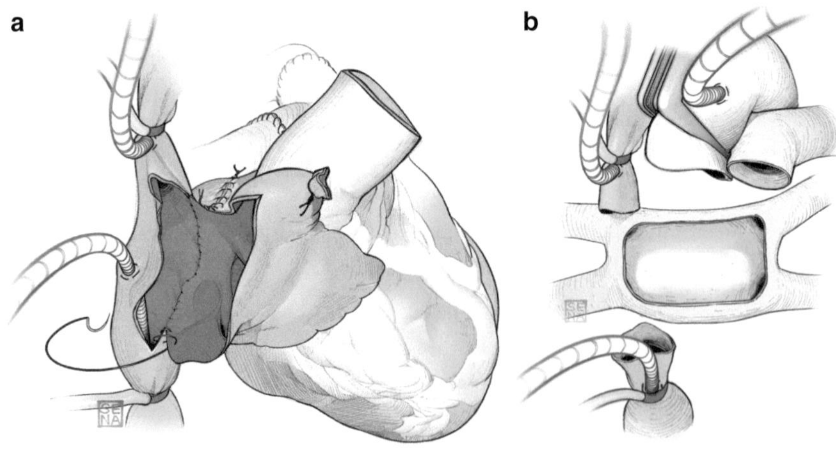

Fig. 11.1 Biatrial (**a**) and bicaval (**b**) anastomosis technique

and the incision is extended toward the base of the left atrial appendage. Excision is completed by extending the left atrial incision while preserving a broad section of the posterior left atrial wall to confirm the openings of the pulmonary veins.

2. *Donor Heart Anastomosis*

The left atrial anastomosis begins at the recipient's left upper pulmonary vein area and the donor's left atrial appendage area. Continuous suturing is performed with 3–0 or 4–0 polypropylene sutures. Suturing is carried downward on the recipient's left side toward the atrial septum junction. The other needle continues suturing from the left atrial dome toward the atrial septum, completing the circumferential anastomosis. Right atrial anastomosis starts near the center of the atrial septum suture line and proceeds caudally toward the IVC (Fig. 11.1a). The other needle continues suturing from the cranial side to the lateral wall, completing the circumferential anastomosis. Pulmonary artery anastomosis follows, with stumps trimmed to avoid kinking. The aorta is similarly trimmed, and anastomosis is performed with continuous 4–0 polypropylene sutures.

3. *Issues with Biatrial Anastomosis Technique*

This method retains both recipient and donor atria, often resulting in an enlarged and distorted atrium with asynchronous contractions. This leads to increasing atrial pressure and reduced cardiac output. Blood stagnation within the atrium increases the risk of thrombus formation [2]. Sinus node dysfunction is a frequent arrhythmia, often necessitating permanent pacemaker implantation in 5.3% of patients compared to 3% with the bicaval technique. Tricuspid regurgitation is more common due to atrial enlargement and twisting. Despite these challenges, long-term survival rates are generally comparable [3, 4].

4. *Indications for Biatrial Anastomosis Technique*

The biatrial anastomosis technique is simple and thus minimizes ischemic and cardiopulmonary bypass time. It may be preferable in cases of significant vena cava mismatch or reoperations with challenging dissection around the right atrium.

11.3 Bicaval Anastomosis Technique (Fig. 11.1b)

The bicaval technique was developed around the 1990s to address the issues associated with the biatrial technique. This method involves individual anastomoses of the SVC and IVC, preserving right atrial volume and morphology. This technique significantly reduces tricuspid regurgitation and sinus node dysfunction, lowering the need for permanent pacemakers.

1. *Recipient Heart Excision*

The procedure setup is similar to the biatrial technique. The SVC is transected at the cavo-atrial junction, and care is taken to preserve a sufficiently large atrial cuff during the IVC excision. If the cuff is too small, venous drainage snares may retract the IVC toward the diaphragm, complicating the anastomosis. After transecting the aorta and pulmonary artery, the recipient's heart is retracted caudally, and the left atrial incision proceeds as in the biatrial technique.

2. *Donor Heart Anastomosis*

In the bicaval technique, the SVC and the IVC are individually anastomosed. For the SVC anastomosis, continuous sutures using 4–0 or 5–0 polypropylene are employed. Using interrupted or interlocking sutures may help reduce the risk of stenosis. Meticulous attention is essential to prevent twisting or kinking at the anastomosis site. The IVC anastomosis involves suturing the donor heart to the recipient's right atrial cuff. As previously noted, a larger atrial cuff facilitates this step, as an IVC snare can retract atrial tissue toward the diaphragm. Alternatively, the open anastomosis method was proposed by Aklog et al. Their approach utilizes vacuum-assisted venous drainage with a long IVC cannula inserted through the femoral vein, thereby eliminating the need for IVC snaring [5].

11.4 Modified Bicaval Anastomosis Technique (Fig. 11.2)

Kitamura and his colleagues introduced the modified bicaval technique, preserving continuity between the SVC and IVC by leaving a strip of the right atrial posterior wall [6]. This prevents shrinkage and retraction of the divided atrial cuffs, which is

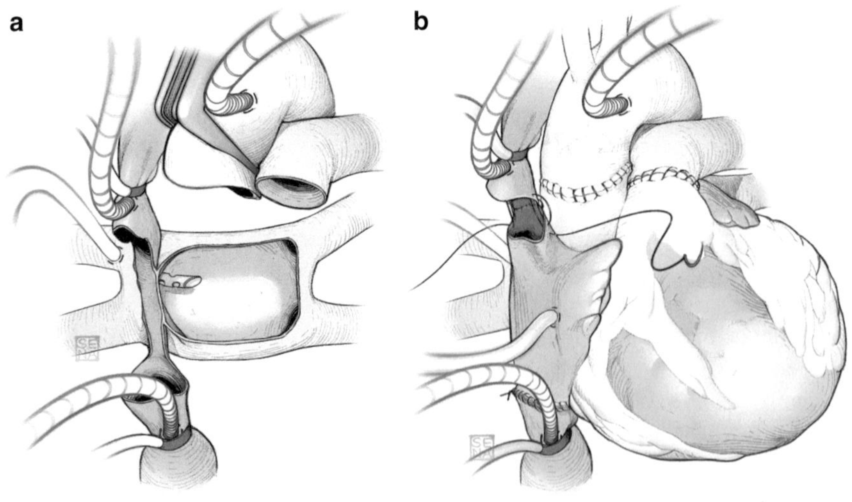

Fig. 11.2 Modified bicaval anastomosis technique. Recipient heart preparation (**a**) and donor heart implantation (**b**)

the Achilles heel of the conventional bicaval technique. Furthermore, anastomotic twisting and stenosis are avoidable. While facilitating optimal donor heart orientation [7]. Hemodynamic studies have shown no pressure differences at the anastomotic sites, even in mismatched transplants [8]. Comparative analyses indicate that the modified technique reduces the risk of anastomotic stenosis [9].

11.5 Order of Donor Heart Suturing

The typical sequence for anastomosis is left atrium, IVC, pulmonary artery, aorta, and SVC. To reduce ischemic time, the left atrial and aortic anastomoses may be completed first, followed by the remaining steps with the heart beating [10]. Poor visualization and retention of the posterior wall of caval cuffs may be a concern of beating heart anastomosis. The modified bicaval technique is also advantageous for this situation.

11.6 Total Heart Transplantation (Fig. 11.3)

Yacoub [11] and Dreyfus [12] and their colleagues proposed another modification of the bicaval technique that involves the complete excision of the recipient's left atrium, leaving two separate left atrial cuffs: one on the right containing the right superior and inferior pulmonary veins, and one on the left containing the left superior and inferior pulmonary veins. Each cuff is individually anastomosed to the

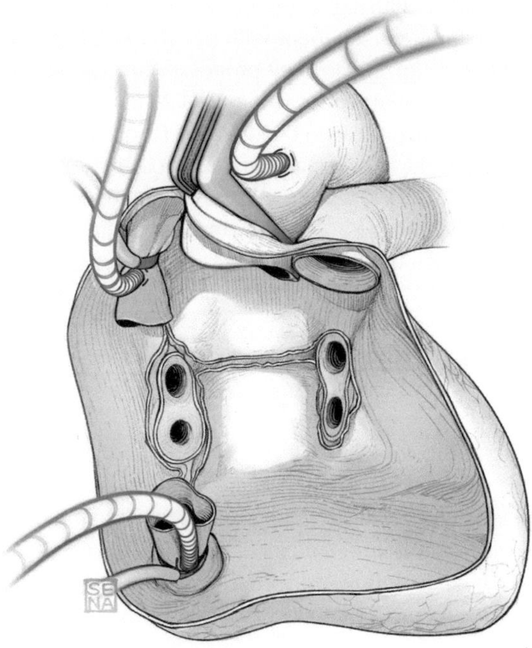

Fig. 11.3 Recipient heart preparation in total heart transplantation

donor's left atrium. This approach aims to preserve physiological geometry and reduce complications such as valve incompetence, rhythm disturbances, thrombus formation, and septal aneurysm.

However, several challenges have limited the adoption of this technique. These include prolonged ischemic time, potential for stenosis at the venous anastomoses, and difficulty in controlling posterior wall bleeding. Furthermore, advancements in lung transplantation often necessitate the donor's intact left atrium, complicating organ retrieval and limiting the feasibility of total heart transplantation. As no significant physiological or clinical advantages over the conventional bicaval approach have been demonstrated, this method remains infrequently utilized. A summary of the recipient's preparation for each transplant technique is shown in Fig. 11.3.

11.7 Special Consideration for Heart Transplantation in Patients with Congenital Heart Anomaly

Heart transplantation for congenital heart diseases (CHD) presents unique challenges, particularly in patients who have undergone previous repair or palliation. Visceral heterotaxy further adds to surgical complexity. Patients with systemic complications of Fontan physiology represent a vulnerable cohort, often suffering from protein-losing enteropathy and hepatic dysfunction.

11.7.1 Heterotaxy (Left Isomerism) and Dextrocardia

Matsuda and his colleagues reported a novel modification of the bicaval anastomosis technique in a patient with heterotaxy, absent inferior vena cava, and dextrocardia [13] (Fig. 11.4). They proposed three key technical points: the left mediastinal space was enlarged to accommodate the donor heart while preserving the phrenic nerve; the hepatic vein conduit was reconstructed using adjacent atrial wall and connected to the donor right atrium, crossing the midline without prosthetic material; and the left SVC was connected to the donor SVC via the donor's innominate vein, routed behind the ascending aorta to ensure an unobstructed pathway. These adjustments made transplantation feasible in this unique congenital anatomy.

11.7.2 Congenitally Corrected Transposition of Great Arteries (ccTGA) (Fig. 11.5)

One of the complete TGAs, ccTGA has been known to develop late systemic right ventricular failure when anatomical correction is not performed, and heart transplantation is indicated when medical and surgical treatment cannot extend the life [14]. In this cohort study of 558 ccTGA patients, age at first visit 36 ++- 14.2 years and median follow-up of 8.7 years, heart transplantation as the primary outcome was found in 12 patients (16%) and mechanical support in 11 patients (3 shifted to

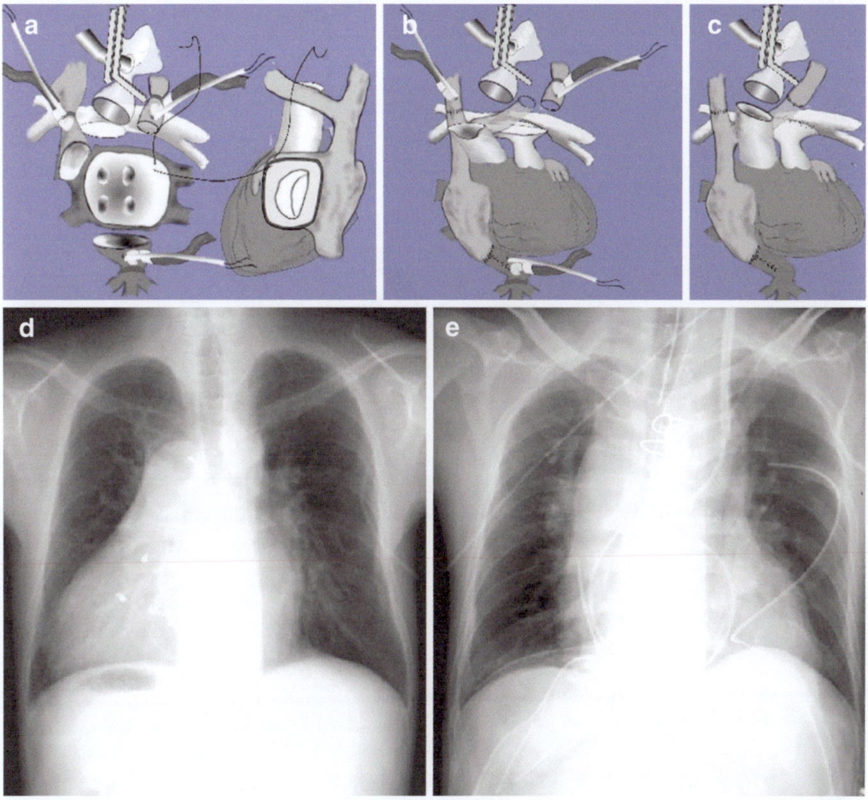

Fig. 11.4 Outline of the operative procedures of orthotopic heart transplantation in a case with heterotaxy, absent inferior vena cava and dextrocardia. (**a**) Schematic drawing of the gross appearance of the heart: dextrocardia, absent inferior vena cava, persistent left superior vena cava. (**b**, **c**): Transplantation was completed by three venous anastomoses, reconstruction of pulmonary artery trunk and ascending aorta. (**d**, **e**): Chest x-rays before and after transplantation. (Source; Ref. 13 with permission)

transplantation). Recently, the VAD application as the bridge to transplantation has been the important strategy to cope with progressive heart failure in ccTGA or post-atrial switch operation [15, 16]. In this group of patients, it requires a specific strategy to cope with repeated thoracotomy, arterial dislocation, and also other lesions such as dextrocardia and anomalous systemic and pulmonary venous abnormalities.

A case, a 45-year-old female with DORV (S,L,L), subpulmonary VSD, infundibular and valvular PS who was supported by VAD for systemic right ventricle as a bridge to transplantation, is presented. She underwent a functional repair with a conduit from left ventricle to pulmonary artery (Hancock Bioprosthetic Valved Conduit, size 18 mm) at the age of 6. Aortic and tricuspid valve replacements were performed at the age of 12 (Fig. 11.5a, b). At the age of 39, the patient developed exertional heart failure. Echocardiography showed systemic right ventricular

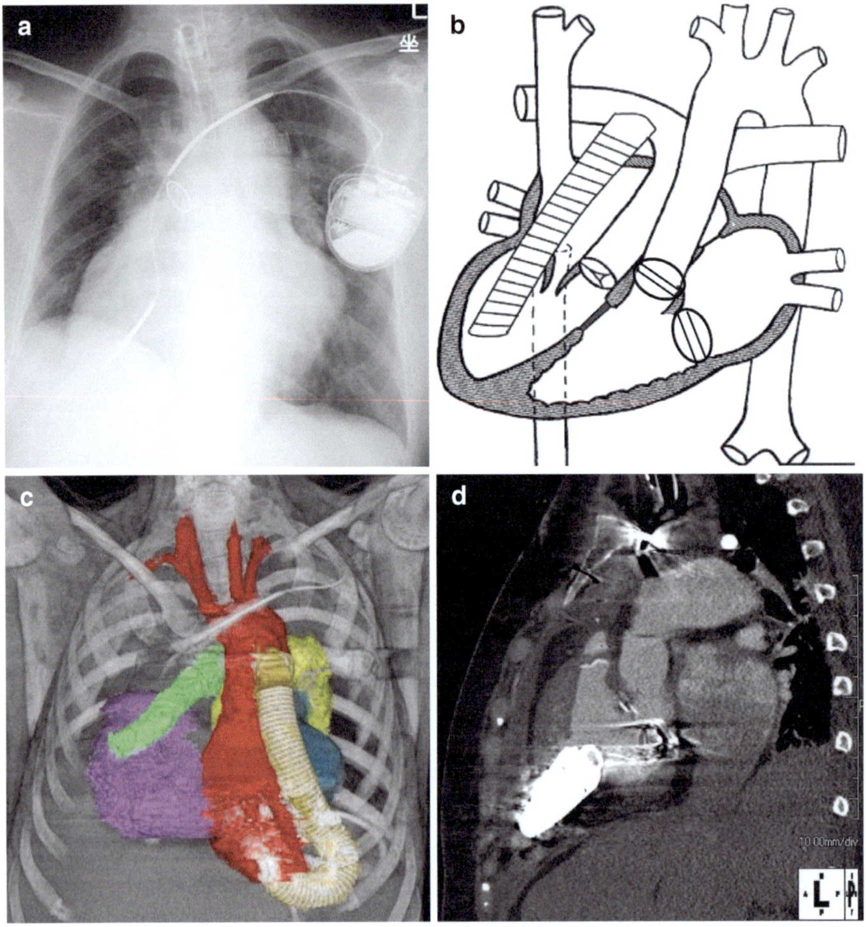

Fig. 11.5 Mechanical circulatory support to an adult patient with congenitally corrected transposition of the great arteries. (**a**, **b**) previously performed surgical intervention. (**c**, **d**) mechanical support with Jarvik 2000 ventricular assist device from anatomical right ventricle to ascending aorta. (Courtesy of Professor Hikaru Matsuda, MD, former Chairmen of the First Department of Surgery, Osaka University)

dysfunction and aortic prosthetic valve stenosis. Cardiac catheterization revealed low cardiac output with a cardiac index of 1.6 L/min/m^2 and diastolic dysfunction of systemic right ventricle with a PCWP of 18 mmHg. She was eventually listed for heart transplantation and underwent aortic valve re-replacement and VAD implantation at the age of 41. The device selected was Jarvik 2000 because of the characteristics of low profile, and the graft was placed on the left chest side and anastomosed to ascending aorta (Fig. 11.5c, d). She had been supported for 3.8 years, but could not reach the transplantation under the severe donor shortage and the allocation system remained as classical Status-1.

11.7.3 Failed Fontan Circulation

Fontan patients present specific anatomical and hemodynamic complexities requiring tailored surgical approaches. Pulmonary artery reconstruction is required in 50–85% of cases due to stenosis, prior stenting, or hypoplasia. Aortic arch reconstruction is often required after Norwood procedures [17]. Rerouting anomalous venous return is critical, ensuring proper blood flow alignment in the transplanted heart. Additional measures include reconstructing or closing systemic-to-pulmonary collateral vessels, ligating arteriovenous malformations, and managing liver dysfunction. Mechanical circulatory support, such as ventricular assist devices (VADs), may be employed for right-sided or bi-ventricular assistance, tailored to the patient's physiology [18, 19]. Cavopulmonary VADs can lower pulmonary vascular resistance and promote pulmonary artery growth, enhancing transplant eligibility. Such support can also help reverse end-organ dysfunction, particularly liver disease, reducing the need for combined organ transplants.

Facing the growing number of adult patients with congenital heart disease (ACHD) who develop progressive heart failure, the needs of HT has been increasing. In such a situation, the importance of preoperative planning, including a comprehensive evaluation of the patient's anatomical and hemodynamic status, as well as the status of end-organ function are critical determinants of postoperative success [20].

11.7.4 Partial Heart Transplantation (Fig. 11.6)

Partial heart transplantation (PHT) has emerged as a novel approach for cases with irreparable truncal valve dysfunction. In PHT, viable donor heart valve structures are transplanted into the recipient's heart, providing living, growing tissue that adapts as the child grows. This approach aims to reduce the need for reoperations associated with non-living valve implants that do not grow with the patient. A notable case involved a neonate with truncus arteriosus and severe truncal valve regurgitation, where PHT was successfully performed. The transplanted valves demonstrated adaptive growth and excellent hemodynamic function during follow-up, suggesting that PHT may offer a promising alternative for complex congenital defects involving the truncal valve [21–23].

PHT may also address donor organ shortages through techniques like domino and split-root procedures [24]. Ongoing research and clinical trials are essential to evaluate the long-term outcomes and broader applicability of PHT in managing CHD.

11.7.5 Persistent Left Superior Vena Cava

Persistent left superior vena cava (PLSVC) is a relatively common congenital vascular anomaly, with an incidence of 0.3–0.5% in the general population. Several case reports have documented orthotopic heart transplantation in patients with

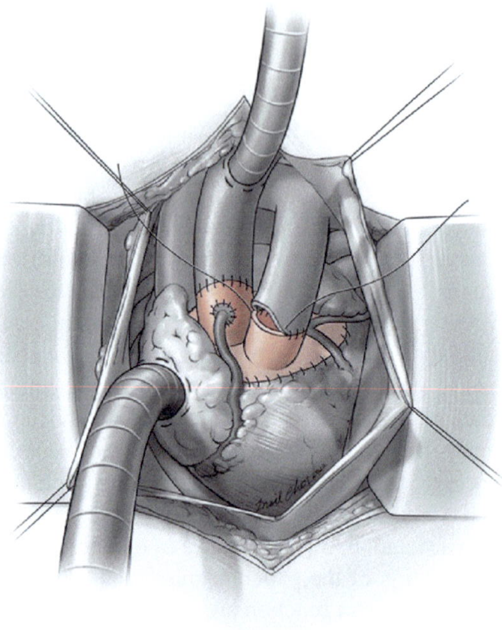

Fig. 11.6 Partial heart transplantation for truncus arteriosus. (Source: Ref. 22 with permission)

PLSVC. Although simple ligation can be performed in some cases, several techniques to reconstruct the PLSVC have been reported, including harvesting the donor heart with a long SVC, which is anastomosed to the PLSVC [25]; or modified recipient's cardiectomy with preservation of the coronary sinus, which is connected to the donor's right atrium [26].

11.8 Advanced Planning Using New Modalities

Three-dimensional (3D) printing and virtual reality (VR) have significantly advanced the planning and execution of surgical procedures for CHD. These technologies enable surgeons to meticulously plan procedures tailored to the patient's unique anatomy, thereby enhancing surgical precision, improving patient outcomes, and facilitating medical education. Fujita et al. reported the efficacy of a 3D replica in the first heart transplantation performed on a patient with corrected transposition of the great arteries in Japan [27] (Fig. 11.7).

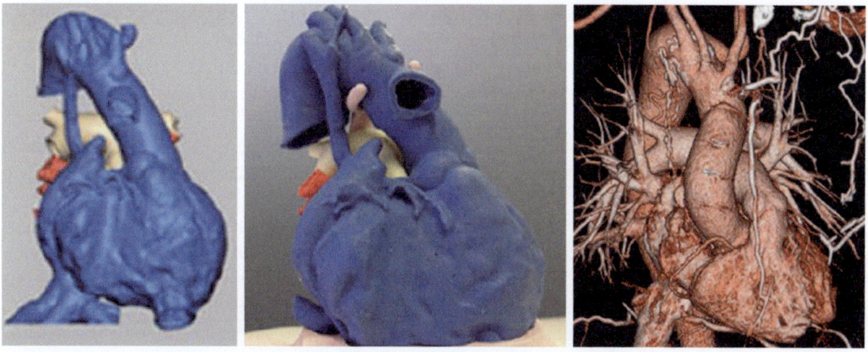

Fig. 11.7 Three-dimensional replica in heart transplantation for congenitally corrected transposition of the great arteries. (Source: Ref. 27 with permission)

11.9 Summary

Advances in heart transplantation techniques have improved surgical outcomes by addressing associated complications. Continued efforts to refine the surgical techniques should be mandated for complex congenital heart disease, bridged patients with long-term implantable assist devices, and donor hearts preserved by mechanical perfusion, and less invasive techniques may also be explored. For further progress in orthotopic heart transplantation, innovative surgical technique combined with advanced heart preservation strategy seems important in the near future.

Advances in heart transplantation techniques have improved surgical outcomes by addressing associated complications. Continued advances in surgical techniques should be mandated for complex congenital heart disease, bridged patients with long-term implantable assist devices, and donor hearts preserved by mechanical perfusion. Less invasive techniques may also be explored. For further progress in orthotopic heart transplantation, innovative surgical technique combined with advanced heart preservation strategy seems to be developed.

References

1. Lower RR, Shumway N. Studies on the orthotopic homotransplantation of the canine heart. Surg Forum. 1960;11:18–9.
2. Fernandez-Gonzales AL, Llorens R, Herreros JM, et al. Intracardiac thrombi after orthotopic heart transplantation: clinical significance and etiologic factors. J Heart Lung Transplant. 1994;13:236–40.
3. Weiss ES, Nwakanma LU, Russell SB, et al. Outcomes in bicaval versus biatrial techniques in heart transplantation: an analysis of the UNOS database. J Heart Lung Transplant. 2008;27:178–83.
4. Jacob S, Sellke F. Is bicaval orthotopic heart transplantation superior to the biatrial technique? Interact Cardiovasc Thorac Surg. 2009;9:333–42.
5. Aklog L, Sepic J, Filsoufi F, et al. Open inferior vena caval anastomosis during bicaval heart transplantation. Ann Thorac Surg. 2002;73:671–2.

6. Kitamura S, Nakatani T, Bando K, et al. Modification of bicaval anastomosis technique for orthotopic heart transplantation. Ann Thorac Surg. 2001;72:1405–6.
7. Kakuta T, Fukushima S, Shimahara Y, et al. Benefits of the modified bicaval anastomosis technique for orthotopic heart transplantation from a size mismatched marginal donor. Circ J. 2019;84:61–8.
8. Kitamura S, Nakatani T, Kato T, et al. Hemodynamic and echocardiographic evaluation of orthotopic heart transplantation with the modified bicaval anastomosis technique. Circ J. 2009;73:1235–9.
9. Kim HR, Jung SH, Kim JJ, et al. Modified bicaval technique in orthotopic heart transplantation – comparison with conventional bicaval technique. Circ J. 2018;83:117–21.
10. Shudo Y, Wang H, Woo YJ. A modified technique for orthotopic heart transplantation to minimize warm ischaemic time. Eur J Cardiothorac Surg. 2018;53:1089–90.
11. Yacoub M, Mankad P, Ledingham S. Donor procurement and surgical techniques for cardiac transplantation. Semin Thorac Cardiovasc Surg. 1990;2:153–61.
12. Dreyfus G, Jebara V, Mihaileanu S, et al. Total orthotopic heart transplantation: an alternative to the standard technique. Ann Thorac Surg. 1991;52:1181–4.
13. Matsuda H, Fukushima N, Ichikawa H, et al. Orthotopic heart transplantation for adult congenital heart disease: a case with heterotaxy and dextrocardia. Gen Thorac Cardiovasc Surg. 2017;65:47–51.
14. van Dissel AC, Opotowsky AR, Burchill LJ, et al. End-stage heart failure in congenitally corrected transposition of the great arteries: a multicentre study. Eur Heart J. 2023;44:3278–91.
15. Michel E, Hernadez EO, Enter D, et al. Bridge to transplantation with long-term mechanical assist devices in adults with transposition of the great arteries. Artif Organ. 2019;43:90–6.
16. Gyoten T, Rojas S, Fox H, et al. Mechanical circulatory support as a bridge to candidacy in adults with transposition of the great arteries and systemic right ventricle. Eur J Cardiothorac Surg. 2020:ezaa373. https://doi.org/10.1093/ejcts/ezaa373. Accessed Jan 15 2025.
17. Konstantinov IE, Schulz A, Buratto E. Heart transplantation after Fontan operation. JTCVS Tech. 2022;13:182–91.
18. Hasegawa M, Tominaga Y, Watanabe T, et al. Successful bridge to transplantation with long-term support using Berlin heart EXCOR in a child with failing Fontan. Gen Thorac Cardiovasc Surg. 2022;70:750–3.
19. Tanimoto K, Kido T, Taira M, et al. A case of truncus arteriosus with severe heart failure and pulmonary stenosis: bridge to transplant candidacy with surgical correction and a ventricular-assist device. J Artif Organs 2024. https://doi.org/10.1007/s10047-024-01456-w. Accessed Jan 15 2025.
20. Matsuda H, Ichikawa H, Ueno T, et al. Heart transplantation for adults with congenital heart disease: current status and future prospects. Gen Thorac Cardiovasc Surg. 2017;65:309–20.
21. Turek JW, Kan L, Overbey DM, et al. Partial heart transplant in a neonate with irreparable truncal valve dysfunction. JAMA. 2024;331:60–4.
22. Rajab TK, Kang L, Hayden K, et al. New operations for truncus arteriosus repair using partial heart transplantation: exploring the surgical design space with 3-dimensional printed heart models. J Thorac Cardiovasc Surg Tech. 2023;18:91–6.
23. Rajab TK, Vogel AD, Alexander VS, et al. The future of partial heart transplantation. J Heart Lung Transplant. 2024;43:863–5.
24. Aykut B, Overbey DM, Medina CK, et al. Partial heart transplantation promotes organ stewardship: domino hearts and split roots. Ann Thorac Surg Short Rep. 2024. https://doi.org/10.1016/j.atssr.2024.07.033.
25. Weymann A, Schmack B, Karck M, et al. Orthotopic heart transplantation in a patient with persistent left superior vena cava. Ann Thorac Cardiovasc Surg. 2012;18:554–6.
26. Rábago G, Martín-Trenor A, López-Coronado JL, et al. Bicaval anastomosis in a heart transplant recipient with left superior vena cava. Ann Thorac Surg. 2002;74:1242–4.
27. Fujita T, Fukushima S, Shiraishi I, et al. Three-dimensional replica of corrected transposition of the great arteries for successful heart transplantation. J Artif Organs. 2017;20:289–91.

Part V

Medical Management of Heart Failure, Update

Therapeutic Strategies for Advanced Heart Failure Related to Heart Transplantation

12

Yasushi Sakata, Fusako Sera, and Yasuhiro Akazawa

Abstract

Currently, there is a worldwide pandemic of heart failure, and its medical management has been targeted in the current era to prevent the progression of the disease and to reduce the number of deaths from advanced heart failure. As the other aspect, the application of ventricular assist devices as a bridge to transplantation or destination therapy has been well accepted, and the paradigm of end-stage heart failure management has been changed.

In this report, we have reviewed the new developments in the treatment of advanced heart failure divided into conventional treatment and how to respond to the issues raised by the advances in diagnostic modalities. Among the newly developed evaluation methods for advanced heart failure, biomarkers such as genetic information, electrocardiogram information (complete left bundle branch block), global longitudinal strain (GLS) on echocardiography, delayed myocardial contrast enhancement on MRI, and BNP are attracting attention. TcMIBI myocardial scintigraphy has been also introduced as the new modality.

Keywords

Advanced heart failure · Medical management · Ventricular assist device · Perfusion SPECT imaging · TcMIBI myocardial scintigraphy · Wellbeing-based heart failure therapy · QALY

Y. Sakata (✉) · F. Sera · Y. Akazawa
Department of Cardiovascular Medicine, The University of Osaka Graduate School of Medicine, Suita, Osaka, Japan
e-mail: sakata.yasushi.med@osaka-u.ac.jp; sera.fusako.med@osaka-u.ac.jp; akazawa.yasuhiro.med@osaka-u.ac.jp

H. Matsuda et al. (eds.), *Heart and Lung Transplantation*,
https://doi.org/10.1007/978-981-96-8810-4_12

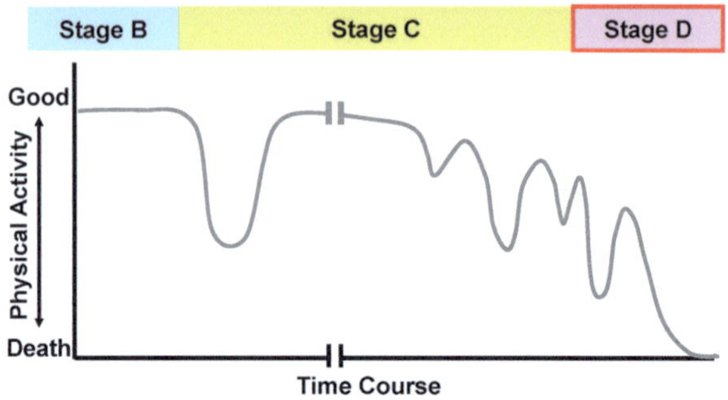

Fig. 12.1 Stages in the development and progression of heart failure

12.1 Introduction

What is advanced heart failure? Heart failure is defined as "a clinical syndrome consisting of dyspnea, malaise, swelling and/or decreased exercise capacity due to the loss of compensation for cardiac pumping function due to structural and/or functional abnormalities of the heart" [1]. Advanced heart failure is expressed as Stage D in the heart failure stage classification (Fig. 12.1). Stage D is defined as "refractory heart failure who have had New York Heart Association (NYHA) Class III or IV heart failure despite all available drug therapy or nonpharmacologic therapy with proven efficacy, and are hospitalized for heart failure at least twice a year" [1]. In other words, the diagnosis of advanced heart failure requires two conditions: frequent hospitalization and treatment resistance. Patients who meet this definition are presenting with end-stage heart failure regardless of their age.

Advanced heart failure has a poor prognosis. The REMATCH trial was a study of 129 patients with advanced heart failure (NYHA functional class IV) who were not eligible for heart transplantation due to their age or other reasons. In this trial, the one-year survival rate for the medical treatment group was 25% [2]. We should provide treatment for patients with a poor prognosis that considers the remainder of their lives.

12.2 New Developments in the Treatment of Advanced Heart Failure

1. Conventional Treatment for Advanced Heart Failure

For patients with stage D heart failure who do not improve from symptoms of NYHA class III or higher even after standard treatment, heart transplantation is considered a treatment that improves prognosis. In the Japanese Circulation Society's guidelines for treating acute and chronic heart failure, it is recommended as Class IIa, Evidence Level C [1]. Although no comparative studies exist, the International Society for Heart and Lung Transplantation registry data shows excellent long-term results. However, heart transplants in Japan currently require a long waiting period. For patients who are eligible for a transplant, waiting in the hospital for an extended period while receiving continuous administration of inotropic drugs is a significant psychological burden. Therefore, it is recommended that patients stay at home with an implantable ventricular assist device (Bridge to transplantation: BTB) (Class IIa, Level of evidence C) [1].

2. Issues in the Treatment of Advanced Heart Failure and How to Respond to Them

There are at least two significant issues in the treatment of advanced heart failure in Japan, which is mainly based on heart transplantation and the use of an artificial heart during the waiting period for a heart transplant. The first is the shortage of heart transplant donors. The 2010 law revision allowed family members to consent to donation. Since then, the number of heart transplants in Japan has increased rapidly. In 2024, after the end of the COVID-19 pandemic, the number of heart transplants exceeded 100 cases. However, the waiting period for patients on the waiting list for heart transplants still exceeds 1500 days. To increase the number of heart transplants, the Japanese Circulation Society and the Japanese Society for Heart Transplantation have been working to raise awareness of heart transplant donors. The second issue is the aging of Japanese society. The number of heart failure patients in Japan is expected to exceed 1.3 million soon [3], and the leading cause of this is the aging of the population. However, it is stipulated that heart transplants are only indicated for patients under the age of 65. Therefore, many patients with advanced heart failure do not qualify for a heart transplant.

For patients who are not eligible for a heart transplant, palliative care should be the first consideration. The Japanese Circulation Society and the Japanese Society of Heart Failure announced the "Statement on Palliative Care in Cardiovascular Diseases" in 2021, proposing the significance of palliative care and the timing when necessary. This proposal states that palliative care should be provided regardless of whether death is inevitable or not. It states that organ failure in heart failure worsens gradually while repeating rapid deterioration and improvement and that palliative care is necessary from the beginning when heart failure symptoms appear.

Furthermore, for patients who are not eligible for transplantation due to their age or other reasons, permanent use of an artificial heart (destination therapy: DT) has been possible since May 2021. The event-free 2-year survival rate for DT patients using the HeartMate III, which is currently used worldwide, is reported to be 73.2% [4]. With the evolution of implantable ventricular assist devices, it is thought that the number of cases will also increase in Japan.

12.3 New Developments in the Evaluation of Advanced Heart Failure

1. What Is Needed in the Evaluation of Advanced Heart Failure?

New means and concepts for treating advanced heart failure require new evaluation methods. Heart failure is a condition that repeatedly goes into remission and worsens. Advanced heart failure worsens rapidly, but it is often unclear to what extent this worsening can be improved. Doctors need to share the patient's progress with the patient and family and understand the patient's outlook on life and the family's thoughts. In other words, doctors cannot provide appropriate treatment to patients and their families unless they are aware of the course of the disease. Conventional assessment of advanced heart failure has focused on functional assessment, such as hemodynamics, and exercise tolerance. In the future, the evaluation that is aware of the passage of time will be necessary to provide more appropriate palliative care, heart transplants, and DT.

2. Evaluation of Cardiac Function with an Awareness of the Passage of Time: Reverse Remodeling Viability

To be aware of the passage of time, doctors need to know whether the changes in the patient are reversible. Cardiologists must at least be able to predict improvements in cardiac function accurately.

The Universal Definition of Heart Failure, published in 2021, defines heart failure with an improved EF as a case in which the left ventricular ejection fraction, less than 40% before treatment, improves by 10% or more to become 40% or more [5]. It has been reported that patients with improved left ventricular ejection fraction have a better prognosis than those without improvement [6]. The degree of improvement in the left ventricular ejection fraction due to appropriate treatment is called reverse remodeling viability, and it is an essential indicator for predicting the course of the disease. Doctors are looking for a method of accurately and efficiently diagnosing reverse remodeling viability. Epidemiologically, it has been reported that women and patients with a short history of heart failure are more likely to show reverse remodeling [7]. We should increase the accuracy by combining several simple indicators.

Currently, biomarkers such as genetic information, electrocardiogram information (complete left bundle branch block), global longitudinal strain (GLS) on echocardiography, delayed myocardial contrast enhancement on MRI, and BNP are attracting attention [8]. We have been conducting research on reverse remodeling viability for some time. We examined the electrocardiographic characteristics of 125 patients with dilated cardiomyopathy who showed reverse remodeling after 12 months and found that it was possible to predict it based on QRS width, presence or absence of splitting, aVR wave height, and QRS axis, and we scored it [9]. In addition, in TcMIBI myocardial scintigraphy, it was shown that cases with a %uptake of less than 40%, which reflects the volume of the defect, are unlikely to show reverse remodeling (Fig. 12.2) [10]. In the future, gathering more cases and searching for predictive factors suited to each population will be necessary.

3. Assessment of Organ Function with an Awareness of the Passage of Time: Liver Stiffness Assessment

The time that has elapsed since the onset of heart failure (HF duration) is a valuable factor for predicting the prognosis of advanced heart failure [11]. However, in many

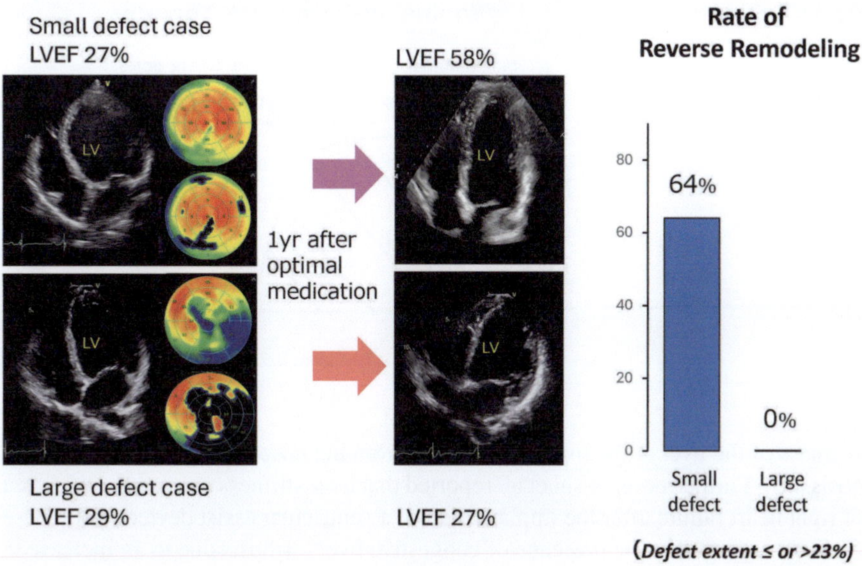

Fig. 12.2 Defect extent of perfusion SPECT imaging is associated with reverse remodeling viability. (Source: Ref. 10 with permission)

cases, the date of onset is unknown. Heart failure is associated with an increase in left atrial pressure, pulmonary hypertension, right atrial pressure, and central venous pressure, and if the duration of these pressure increases is long, the pressure "remains in the memory" of several organs. An increase in left atrial pressure contributes to left atrial enlargement. Since left atrial enlargement reflects the degree and duration of left atrial pressure increase, left atrial enlargement can predict the prognosis of heart failure independently of left ventricular function [12].

As with an increase in left atrial pressure, an increase in right atrial pressure or central venous pressure also indicates the severity of heart failure. Liver stiffness can be expected to reveal the "memory" of an increase in right atrial or central venous pressure. The stiffness of living tissue is related to the pathology of that tissue. A stiff liver indicates liver fibrosis and is a predictor of the progression of cirrhosis and the development of liver cancer. Traditionally, this has been assessed by palpation, but methods have been developed to image tissue stiffness more quantitatively using ultrasound and MRI (elastography) to make it more quantitative and objective. Among these, ultrasound elastography, which uses ultrasound, is widely used in clinical practice because it can evaluate tissue stiffness in real-time and easily. However, it has been revealed that the stiffness of the liver evaluated by elastography is not only determined by liver fibrosis but also by central venous pressure [13], and in heart failure patients without underlying liver disease such as hepatitis, central venous pressure (right atrial pressure) is thought to determine liver stiffness strongly.

In addition to the fact that right atrial pressure and liver stiffness as assessed by elastography correlate in heart failure patients [14], we have also found that the

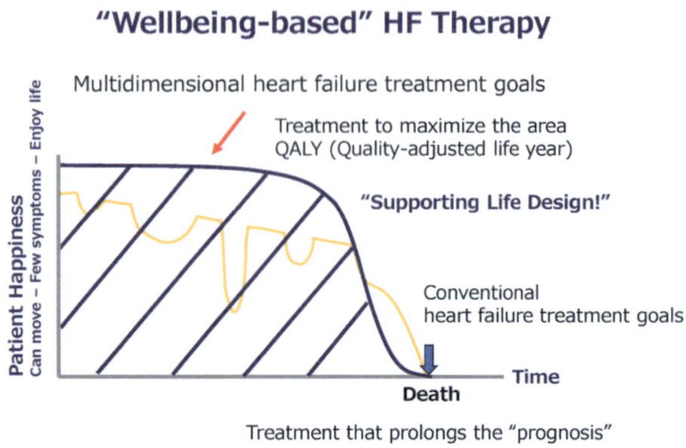

Fig. 12.3 Schematic figure about "Wellbeing-based heart failure therapy"

stiffness of the liver at the time of discharge from the hospital is predictive of prognosis [15]. Furthermore, Nishi et al. reported that liver stiffness can predict the onset of right heart failure after the implantation of a ventricular assist device [16]. These findings suggest that the presence of congestive liver cirrhosis due to an increase in right atrial pressure may predict the prognosis of heart failure, and similar reports have been obtained from Japan and other countries [17].

12.4 Creating New Outcomes

In the past, prognosis, particularly survival rate, has been considered a vital treatment indicator in cardiovascular medicine. In an aging society, it is thought that the outcomes sought by patients will also become more diverse. As shown in Fig. 12.3, in addition to the survival age on the horizontal axis, "happiness" is placed on the vertical axis, and treatment that maximizes the area is sought. This is the concept of QALY (quality-adjusted life years), which is conventionally used in cost-effectiveness evaluations. Quality of life (QOL) has been quantified using cross-sectional questionnaires. Still, with the advent of the Internet of Things (IoT), we have entered an era in which it can be evaluated more continuously and objectively. I think that treatments based on patients' various "feelings of happiness," such as patient-reported outcomes (PROs), will be provided using IoT.

References

1. Tsutsui H, Isobe M, Ito H, et al. JCS 2017/JHFS 2017 guideline on diagnosis and treatment of acute and chronic heart failure – digest version. Circ J. 2019;83(10):2084–184.
2. Rose EA, Gelijns AC, Moskowitz AJ, et al. Long-term use of a left ventricular assist device for end-stage heart failure. N Engl J Med. 2001;345(20):1435–43.
3. Okura Y, Ramadan MM, Ohno Y, et al. Impending epidemic: future projection of heart failure in Japan to the year 2055. Circ J. 2008;72(3):489–91.

4. Goldstein DJ, Naka Y, Horstmanshof D, et al. Association of clinical outcomes with left ventricular assist device use by bridge to transplant or destination therapy intent: the Multicenter Study of MagLev Technology in Patients Undergoing Mechanical Circulatory Support Therapy with HeartMate3 (MOMENTUM3) randomized clinical trial. JAMA Cardiol. 2020;5(4):411–9.
5. Bozkurt B, Coats AJ, Tsutsui H, et al. Universal definition and classification of heart failure: a report of the Heart Failure Society of America, Heart Failure Association of the European Society of Cardiology, Japanese Heart Failure Society and Writing Committee of the Universal Definition of Heart Failure. J Card Fail. 2021;23(3):352–80.
6. Abe S, Yoshihisa A, Ichijo Y, et al. Recovered left ventricular ejection fraction and its prognostic impacts in hospitalized heart failure patients with reduced ejection fraction. Int Heart J. 2020;61(2):281–8.
7. Aimo A, Gaggin HK, Barison A, et al. Imaging, biomarker, and clinical predictors of cardiac remodeling in heart failure with reduced ejection fraction. JACC Heart Fail. 2019;7(9):782–94.
8. Wilcox JE, Fang JC, Margulies KB, et al. Heart failure with recovered left ventricular ejection fraction: JACC Scientific Expert Panel. J Am Coll Cardiol. 2020;76(6):719–34.
9. Konishi S, Ohtani T, Mizuno H, et al. Simple electrocardiographic score can predict left ventricular reverse remodeling in patients with non-ischemic cardiomyopathy. Circ Rep. 2019;1(4):171–8.
10. Chimura M, Ohtani T, Sera F, et al. Focal severe decrease in myocardial technetium-99 m sestamibi uptake indicates ventricular irreversibility in patients with dilated cardiomyopathy. Ann Nucl Med. 2021;35(8):881–8.
11. Lupon J, Gaggin HK, de Antonio M, et al. Biomarker-assist score for reverse remodeling prediction in heart failure: the ST2-R2 score. Int J Cardiol. 2015;184:337–43.
12. Rossi A, Temporelli PL, Quintana M, et al. Independent relationship of left atrial size and mortality in patients with heart failure: an individual patient meta-analysis of longitudinal data (MeRGE heart failure). Eur J Heart Fail. 2009;11(10):929–36.
13. Millonig G, Friedrich S, Adolf S, et al. Liver stiffness is directly influenced by central venous pressure. J Hepatol. 2010;52(2):206–10.
14. Taniguchi T, Sakata Y, Ohtani T, et al. Usefulness of transient elastography for noninvasive and reliable estimation of right-sided filling pressure in heart failure. Am J Cardiol. 2014;113(3):552–8.
15. Taniguchi T, Ohtani T, Kioka H, et al. Liver stiffness reflecting right-sided filling pressure can predict adverse outcomes in patients with heart failure. JACC Cardiovasc Imaging. 2019;12(6):955–64.
16. Nishi H, Toda K, Miyagawa S, et al. Novel method of evaluating liver stiffness using transient elastography to evaluate perioperative status in severe heart failure. Circ J. 2015;79(2):391–7.
17. Wang Q, Song Y, Wu Q, et al. Liver stiffness for predicting adverse cardiac events in Chinese patients with heart failure: a two-year prospective study. BMC Cardiovasc Disord. 2022:51. https://bmccardiovascdisord.biomedcentral.com/articles/10.1186/s12872-022-02497-w. Accessed 15 Feb 2025.

Medical and Surgical Management of Adult Congenital Heart Disease

13

Fusako Sera and Yasushi Sakata

Abstract

The growing population of adults with congenital heart disease (ACHD) highlights the urgent need for specialized care. Most congenital heart surgeries are palliative rather than curative, resulting in residual lesions, complications such as heart failure and arrhythmias, and non-cardiac issues requiring lifelong management. Unique pathophysiological features, such as systemic right ventricle and Fontan circulation, differentiate ACHD from acquired cardiovascular diseases, posing challenges in applying existing evidence-based treatments. Heart failure is a leading cause of mortality in ACHD, necessitating tailored management strategies, including emerging pharmacological treatments like ARNI and SGLT-2 inhibitors, as well as non-pharmacological options like cardiac resynchronization therapy and heart transplantation. Arrhythmias, including atrial tachycardia and ventricular arrhythmias, are major causes of morbidity and mortality, emphasizing the importance of timely evaluation and intervention, such as catheter ablation. Surgical management demands precise risk assessment and a multidisciplinary team approach. End-of-life care is particularly complex, as ACHD patients often struggle with disease awareness and decision-making due to lifelong medical dependence. Collaboration among specialists, including cardiologists, pediatricians, and palliative care providers, is essential to address these challenges.

F. Sera (✉) · Y. Sakata
Department of Cardiovascular Medicine, The University of Osaka Graduate School of Medicine, Suita, Osaka, Japan
e-mail: sera.fusako.med@osaka-u.ac.jp; sakata.yasushi.med@osaka-u.ac.jp

H. Matsuda et al. (eds.), *Heart and Lung Transplantation*,
https://doi.org/10.1007/978-981-96-8810-4_13

Keywords

Adult congenital heart disease (ACHD) · Heart failure · Arrhythmia · Fontan circulation · Systemic right ventricle · Palliative surgery · Multidisciplinary team · Transition of care · End-of -life care · Heart transplantation

13.1 Introduction

More than 90% of individuals born with congenital heart disease (CHD) now reach adulthood, and the number of patients with adult congenital heart disease (ACHD) is continuing to increase [1]. Most surgeries for CHD are palliative rather than curative, leading to various postoperative residual lesions and complications. Over time, complications such as heart failure and arrhythmia often emerge later in life, and in many cases, medical treatment and repeated surgery are required. In addition, there are often psychosocial problems and non-cardiac complications of other organs, requiring lifelong medical care and follow-up.

13.2 Current Status and Challenges in ACHD

In Canada, as of 2010, the number of adult patients with congenital heart disease greatly exceeded the number of pediatric patients, accounting for two-thirds of the total, and it has been reported that the number of adult patients with complex CHD also exceeds the number of pediatric patients [2] (Fig. 13.1).

A similar trend has also been observed in Japan [3]. In Japan, the Japanese Network of Cardiovascular Department for Adult Congenital Heart Disease (JNCVD-ACHD) was founded in 2011, and the disease profiles of 24,048 patients were collected from 50 facilities in Japan where cardiologists provide ACHD medical care [4]. The average age of patients with ACHD was 37.6 ± 17.1 years, and the most common underlying heart diseases were atrial septal defect (20.5%), ventricular septal defect (20.5%), tetralogy of Fallot (12.9%), and single ventricle (6.6%). Patients with ACHD who had not undergone biventricular repair accounted for 37.0%. Systemic right ventricle cases accounted for 2.8%, and Fontan circulation cases accounted for 6.0%, indicating that the transition from pediatric to adult cardiology departments is gradually taking place in Japan, even for moderate-to-severe CHD cases [4].

Patients with ACHD present with a complex and diverse pathophysiology, as underlying heart diseases vary widely, and coexisting diseases and repair surgeries differ from case to case. In addition, systemic right ventricle and Fontan circulation are specific to ACHD and are not seen in acquired cardiovascular diseases. It is challenging to directly apply existing evidence and practices from general cardiovascular diseases to ACHD patients. There is a growing need for adult cardiologists to become more actively involved in the management of ACHD. However, one of the primary obstacles is the lack of fully established effective treatments and guidelines for managing these patients.

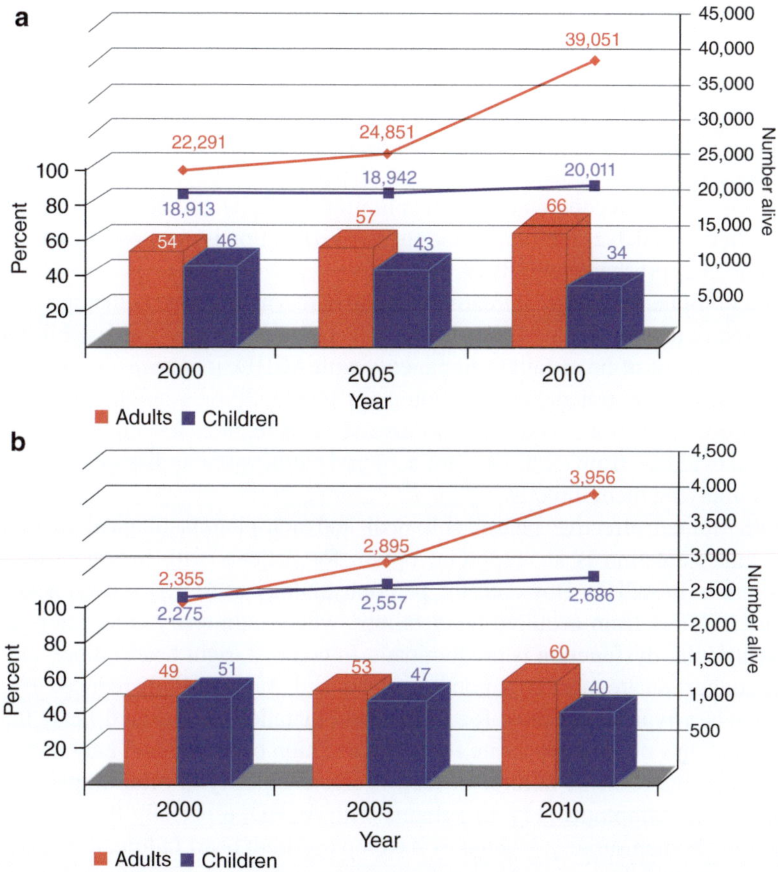

Fig. 13.1 The numbers and proportions of adults and children with congenital heart disease in Quebec, Canada. (**a**) All included. (**b**) Severe case. (Source: Ref. 2 with permission)

13.3 Medical Management of ACHD

1. *Heart Failure*

Heart failure is a major cause of death in ACHD, accounting for 20–30% of all deaths [5–7]. Patients with underlying heart diseases such as tetralogy of Fallot, post-Fontan surgery, and systemic right ventricle exhibit a high risk of heart failure, and the risk of developing heart failure increases with age [8]. Considering the increasing age of ACHD patients, the management of heart failure is expected to become increasingly important.

In clinical practice, treatment for heart failure in patients with ACHD, who have biventricular circulation and impaired systemic ventricular function, is carried out by applying the general guidelines for acquired heart failure. However, although the efficacy of beta-blockers and renin-angiotensin-aldosterone system inhibitors in improving the prognosis of acquired heart failure has been established, and they form the core of GDMT for heart failure, the efficacy of these heart failure treatments in ACHD has not been established. In recent years, several promising results have been reported in small-scale studies of patients with systemic right ventricle using angiotensin receptor neprilysin inhibitors (ARNI) and sodium-glucose co-transporter 2 (SGLT-2) inhibitors, and further verification is awaited in studies such as multicenter prospective trials [9, 10].

As a non-pharmacological treatment, cardiac resynchronization therapy has also been tried in patients with ACHD, but its effectiveness has not been established. In the management of heart failure in patients with ACHD, it is necessary to develop tailored treatment strategies that account for the condition's unique complexities and its differences from acquired heart disease. This requires leveraging the experience and evidence from treatments for acquired cardiovascular diseases, rather than simply applying them directly.

With limited effective pharmacological and non-pharmacological treatments, heart transplantation is an important option for patients with treatment-resistant heart failure in ACHD. However, the pathophysiology of ACHD-related heart failure often differs from acquired heart failure, where pulmonary congestion due to left ventricular dysfunction is predominant. In contrast, right heart failure and systemic congestion are more common in patients with ACHD. While reduced exercise capacity is a typical indicator for heart transplantation in acquired heart failure, ACHD patients often compensate for their condition over time and may not recognize symptoms of heart failure. In fact, exercise capacity is often impaired even without overt symptoms [11]. In patients with ACHD, especially those who have undergone Fontan surgery, when they develop apparent heart failure, they may also have concomitant hepatic and renal dysfunction due to systemic congestion, which may exclude them from being eligible for heart transplantation.

Determining the timing for assessing the necessity of heart transplantation and evaluating eligibility is critical for patients with ACHD. Unlike acquired heart failure, where indications are often more straightforward, decisions for those with ACHD require careful consideration of their unique pathophysiology and lifelong disease course. Many individuals with ACHD may not fully understand their condition or recognize the severity of their symptoms, which can delay timely evaluations and decision-making. Additionally, managing the long waiting period for transplantation despite their complex condition is one of the major challenges in heart transplantation for this population. Addressing these challenges is essential to ensure they are properly assessed and considered for transplantation at the appropriate time.

2. *Arrhythmia and Sudden Death*

Arrhythmia is an important factor associated with hospitalization and death in patients with ACHD, with sudden cardiac death accounting for 7–23% of deaths in these patients [5, 7]. Implantable cardioverter-defibrillators are considered a means of preventing sudden death, although primary prevention with ICDs has not been established for single ventricle or systemic right ventricle cases.

Atrial tachycardia is frequently observed as a type of tachyarrhythmia. Antiarrhythmic drugs often have negative inotropic and conduction effects. Therefore, the latest ESC guidelines recommend catheter ablation as the first-line treatment for treatable local substrates, prioritizing it over long-term drug therapy [12]. The development of arrhythmia is often linked to hemodynamic deterioration caused by residual or secondary complications. Therefore, timely medical evaluation and surgical intervention are crucial, rather than solely focusing on arrhythmia management.

13.4 Surgical Management of ACHD

Patient-specific factors play a major role in determining the risks associated with cardiac surgery in patients with ACHD. The conventional risk scores used for acquired heart disease are insufficient for this population, and the utility of risk scores tailored specifically for ACHD patients has been demonstrated [13]. The timing of surgical intervention is another critical aspect, requiring precise assessment of anatomical and hemodynamic changes.

In recent years, percutaneous catheter-based treatments have gained widespread adoption as alternatives to conventional open-heart surgery. Determining the appropriate indications and ensuring their effective implementation require a multidisciplinary team that includes specialists in cardiothoracic surgery, adult cardiology, and pediatrics.

13.5 End-of-Life Care

Patients with ACHD often undergo multiple surgeries from childhood to adulthood and live with residual disease and complications. Unlike patients with acquired heart disease, who can relate the severity and progression of their condition to their pre-disease health and lifestyle, ACHD patients often perceive living with heart disease as a normal part of their daily life. As a result, they may struggle to recognize the severity or progression of their condition and to consider end-of-life planning.

In childhood, decision-making is typically managed by parents, and even in adulthood, some ACHD patients may feel unprepared to make independent decisions about their care. Therefore, explaining the patient's condition and supporting decision-making toward the end of life should be done carefully, considering their general and psychological condition, and in collaboration with a palliative care team and clinical psychologists. Many existing support tools for advance care planning and decision-making in heart failure are designed for patients with acquired heart disease. These tools often require adaptation to meet the unique needs of patients with ACHD. A multidisciplinary approach is essential to support decision-making in this population, addressing their specific conditions and challenges (Table 13.1).

Table 13.1 Comparison of ACHD-related heart failure vs. acquired heart failure

Aspect	ACHD-related heart failure	Acquired heart failure
Predominant pathophysiology	Right heart failure and systemic congestion are key features	Left ventricular dysfunction and pulmonary congestion are dominant
Symptom recognition	May not recognize symptoms due to lifelong adaptation; reduced exercise capacity can occur without noticeable symptoms	Symptoms such as reduced exercise capacity, fatigue, and dyspnea are more clearly linked to disease progression
Treatment guidelines	Limited evidence for standard treatments, requiring a tailored approach	Guideline-directed medical therapy (GDMT) is well-established and proven effective
Heart transplantation challenges	Systemic congestion, organ dysfunction, and unique pathophysiology complicate timing and eligibility assessment	Clearer indications for transplantation, with eligibility based on exercise capacity and straightforward metrics
Patient perception	Perceive heart disease as a normal part of life, making it difficult to recognize severity or plan for advanced care.	Can compare current health with pre-disease levels, aiding recognition of severity and end-of-life planning

13.6 Conclusion

The growing population of ACHD patients highlights the critical need for seamless care transitions, facilitated by effective collaboration between pediatricians and adult cardiologists. These patients require comprehensive lifelong support to manage complications such as heart failure and arrhythmia, pregnancy-related risks, and end-of-life care. To provide timely and appropriate medical care, a multidisciplinary support team involving specialists from various fields and professions is essential. Furthermore, accumulating robust data and establishing evidence-based approaches are crucial for improving treatment outcomes for the diverse and complex conditions associated with ACHD.

References

1. Gilboa SM, Devine OJ, Kucik JE, et al. Congenital heart defects in the United States: estimating the magnitude of the affected population in 2010. Circulation. 2016;134(2):101–9.
2. Marelli AJ, Ionescu-Ittu R, Mackie AS, et al. Lifetime prevalence of congenital heart disease in the general population from 2000 to 2010. Circulation. 2014;130(9):749–56.
3. Shiina Y, Toyoda T, Kawasoe Y, et al. Prevalence of adult patients with congenital heart disease in Japan. Int J Cardiol. 2011;146(1):13–6.
4. Yao A, Inuzuka R, Mizuno A, et al. Status of adult outpatients with congenital heart disease in Japan: The Japanese Network of Cardiovascular Departments for Adult Congenital Heart Disease Registry. J Cardiol. 2022;80(6):525–31.
5. Engelings CC, Helm PC, Abdul-Khaliq H, et al. Cause of death in adults with congenital heart disease – an analysis of the German National Register for Congenital Heart Defects. Int J Cardiol. 2016;211:31–6.

6. Yu C, Moore BM, Kotchetkova I, et al. Causes of death in a contemporary adult congenital heart disease cohort. Heart. 2018;104(20):1678–82.
7. Diller GP, Kempny A, Alonso-Gonzalez R, et al. Survival prospects and circumstances of death in contemporary adult congenital heart disease patients under follow-up at a large tertiary centre. Circulation. 2015;132(22):2118–25.
8. Norozi K, Wessel A, Alpers V, et al. Incidence and risk distribution of heart failure in adolescents and adults with congenital heart disease after cardiac surgery. Am J Cardiol. 2006;97(8):1238–43.
9. Zandstra TE, Nederend M, Jongbloed MRM, et al. Sacubitril/valsartan in the treatment of systemic right ventricular failure. Heart. 2021;107(21):1725–30.
10. Neijenhuis RML, Nederend M, Jongbloed MRM, et al. The potential of sodium-glucose cotransporter 2 inhibitors for the treatment of systemic right ventricular failure in adults with congenital heart disease. Front Cardiovasc Med. 2023;26(10):1093201.
11. Diller GP, Dimopoulos K, Okonko D, et al. Exercise intolerance in adult congenital heart disease: comparative severity, correlates, and prognostic implication. Circulation. 2005;112(6):828–35.
12. Baumgartner H, De Backer J, Babu-Narayan SV, et al. 2020 ESC guidelines for the management of adult congenital heart disease. Eur Heart J. 2021;42(6):563–645.
13. Hörer J, Roussin R, LeBret E, et al. Validation of the grown-ups with congenital heart disease score. Heart. 2018;104(12):1019–25.

Social Reintegration in Survivors of Pediatric Heart Transplantation

14

Hidekazu Ishida, Kaori Kubota, Ryo Ishii, Masaki Hirose, Fusako Sera, and Jun Narita

Abstract

Advancements in medical management have improved the survival rate of pediatric heart transplant recipients. However, social reintegration among these patients remains unclear. This retrospective study examined 61 patients who underwent heart transplantation under 18 years of age between 2000 and 2019. The cohort consisted of 29 males and 32 females, with a median age at transplantation of 7 years (interquartile range [IQR], 2–13). The median follow-up duration was 10 years (IQR, 7–15.5). 5-year, 10-year, and 15-year survival rates were 91%, 91%, and 83%, respectively. Excluding three patients who died before reaching school age, stable school attendance was achieved in 56 of 58 patients (97%). Among the 38 patients aged 18 years or older, 15 (39%) were employed, 13 (34%) were enrolled in higher education, and 10 (26%) were neither employed nor enrolled in education. Univariate analysis revealed that neurological disorders significantly hindered educational and occupational outcomes ($P = 0.002$).

H. Ishida (✉) · R. Ishii · M. Hirose · J. Narita
Department of Pediatrics, The University of Osaka Graduate School of Medicine, Suita, Osaka, Japan
e-mail: hideishi@ped.med.osaka-u.ac.jp; i-ryo@ped.med.osaka-u.ac.jp; mhirose@ped.med.osaka-u.ac.jp; junn21@ped.med.osaka-u.ac.jp

K. Kubota
Department of Transplant Medicine, The University of Osaka Hospital, Suita, Osaka, Japan
e-mail: k-kubota@hp-trpmed.med.osaka-u.ac.jp

F. Sera
Department of Cardiovascular Medicine, The University of Osaka Graduate School of Medicine, Suita, Osaka, Japan
e-mail: sera.fusako.med@osaka-u.ac.jp

H. Matsuda et al. (eds.), *Heart and Lung Transplantation*,
https://doi.org/10.1007/978-981-96-8810-4_14

While compulsory educational outcomes were favorable among pediatric heart transplant recipients, 26% of patients above age 18 were neither employed nor enrolled in education. Neurological complications emerged as a key risk factor for social outcomes.

Keywords

Heart transplantation · Pediatric · Social · Reintegration · Achievement · Outcome · Cardiomyopathy · Heart failure

14.1 Introduction

Heart transplantation is the definitive treatment for severe heart failure unresponsive to multidisciplinary medical therapies [1]. While advancements in pharmacological treatments for heart failure have been well-documented in adults, evidence for their efficacy in pediatric populations remains limited [2–4]. The primary etiologies of severe heart failure in children include cardiomyopathies such as dilated cardiomyopathy (DCM) and, increasingly, congenital heart diseases (CHD). Pediatric heart failure patients often experience reduced quality of life due to activity restrictions, strict fluid intake limitations, and recurrent hospitalizations, necessitating comprehensive psychological, physical, and social support [5, 6]. In Japan, the 2010 revision of the Organ Transplant Act, which legalized brain death in children, enabled the possibility of pediatric heart transplantation domestically. Despite this, the number of pediatric brain-dead donors remained low, surpassing five annual transplants in 2017. However, little is known about the social reintegration of pediatric heart transplant recipients in Japan, including their educational and occupational outcomes. Therefore, this study aimed to elucidate the current status of social reintegration among pediatric heart transplant recipients followed at Osaka University Hospital through a retrospective analysis.

14.2 Subjects and Methods

This retrospective observational study was conducted with approval from the Osaka University Clinical Research Review Committee (IRB No. 15211-8).

14.2.1 Study Population and Clinical Profiles

The study included pediatric patients who underwent heart transplantation before the age of 18 between 2000 and 2019, and were followed postoperatively at Osaka University Hospital. Data on patient characteristics, including sex, primary heart failure diagnosis, age at onset, age at analysis, age at transplantation, transplant location, ventricular assist device (VAD) usage, pre- and post-transplant complications, and educational/occupational status, were retrospectively extracted from the medical records at September 2024.

14.2.2 Statistical Analysis

Statistical analyses were conducted using JMP Pro 16. Risk factors for educational and occupational outcomes were assessed using univariate analysis, with a *P*-value of <0.05 considered statistically significant.

14.3 Results

14.3.1 Clinical Status of the Study Cohort

The cohort enrolled 61 pediatric heart transplant recipients, consisting of 29 males and 32 females (Table 14.1). The primary indications for transplantation were dilated cardiomyopathy (DCM) in 36 cases (59%), restrictive cardiomyopathy in 17 cases (28%), congenital heart disease in 2 cases (3%), and other etiologies in 6 cases (10%). The median age at heart failure onset was 1 year (interquartile range [IQR], 0–6). Pre-transplant VAD use was reported in 29 patients (48%), with 17 cases (28%) requiring extracorporeal devices (e.g., EXCOR) and 12 cases (20%) utilizing implantable VADs. The median age at transplantation was 7 years (IQR, 2–13), and the median follow-up period was 9 years (IQR, 7–15.5). Transplants were performed domestically in 26 cases (43%) and abroad in 35 cases (57%), including 33 in the United States and 2 in Germany. Ten deaths occurred during the observation period, with 5-, 10-, and 15-year survival rates of 91%, 91%, and 83%, respectively (Fig. 14.1).

Post-transplant complications included 14 cases (23%) of acute cellular rejection and antibody-mediated rejection requiring intensified immunosuppression, 13 cases (22%) of post-transplant lymphoproliferative disease (PTLD), 5 cases (8%) of chronic kidney disease, 5 cases (8%) of coronary artery vasculopathy (CAV), and 13 cases (22%) of opportunistic infections.

14.3.2 Social Reintegration

A flow chart of the analysis for social integration is shown in Fig. 14.2. Excluding three patients who died before reaching school age, stable enrollment in primary school, junior high school, or high school was achieved in 56 of 58 (97%) patients (Fig. 14.3a). Of the 38 patients who reached 18 years of age during the follow-up period, 15 (39%) were employed, 13 (34%) were pursuing higher education (university or vocational college), and 10 (26%) were neither employed nor enrolled in education (Fig. 14.3b).

Table 14.1 Clinical characteristics and outcomes of 61 patients enrolled for the study

	N = 61 (*n*, [%]; median, [IQR])
Male: Female	29 [48%]: 32 [52%]
Primary diagnosis	
DCM	36 [59%]
RCM	17 [28%]
CHD	2 [3%]
Others	6 [10%]
VAD implantation	
None	32 [52%]
Extracorporeal	17 [28%]
Implantable	12 [20%]
Age at diagnosis	1 years old [0–6]
Age at heart transplantation	7 years old [2–13]
Age at analysis	20 years old [12–22.5]
Years after transplantation	10 years [7–15.5]
Transplant location	
Domestic	26 [43%]
Abroad	35 [57%]
Outcome	
Alive	51 [84%]
Dead	10 [16%]
Post-transplant complications	
Rejection (ACR and/or AMR)	14 [23%]
PTLD	13 [22%]
Kidney dysfunction	5 [8%]
CAV	5 [8%]
Infection	13 [22%]

DCM dilated cardiomyopathy, *RCM* restrictive cardiomyopathy, *CHD* congenital heart disease, *VAD* ventricular assist device, *ACR* acute cellular rejection, *AMR* antibody mediated rejection, *PTLD* post-transplant lymphoproliferative disease, *CAV* coronary artery vasculopathy, *IQR* inter-quartile range

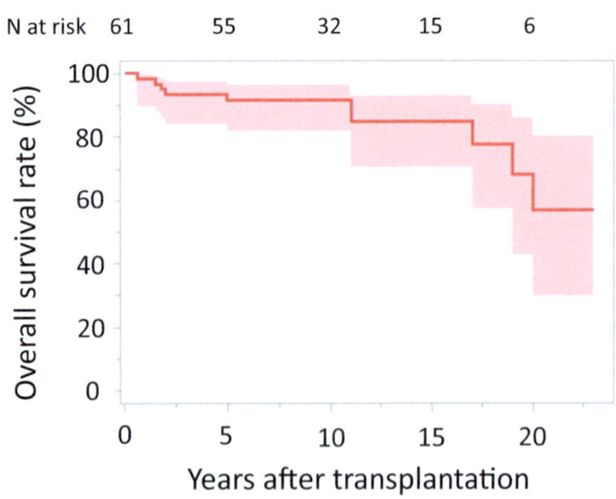

Fig. 14.1 Overall survival rate after heart transplantation in our cohort. The 5-, 10-, and 15-year survival rates of 91%, 91%, and 83%, respectively

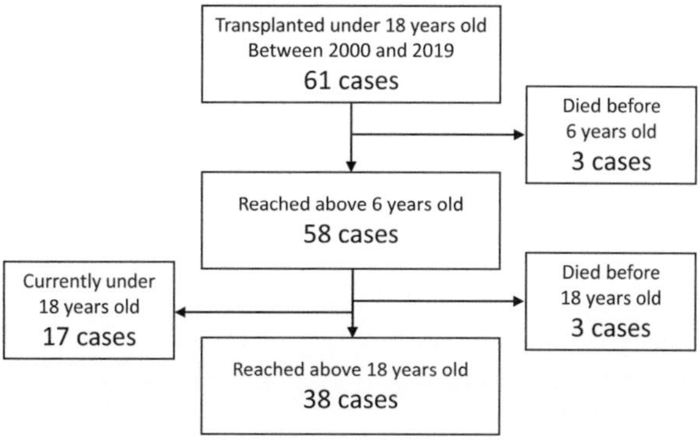

Fig. 14.2 Flow chart of the analysis for social reintegration after pediatric heart transplantation

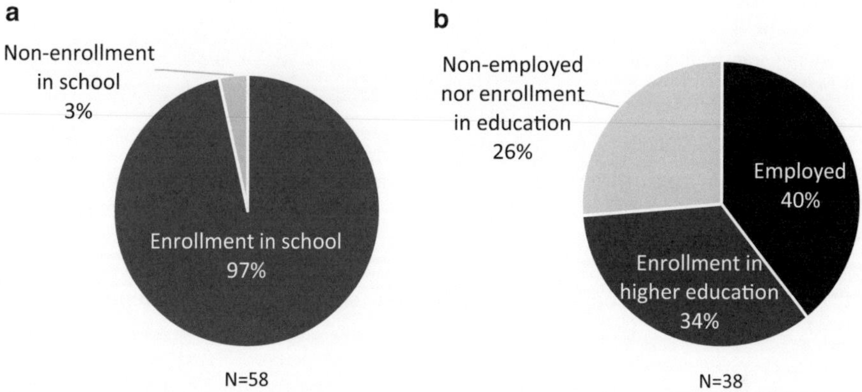

Fig. 14.3 The ratio of social reintegration in our cohort. (**a**) The ratio of stable enrollment in school during primary, junior-high, and high school ages. (**b**) The ratio of employed and enrollment in higher education at the age of 18 in survivors of pediatric heart transplant recipients

Among the 10 patients classified as neither employed nor in education, 7 exhibited neurological complications attributed to pre-transplant factors, such as cerebrovascular events related to mechanical circulatory support, autism spectrum disorder, or developmental delay. Post-transplant complications were identified in 8 patients, including allograft rejection (2 cases), PTLD (3 cases), kidney transplant (3 cases), CAV (1 case), and opportunistic infections (3 cases).

Univariate analysis identified pre-transplant neurological comorbidities, such as cerebrovascular events and developmental disorders, as significant risk factors for non-employment and non-enrollment in education at 18 years of age (14% vs. 70%; $P = 0.002$; Table 14.2). While not statistically significant, earlier age at heart failure onset showed a trend toward association with non-employment and non-enrollment in education at 18 years of age (median; 5 years old vs. 0 years old; $P = 0.093$). Additionally, a higher proportion of patients with post-transplant complications were found in the non-employment/non-enrollment in education group (80% vs.

Table 14.2 Univariate analysis of risk factors for social reintegration at 18 years old in post-pediatric heart transplant recipients

	Employment or enrollment in education (*N* = 28)	Non-employment or non-enrollment in education (*N* = 10)	*P*-value
Male (*n*, %)	13 (46%)	3 (30%)	0.469
Age at onset (y.o., IQR)	5 (1–9.5)	0 (0–6.5)	0.093
Age at transplantation (y.o., IQR)	12 (4.25–14)	10 (1–14.5)	0.605
VAD implantation (*n*, %)	12 (43%)	5 (50%)	0.893
Pre-transplant neurological complications (*n*, %)	4 (14%)	7 (70%)	0.002*
Any post-transplant complications (*n*, %)	13 (48%)	8 (80%)	0.137
ACR/AMR (*n*, %)	9 (33%)	2 (20%)	0.688
PTLD (*n*, %)	3 (11%)	2 (20%)	0.313
Kidney transplant/hemodialysis (*n*, %)	2 (7%)	3 (30%)	0.110
CAV (*n*, %)	3 (11%)	1 (10%)	1.00
Opportunistic infections (*n*, %)	1 (4%)	3 (30%)	0.052

**IQR* interquartile range, *VAD* ventricular assist device, *ACR* acute cellular rejection, *AMR* antibody-mediated rejection, *PTLD* post-transplant lymphoproliferative disease, *CAV* coronary artery vasculopathy

48%; $P = 0.137$), with opportunistic infections showing a notable trend (30% vs. 4%; $P = 0.052$).

14.4 Discussion

Pediatric heart transplant recipients in Japan exhibit favorable survival outcomes compared to international registry data. However, their social reintegration status, particularly concerning educational and occupational outcomes, has remained poorly characterized. A recent single-center study from Columbia University reported that approximately 30% of adult survivors of pediatric heart transplantation were either unemployed or unable to work [7]. This study primarily evaluated quality of life (QOL) metrics, finding no significant differences based on the primary heart failure diagnosis, transition to adult care, or transplantation era. However, it did not analyze risk factors influencing employment outcomes. Another single-center survey conducted at Loma Linda University revealed that while 95% of survivors who underwent pediatric heart transplantation graduated from high school, only 40% were employed. This employment rate was notably lower than that of the general population in the United States [8].

The other QOL studies for post-pediatric transplant recipients also reported the rate of unemployment was approximately 20–40% [9, 10]. Furthermore, a randomized controlled trial assessing an intensive patient education program (focusing on medical knowledge, self-care, self-advocacy, and social support) versus standard care showed no significant impact on patient adherence or employment and educational outcomes [11]. These findings underscore that even in countries with a higher volume of pediatric heart transplant recipients, optimal social reintegration support programs remain inadequately defined. Research on the social outcomes of pediatric transplant recipients is further complicated by cross-national differences in educational systems, higher education policies, and labor laws, emphasizing the importance of context-specific studies. This highlights the significance of the present study, the first to explore the social reintegration of pediatric heart transplant recipients in Japan.

Our findings show that most pediatric heart transplant recipients in Japan successfully achieve stable school attendance. This outcome is likely facilitated by enhanced educational support programs tailored for children requiring medical care and local government initiatives promoting school inclusion for children with disabilities. Nevertheless, significant challenges remain in higher education after high school graduation and employment, particularly among individuals with pre-transplant neurological complications or multiple post-transplant complications.

Addressing these challenges necessitates a holistic approach. Beyond employment support programs for individuals with cardiac conditions, systemic enhancements to Japan's disability employment framework are essential. Tailored vocational training programs, inclusive workplace policies, and robust societal support systems are critical for improving the social reintegration of these patients.

This study provides valuable insights into the current state of social reintegration among pediatric heart transplant recipients in Japan, highlighting critical areas for intervention and systemic reform. Future research should focus on developing multidisciplinary, longitudinal support strategies to optimize long-term social and functional outcomes for this vulnerable population.

14.5 Limitations

The retrospective design and relatively small sample size may limit generalizability. Prospective, multicenter studies are warranted to validate these findings and explore additional risk factors.

14.6 Conclusion

Pediatric heart transplant recipients in our hospital demonstrate high survival rates and favorable early educational integration. However, one in four faces significant challenges in higher education or employment by age 18, largely due to pre- and post-transplant neurological complications. Comprehensive, multidisciplinary interventions are essential to improve long-term social reintegration in this population.

Conflicts of Interest Disclosure The authors declare no conflicts of interest related to this study.

Funding This study has no funding support.

References

1. Singh TP, Cherikh WS, Hsich E, et al. The International Thoracic Organ Transplant Registry of the International Society for Heart and Lung Transplantation: twenty-fifth pediatric heart transplantation report-2022; focus on infant heart transplantation. J Heart Lung Transplant. 2022;41:1357–65.
2. McDonagh TA, Metra M, Adamo M, et al. 2021 ESC guidelines for the diagnosis and treatment of acute and chronic heart failure. Eur Heart J. 2021;42:3599–726.
3. Heidenreich PA, Bozkurt B, Aguilar D, et al. 2022 AHA/ACC/HFSA guideline for the management of heart failure: a report of the American College of Cardiology/American Heart Association Joint Committee on clinical practice guidelines. Circulation. 2022;145:e895–1032.
4. Bogle C, Colan SD, Miyamoto SD, et al. Treatment strategies for cardiomyopathy in children: a scientific statement from the American Heart Association. Circulation. 2023;148:174–95.
5. Wernovsky G. Outcomes regarding the central nervous system in children with complex congenital cardiac malformations. Cardiol Young. 2005;1:132–3.
6. Gold A, Bondi BC, Ashkanase J, et al. Early school-age cognitive performance post-pediatric heart transplantation. Pediatr Transplant. 2020;24:e13832.
7. Stanford NT, McAllister J, Gibbons M, et al. Quality of life and lifetime achievement in adult survivors of pediatric heart transplant. Pediatr Transplant. 2022;26:e14370.
8. Copeland H, Razzouk A, Beckham A, et al. Social framework of pediatric heart recipients who have survived more than 15 post-transplant years: a single-center experience. Pediatr Transplant. 2017;21:e12853.
9. Hollander SA, Chen S, Luikart H, et al. Quality of life and metrics of achievement in long-term adult survivors of pediatric heart transplant. Pediatr Transplant. 2015;19:76–81.
10. Sepke M, Ferentzi H, Disselhoff VSU, et al. Exploring the developmental tasks of emerging adults after paediatric heart transplantation: a cross-sectional case control study. BMJ Open. 2018;8:e022461.
11. Grady KL, Andrei AC, Shankel T, et al. Pediatric heart transplantation: transitioning to adult care (TRANSIT): feasibility of a pilot randomized controlled trial. J Card Fail. 2019;25:948–58.

Part VI

Future Perspectives

Pediatric Heart Failure Management with Ventricular Assist Device and Heart Transplantation

15

Takayoshi Ueno, Masaki Taira, Takashi Kido, Takuji Watanabe, and Shigeru Miyagawa

Abstract

The role of pediatric ventricular assist devices (VADs) in the treatment of severe heart failure in children is expected to become increasingly important. Currently, the only durable VAD available for infants and small children is the Berlin Heart EXCOR® (EXCOR), and experience with its use is beginning to accumulate. In Japan, it has been about 10 years since the start of this pediatric VAD, and a total of 133 implantations were performed as of 2024.

Out of these, 59 cases (44.4%) have reached heart transplantation. Thus, EXCOR has an exclusive role in pediatric heart failure treatment especially aiming for transplantation. At Osaka University, a total of 37 patients received EXCOR support and its demographics showed the age range from 4 months to 11 years, and the duration of support 45 to 1421 days. Among these, 15 patients have reached heart transplantation.

Keywords

Heart failure in children · Pediatric VAD · Pediatric heart transplantation · Bridge to transplantation · Bridge to recovery · EXCOR · Biventricular support

T. Ueno (✉)
Division of Health Sciences, The University of Osaka Graduate School of Medicine, Suita, Osaka, Japan
e-mail: uenotm@sahs.med.osaka-u.ac.jp

M. Taira · T. Kido · T. Watanabe · S. Miyagawa
Department of Cardiovascular Surgery, The University of Osaka Graduate School of Medicine, Suita, Osaka, Japan
e-mail: miyagawa.shigeru.med@osaka-u.ac.jp

H. Matsuda et al. (eds.), *Heart and Lung Transplantation*,
https://doi.org/10.1007/978-981-96-8810-4_15

15.1 Introduction

In recent years, advances in the treatment of severe heart failure in children have led to active discussions about strategies aimed at heart transplantation, the golden standard treatment. Mechanical circulatory support occupies a crucial position within these discussions, and its use has dramatically increased since the 2000s [1]. According to the 2021 statistics from the International Society of Heart and Lung Transplantation (ISHLT), among 5307 pediatric heart transplants performed between 2010 and 2018, approximately one-quarter of the cases involved heart transplantation under ventricular assist device (VAD) support [2]. In contrast, in Japan, data from the Japanese Society for Heart Transplant Registry indicates that about 79% of pediatric cases that reached heart transplantation received VAD implantation, highlighting its particular importance in Japan. As the significance of VADs in the treatment of severe pediatric heart failure increases, the expanded application of the Berlin Heart EXCOR (Berlin Heart, AG, Berlin, Germany), the only device available for infants, has allowed for safer heart transplantation support.

15.2 Ventricular Assist Device for Children

As the currently available pediatric VAD, the Berlin Heart EXCOR® (Berlin Heart GmbH; Berlin, Germany) (EXCOR) has been the device of choice for bridging to transplantation. The first implantation of EXCOR in small children was performed in an 8-year-old child in Germany in 1990 (50 mL pump) [3], and with the miniaturization of the pump, a 10 mL pump was implanted in an infant in 1992 [4]. Following FDA approval in the United States in 2011, the number of implantations exploded, and subsequently the number of patients bridged to heart transplantation with the Berlin Heart increased [5]. In this report analyzing UNOS data, between 2004 and 2022, 806 patients under 18 years of age received heart transplantation bridged by Berlin Hearts, and 233 patients had congenital heart disease. The annual trend of congenital cases showed a steep increase from less than 10 in 2015 to 46 in 2022 per year.

Regarding the survival curves after heart transplantation analyzed from this UNOS data [5], the cohort of congenital heart disease showed a 3-year survival estimate was 79.6% compared to 89.3% of the acquired group. This shows the inferiority of survival rate in the congenital group, but for those who survived 1 year, the later survival rate is expected to be comparable to the level of the acquired group.

In Japan, physician-led clinical trials for pediatric VAD (EXCOR) began in 2011, and after its approval in 2015, EXCOR implantation has been carried out in infants and small children weighing over 3 kg using wide-ranged pump sizes (Fig. 15.1). The pump's drive unit is called Ikus, and one drive unit can be applied in left ventricular assist (LVAD), right ventricular assist (RVAD), and biventricular assist (BiVAD). It is equipped with a battery to allow mobility. The guaranteed battery drive time is 30 min.

Currently, there are 14 hospitals in Japan that perform pediatric EXCOR implantations, and as of the end of September 2024, a total of 133 implantations have been

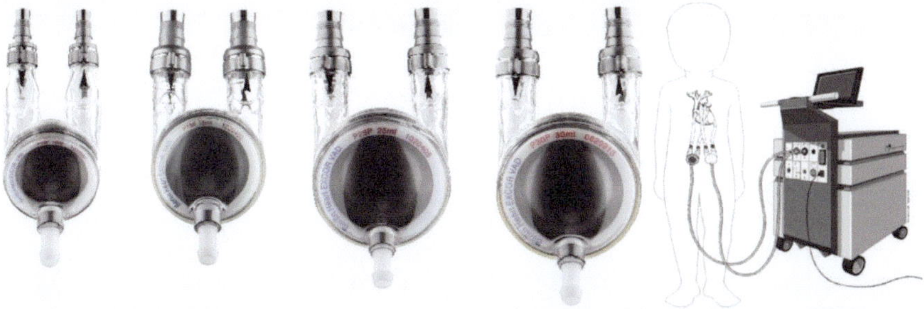

Fig. 15.1 Berlin Heart EXCOR pneumatic-driven blood pumps and console system. Size (left side): from left to right: 10-, 15-, 25-, and 30-mL pumps. Right: console system. (Permission from Berlin Heart GmbH)

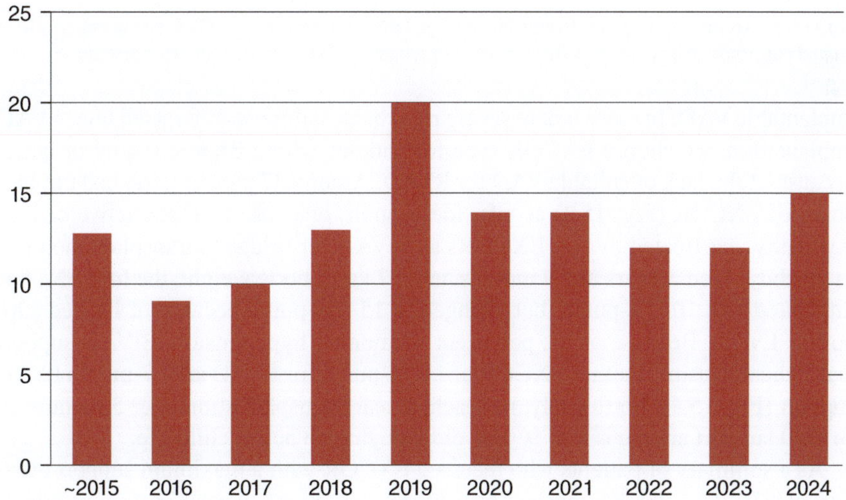

Fig. 15.2 Annual number of Berlin Heart EXCOR implantations in Japan

performed (9 of which were clinical trial cases) [6] (Fig. 15.2). The outcome of the EXCORs has been relatively good, with 59 cases (44.4%) reaching transplantation, 25 cases (18.8%) bridge to recovery, and 14 cases (10.5%) resulting in death during support.

15.3 Osaka University Experience of Pediatric VADs

Our department has participated in the EXCOR physician-led clinical trial since 2012 and granted use in 2015 [7]. For cases that can be managed with left ventricular assist alone, we use EXCOR for patients with a body surface area (BSA) of approximately 0.8 to 1.0 m^2 or less, and for larger patients, we consider an

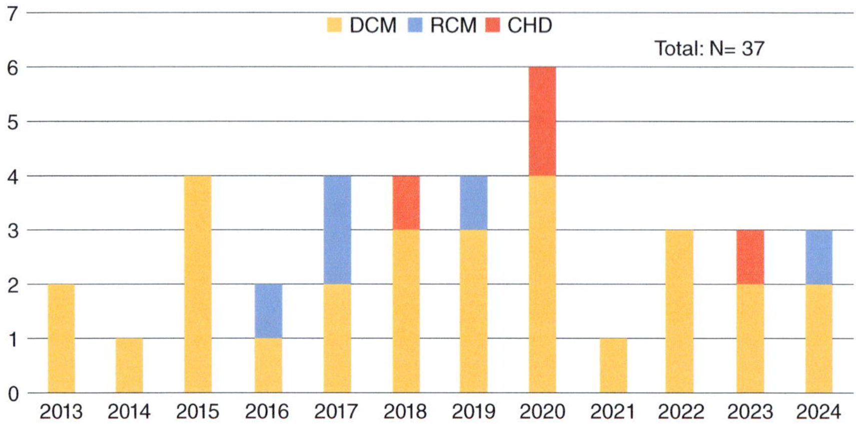

Fig. 15.3 Annual number of Berlin Heart EXCOR implantations at Osaka University. *DCM* dilated cardiomyopathy, *RCM* restrictive cardiomyopathy, *CHD* congenital heart disease

implantable VAD. In cases where severe right heart failure is anticipated after LVAD implantation, we choose EXCOR even for patients with a BSA of 0.8 m^2 or larger because of the lack of suitable VAD for RVAD. Among 37 patients who had implantation of EXCOR (Fig. 15.3) as left-side support, one case with restrictive cardiomyopathy was treated by two EXCORs as BiVAD for bridge to transplantation [8]. In this boy, aged 3 years and 9 months and 9.7 kg of body weight, the first EXCOR implanted was 10 mL-pump, but changed to 15 mL-pump because of limited support as LVAD. Because of the persistent pulmonary hypertension, BiVAD support was indicated using another EXCOR of 15 ml-pump for RVAD after 7-month LVAD support (Fig. 15.4). Fortunately, he reached heart transplantation after 5 months on BiVAD support and he is now 9-year-old enjoying an active child life.

As a summary of patients who received EXCOR with a maximum support duration of 850 days, 44.4% reached transplantation, 38.9% weaned off as bridge to recovery with a mortality rate of 5.6%. This indicates that EXCOR is a highly important medical device for VAD in small children with severe heart failure (Fig. 15.5). It is noteworthy that the proportion of patients who were able to be weaned was high, which indicates that the bridge to recovery strategy using a VAD may be considered in selected patients [9].

Recently, with technological advancements, the application of implantable VADs in children has expanded, and currently, the HeartMate3 (HM3, Abbott, Chicago, IL, USA) is used in children with a BSA of approximately 1.0 m^2 or larger. The HM3 is a magnetically levitated centrifugal continuous-flow pump that was approved in Japan in 2019, and implantation has begun. As a new device, the number of cases is still limited, and reports only cover short support periods, but it is expected to play a significant role in pediatric care in the future.

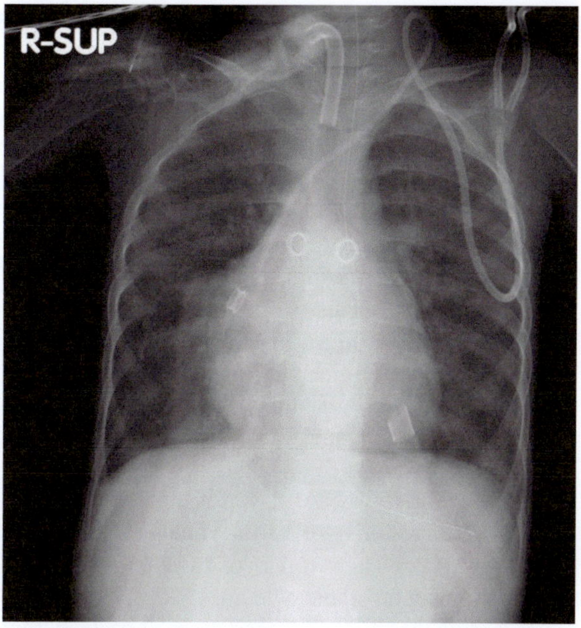

Fig. 15.4 Chest X-ray of a 4-year-old boy with restrictive cardiomyopathy on biventricular support with two EXCORs

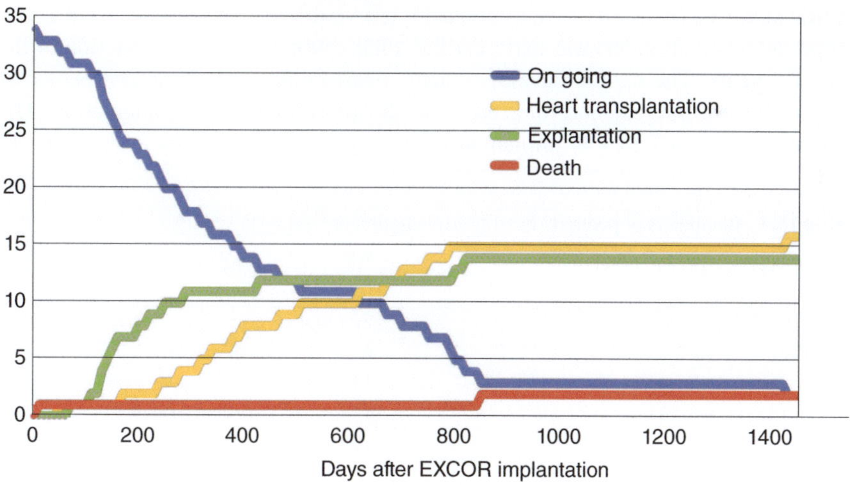

Fig. 15.5 Competing outcomes after EXCOR implantation: Osaka University experience

15.4 Pediatric Heart Transplantation at Osaka University

In 2000, we performed a pediatric heart transplantation for a 10-year-old from an adult donor, and in 2011, we performed the first pediatric heart transplantation using a pediatric donor heart in Japan [10]. As of September 2024, we performed 45 pediatric heart transplants on patients under 18 years old (Table 15.1). Before the revision of the Organ Transplant Law, there were 2 cases, but from the revision until 2019, there were 25 cases, and 18 cases since 2020, showing an increasing trend year by year. The age at transplantation ranged from 10 months to 17 years, with a median age of 13.3 years.

The number of bridged transplantations with VADs was 30, and with catecholamines 14, and the remaining patients had no support. The waiting period after registration with the organ transplant network ranged from 117 to 1764 days, with a median of 694 days, and the waiting period with status 1 ranged from 117 to 1532 days. Among 24 cases under 10 years of age, the average waiting period was 533 days, while it was 861 days for those 11 years and older, indicating a significantly shorter waiting period for younger children. The median follow-up period was 6.2 years (with a maximum of 15 years), with three deaths during the follow-up period, showing favorable outcomes.

Regarding the congenital heart cases of bridged transplant by EXCOR, our experience was limited in two patients. One of the patients had univentricular physiology (mitral stenosis, aortic stenosis, hypoplastic left ventricle, and muscular ventricular septal defect) and underwent extra-cardiac total cavopulmonary connection at the age of 2 years. The patient developed acute heart failure following gastroenteritis 1 year after the surgery and referred to our hospital for heart transplantation. The patient underwent EXCOR implantation as a systemic circulatory assist and was

Table 15.1 Recipients of pediatric heart transplantation at Osaka University

Age at heart transplantation (years)	0.8 ~ 17.7y, median 13.3y
Follow up (years)	0.1 ~ 15.6y, median 6.2y
Male (%)	20 (44.4%)
BW (kg)	6.6 ~ 55.4, median 27.8
Waiting period (days)	117 ~ 1764, median 694
Status 1 (days, $n = 44$)	117 ~ 1532, median 615
Mechanical circulatory support (%)	30 (66.6%)
Diagnosis (%)	
DCM	22 (48.9%)
RCM	13 (28.9%)
NCLV	3 (6.7%)
CHD	2 (4.4%)
ICM	2 (4.4%)
Others	3

$N = 45$

Status 1: on catecholamine or ventricular assist device

DCM dilated cardiomyopathy, *RCM* restrictive cardiomyopathy, *NCLV* non-compaction cardiomyopathy, *CHD* congenital heart disease, *ICM* ischemic cardiomyopathy successfully bridged to heart transplantation after 450 days of EXCOR support. The other patient was 3 years old, had an anomalous aortic origin of the left coronary artery, and underwent repair surgery with unroofing technique at the referring hospital. Due to severe cardiac dysfunction, the patient was bridged to heart transplantation with EXCOR support at our hospital.

15.5 Discussion

VAD treatment has been making daily progress as experience accumulates, and recent reports indicate that the mortality rate during the waiting period has been decreasing year by year due to proactive VAD introduction [11]. In Japan, where the waiting period for heart transplantation is expected to become increasingly long, it is essential to actively consider VAD treatment as part of the treatment strategy, given the increasing importance of VAD in heart failure treatment. Additionally, it is well-documented in the ISHLT registry, mentioned earlier, that more children than adults can recover cardiac function and be weaned off VADs, and about 30% of cases in our EXCOR results were weaned off the device. The potential for cardiac function recovery using VAD could emerge as a new treatment strategy for severe pediatric heart failure in the future.

Currently, heart transplantation remains the final treatment option for severe heart failure in children, but even after the revision of the Organ Transplant Law in Japan in 2010, it must be said that transplantation remains a very limited medical option. As mentioned earlier, we have only had experience with 45 cases of pediatric heart transplants, and we have followed up on 6 cases for more than 10 years after the transplant. However, we believe that the outcome has been relatively good (Fig. 15.6). In this situation, six cases required mechanical circulatory support postoperatively, and risk factors such as the duration of cardiac arrest of the donor heart and the age difference between donor and recipient were identified. As there are still many unresolved issues, further research to overcome these risk factors and further improvements in the allocation system are necessary at the national level.

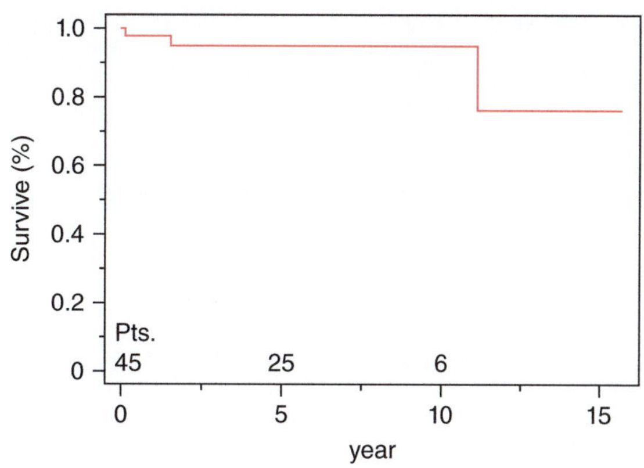

Fig. 15.6 The survival rate in pediatric heart transplantation at Osaka University ($N = 45$)

15.6 Conclusion

The treatment of severe heart failure in children is still developing. In this situation, heart failure treatment using VADs holds various possibilities, including temporary support aimed at recovery during acute exacerbations, collaboration with regenerative medicine, and destination therapy where VAD support leads to end-of-life care, beyond the current application limited to bridge-to-transplant. Furthermore, by analyzing the specific risk factors associated with pediatric heart transplantation and improving transplantation outcomes through technological advancements, new treatment strategies may be developed.

References

1. Morales DLS, Rossano JW, VanderPluym C, et al. Third annual pediatric interagency registry for mechanical circulatory support (Pedimacs) report: preimplant characteristics and outcomes. Ann Thorac Surg. 2019;107:993–1004.
2. Singh TP, Cherikh WS, Hsich E, et al. The International Thoracic Organ Transplant Registry of the International Society for Heart and Lung Transplantation: twenty-fourth pediatric heart transplantation report-2021; focus on recipient characteristics. J Heart Lung Transplant. 2021;40:1050–9.
3. Warnecke H, Berdjis F, Hennig E, et al. Mechanical left ventricular support as a bridge to transplantation. Eur J Cardiothorac Surg. 1991;5:330–3.
4. Hennig E. Design criteria for pediatric mechanical circulatory support systems (PMCSS). In: Ferrazzi P, Parenzan L, editors. Annals of the concerted action HEART 1991–1992. Bergamo: Commission of the European Communities; 1991. p. 39–43.
5. Bilgili A, Sharaf OM, Verzwyvelt Z, et al. Analysis of UNOS: Berlin heart bridged to transplant in acquired vs congenital heart. Ann Thorac Surg. 2024. S0003-4975(24)00782-3.
6. Kido T, Komori M, Taira M, et al. Bridging treatment to Berlin Heart EXCOR implantation: first 10-year experience in two tertiary centers in Japan. Presented in 30th congress of the International Society for Mechanical Circulatory Support, Utsunomiya, Japan, 14 Nov 2024.
7. Kanaya T, Ueno T, Taira M, et al. Impact of long-term support with Berlin Heart EXCOR in pediatric patients with severe heart failure. Pediatr Cardiol. 2019;40:1126–33.
8. Araki K, Ueno T, Taira M, et al. Pediatric patient with restrictive cardiomyopathy on staged biventricular assist device support with Berlin Heart EXCOR underwent heart transplantation successfully: the first case in Japan. J Artif Organs. 2021;24:269–72.
9. Tominaga Y, Ueno T, Kido T, et al. Bridge to recovery with Berlin Heart EXCOR in children <10 kg with dilated cardiomyopathy: a histological analysis. Eur J Cardiothorac Surg. 2020;58:253–60.
10. Ueno T, Fukushima N, Sakaguchi T, et al. First pediatric heart transplantation from a pediatric donor heart in Japan. Circ J. 2012;76:752–4.
11. Zafar F, Castleberry C, Khan MS, et al. Pediatric heart transplant waiting list mortality in the era of ventricular assist devices. J Heart Lung Transplant. 2015;34:82–8.

Ventricular Assist Device for Children: State of the Art and Future Directions

16

Junsang Cho and Iki Adachi

Abstract

The increasing awareness of pediatric heart failure in the setting of limited cardiac donor organ availability has led to substantial growth in pediatric ventricular assist devices. Despite major advancements witnessed over the last decade in the field, however, many challenges persist, particularly in addressing device-size mismatch and anatomical complexities in the pediatric population. This chapter reviews recent breakthroughs in real-world applications of mechanical circulatory support, including catheter-based techniques and targeted solutions for single-ventricle circulation. Further discussion is added to highlight newer devices on the horizon, particularly total artificial heart systems, that hold promise for addressing the current unmet needs in the management of pediatric heart failure.

Keywords

Pediatric heart failure · Mechanical circulatory support · Ventricular assist device · Temporary ventricular assist device support · Durable ventricular assist device support · Extracorporeal membrane oxygenation · Congenital heart disease · Single ventricle disease · Fontan failure · Total artificial heart

16.1 Introduction

The field of pediatric ventricular assist devices (VADs) has seen remarkable advancements over the years, reflecting the progress seen in the management of adult heart failure. VAD therapy has now solidified its role as a standard treatment

J. Cho · I. Adachi (✉)
Congenital Heart Surgery, Texas Children's Hospital, Michael E. DeBakey Department of Surgery, Baylor College of Medicine, Houston, TX, USA
e-mail: junsang.cho@bcm.edu

H. Matsuda et al. (eds.), *Heart and Lung Transplantation*,
https://doi.org/10.1007/978-981-96-8810-4_16

option for children with severe heart failure, driven by significant progress in both clinical management and device technology. Such progress has translated into substantially improved clinical outcomes, contributing to a steady rise in pediatric VAD implantations [1, 2]. Alongside this rapid growth, however, the field continues to face unique challenges, particularly in addressing complex anatomies such as single ventricle hearts. This chapter examines the evolution of pediatric VAD support over the past decade, providing an overview of current device options and discussing future innovations on the horizon.

16.2 Evolving Trends of Heart Failure Management

In the past two decades, VADs have become a cornerstone in the treatment of adults with end-stage heart failure. A key advancement arose with the advent of implantable, continuous-flow second-generation devices, including the HeartMate II® (Abbott, North Chicago, IL) and HeartWare HVAD® (Medtronic, Minneapolis, MN), enabling outpatient care with significant improvements in quality of life. The progression to the third-generation device, the HeartMate 3™ (Abbott, North Chicago, IL), characterized by full-magnetic levitation technology, significantly enhanced hemocompatibility and elevated the overall efficacy of VAD therapy. This technological evolution, paired with improved clinical outcomes and reduced morbidity, has shifted clinical practice to favor earlier device implantation over prolonged reliance on further escalation of medical therapy [3]. VADs are now routinely employed not only as a bridge to heart transplantation but also as a destination therapy for patients who are deemed unsuitable for cardiac transplantation. Notably, nearly 70% of adult VAD implants are now performed as destination therapy [4]. As VAD technology continues to evolve, there is growing momentum in the medical community that these devices will be regarded as the primary alternative to heart transplantation [5, 6].

While the third-generation VAD (i.e., HeartMate 3) has undoubtedly brought substantial benefits in patient care, it has also brought inadvertent challenges for the pediatric population. The rise in its use prompted the manufacturer to discontinue the second-generation HeartWare HVAD in June 2021 [7]. This withdrawal had a particularly pronounced impact on pediatric care, as the HVAD's smaller size and design had made it the primary implantable, continuous-flow VAD for children. With this change, the threshold for offering continuous-flow VADs in pediatric patients has been redefined. As a result, the Berlin EXCOR® system (Berlin Heart, Berlin, Germany), a more traditional pediatric-specific device, has seen markedly increased utilization, which will be discussed in greater detail later in this chapter.

16.3 Candidate Selection

Currently, there is no universal consensus on the indications for initiating VAD support. In general, VAD therapy is considered when the anticipated benefits outweigh the associated risks. The risk-to-benefit ratio is significantly influenced by factors such as the patient's clinical status, institutional experience, and the types of devices available. Consequently, decisions regarding VAD support must be highly individualized and carefully tailored by the clinical team.

Historically, VADs were reserved as a last-resort option for cases unmanageable by medical therapy. Over time, however, growing confidence in achieving consistent and positive outcomes has progressively lowered the threshold for their use in adults. Data from the Interagency Registry for Mechanically Assisted Circulatory Support (INTERMACS) consistently underscores the critical impact of preoperative clinical status on post-VAD outcomes, with a trend toward earlier implantation leading to notable improvements in survival and recovery [4, 6]. In contrast, pediatric practitioners often adopt a more cautious approach, driven by limited institutional experience and the technical challenges of supporting smaller children. VAD support in pediatric patients, particularly those within the smallest cohort, relies almost exclusively on pulsatile, extracorporeal devices (i.e., Berlin Heart EXCOR), which carry higher risk profiles compared to implantable continuous-flow devices [8].

While early intervention may improve survival in some cases, initiating support too soon can lead to increased device-related complications, underscoring the delicate balance required in these decisions. This complexity is further compounded by a range of contraindications, including extreme prematurity, low body weight (<2.0 kg), pre-existing neurological injuries, and severe congenital or chromosomal anomalies with poor prognoses. Each of these factors introduces unique risks, making the decision-making process in pediatric patients particularly challenging. Again, individual assessment of the patient's risk profile is of critical importance to navigating these complexities and tailoring the approach to each case. Although multisystem end-organ injury is a relative contraindication to VAD support, it does not necessarily preclude its use, particularly when improved cardiac output is expected to facilitate organ recovery.

Figure 16.1 provides an overview of pediatric VAD utilization at Texas Children's Hospital (TCH), showing a steady increase in implant volume over the past decade (A), as well as the distribution of underlying diagnoses (B). Historically, at TCH, the Berlin Heart EXCOR was primarily reserved for critically ill children in cardiogenic shock or those with severe end-organ dysfunction (i.e., INTERMACS profiles 1 or 2) [9]. However, with the recent favorable changes in outcomes, we now consider offering EXCOR support with broader indications, extending to patients with more stable conditions (i.e., INTERMACS profile 3). For older children who meet the anatomical and physiological criteria for adult-sized implantable device (i.e., HeartMate 3), we typically initiate VAD support at INTERMACS profiles 2 or 3. The lower risk profile of implantable devices, combined with their feasibility for outpatient management, justifies this shift toward earlier initiation of VAD therapy.

Another critical consideration in pediatric VAD support is the anatomical complexity frequently encountered in children with congenital heart disease (CHD). Structural abnormalities, such as abnormal aortic size or position, anomalous coronary artery origins, or irregularly shaped systemic ventricles, pose significant challenges to the proper placement of inflow and outflow cannulas. As most implantable

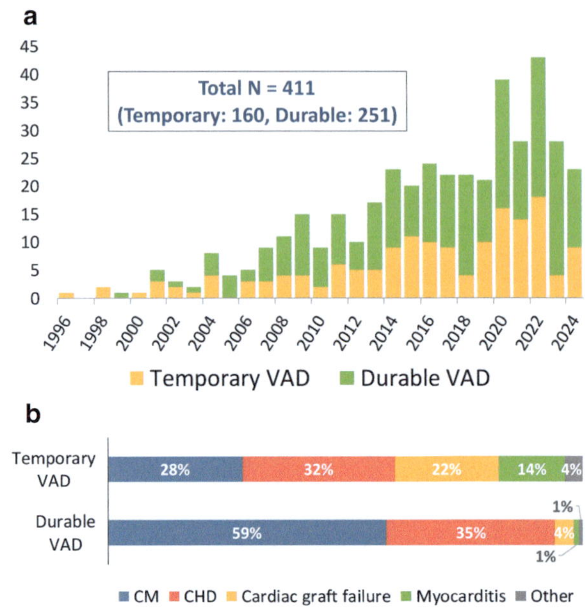

Fig. 16.1 Overview of pediatric ventricular assist device (VAD) utilization at Texas Children's Hospital. (**a**) Annual implant volume; (**b**) Distribution of underlying diagnoses among VAD recipients. Total $N = 411$. Data for 2024 includes cases through October. Image, courtesy of Texas Children's Hospital, 2025. Abbreviations: *CM* cardiomyopathy, *CHD* congenital heart disease

VADs are designed for structurally normal hearts, achieving a proper fit in anatomically malformed hearts can be a complex challenge. Previous palliative surgeries, such as Glenn or Fontan procedures or systemic-to-pulmonary artery shunts, further complicate VAD implantation by altering both anatomy and circulatory physiology. These technical hurdles are compounded by the unique pathophysiologic characteristics of CHD, particularly in patients with single-ventricle physiology, where device selection and timing must be carefully customized. The specific challenges and considerations inherent to VAD implantation in this population will be discussed in detail in a later section of this chapter.

Finally, psychosocial and family counseling are essential, particularly for patients eligible for home discharge with implantable VADs. Comprehensive preparation is critical to ensuring the success of outpatient management and optimizing overall outcomes.

16.4 Device Selection

Determining the appropriate type of mechanical circulatory support (MCS) depends on two key factors: the anticipated duration of support and whether univentricular or biventricular support is required. The duration of support is largely dependent on the underlying etiology of heart failure, whether it is acute in nature (e.g., viral myocarditis) or a chronic condition (e.g., dilated cardiomyopathy) (Fig. 16.1b). Short-term support is typically offered to patients with acute-type or uncertain etiologies, or if transplant candidacy has not yet been established. The goal of support

Table 16.1 Modes of mechanical circulatory support and current devices for use in children

Extracorporeal membrane oxygenation
Short-term ventricular assist devices
Central cannulation
CentriMag™ (centrifugal)
PediMag™ (centrifugal)
Rotaflow® II (centrifugal)
Peripheral cannulation
Impella® (axial)
Long-term ventricular assist devices
Pulsatile
Berlin Heart EXCOR®
Continuous-flow
HeartMate 3™ (centrifugal)

is to stabilize hemodynamics and to provide time for additional diagnostic investigation to guide further management decision-making (bridge-to-decision). If, at this point, long-term support is deemed necessary either as a bridge to transplant or to facilitate potential cardiac recovery, temporary MCS can be transitioned to a durable VAD (bridge-to-bridge). The second factor involves determining whether left ventricular support (LVAD), right ventricular support (RVAD), or simultaneous support for both ventricles (BiVAD), is needed. Table 16.1 outlines the different modes of support and provides an overview of devices currently available for pediatric use.

16.4.1 Short-Term Ventricular Assist Device

Short-term VADs are increasingly being adopted as the preferred MCS option for managing acute heart failure, particularly in cases where cardiac recovery is anticipated within a short timeframe (i.e., 2 weeks or less). In many pediatric centers, however, extracorporeal membrane oxygenation (ECMO) remains the first-line strategy, even with intact pulmonary function requiring circulatory support alone. The primary MCS philosophy at TCH is being a "minimalist", prioritizing support for only the system in need. As such, ECMO is reserved for cases requiring pulmonary support, such as severe pulmonary edema due to ventricular dysfunction, pulmonary hypertension, or other conditions threatening pulmonary function [10, 11]. For short-term circulatory support alone, VADs are the preferred choice.

A significant advantage of VADs over ECMO lies in their ability to directly decompress the left heart, which provides optimal conditions for myocardial and pulmonary recovery. ECMO, by contrast, relies on venous inflow cannulation on the right side of the heart, which only indirectly unloads the left ventricle and often is insufficient. When ECMO cannulation is performed percutaneously, the size of the venous cannula is often limited, exacerbating this issue.

Inadequate left heart unloading is a key concern with ECMO use, particularly in patients with severely depressed systemic ventricular function. ECMO inherently increases afterload on the failing ventricle, which can further impair myocardial

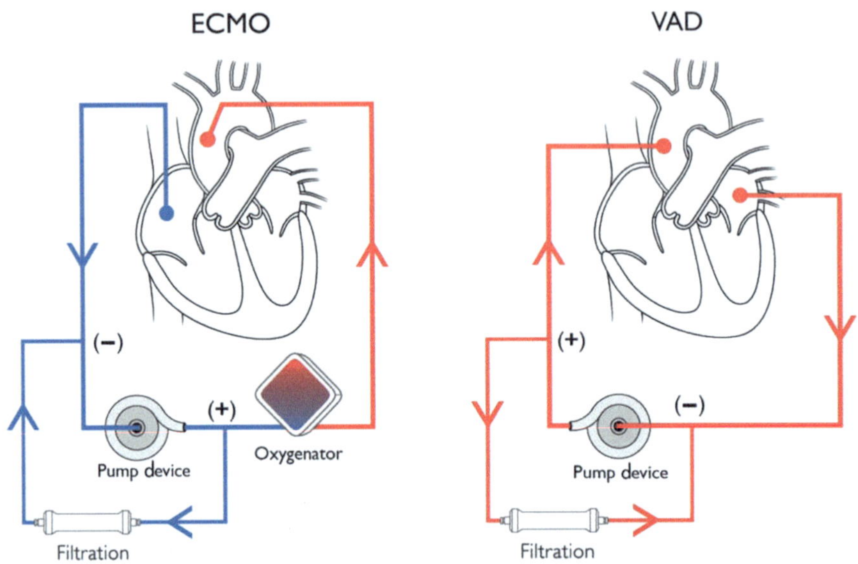

Fig. 16.2 Circuit configurations for extracorporeal membrane oxygenation (ECMO) and short-term ventricular assist device (VAD). The major differences are the location of the inflow cannula and the presence (or absence) of an oxygenator. (Image, courtesy of Texas Children's Hospital, 2014)

contractility [12]. If the myocardium lacks sufficient reserve to manage this elevated afterload, intraventricular pressures rise, resulting in increased left atrial and pulmonary venous pressures [13]. This cascade can lead to pulmonary edema, particularly when volume unloading is inadequate, which is often the case with ECMO support. This makes left heart decompression a critical consideration when using ECMO for patients with compromised cardiac function [14].

16.4.1.1 Extracorporeal Short-Term Ventricular Assist Device

An extracorporeal short-term VAD system typically comprises a pump head and console, circuit tubing, and inflow and outflow cannulas (Fig. 16.2). Many centers employ centrifugal pumps, such as the CentriMag™ (flow range up to 10 L/min) or PediMag™ (flow range 0.4–1.7 L/min) (Abbott, North Chicago, IL), as well as the Rotaflow® II (Getinge AB, Göteborg, Sweden). While LV apical cannulation is an alternative option [15], our preferred approach is to place the inflow cannula in the left atrium. This is achieved through Waterston's groove (preferred) or via the left atrial appendage (as an alternative). By avoiding direct cannulation of the already compromised LV, this approach ensures stable inflow dynamics and reduces the risk of further ventricular injury. Although left atrial cannulation carries a potential risk of left ventricular thrombus formation, such complications have been exceedingly rare in our experience.

One drawback often cited against short-term VADs is the necessity for a sternotomy, particularly when compared to ECMO, which allows for percutaneous cannulation. However, in our opinion, the central approach provides unparalleled advantages by allowing the insertion of larger cannulas for optimal left heart drainage, resulting in better pulmonary protection. This is particularly advantageous in pediatric cases with increased cardiac return, such as those with systemic-to-pulmonary artery collaterals. On the other hand, the same degree of decompression cannot be achieved with peripheral ECMO, of which a smaller inflow cannula is placed in the right-sided cardiac chamber. For the outflow cannula, the ascending aorta is the standard insertion site. When transitioning to a long-term VAD support (bridge-to-bridge) is anticipated, the outflow cannula for the short-term VAD should be inserted into the distal ascending aorta or even into the proximal arch, ensuring sufficient space in the proximal ascending aorta for a future long-term VAD outflow cannula.

16.4.1.2 Catheter-Based Short-Term Ventricular Assist Device

Catheter-based VADs provide a significant advantage of delivering rapid circulatory support without necessitating sternal access. This is particularly beneficial for children with hemodynamic instability, especially those with a history of prior sternotomies. Among the currently available options, the Impella® (Abiomed, Danvers, MA) has shown success in the pediatric population. Its minimally invasive axial flow pump design, along with availability in multiple sizes, makes it a versatile option [16].

The choice of a catheter-based VAD is primarily determined by patient-specific factors, including anatomical considerations, vessel size, and the urgency of deployment. In patients with CHD, a detailed assessment of cardiac anatomy is essential. This includes an assessment of the aortic arch's size and laterality, as well as valvular and ventricular morphology, to ensure successful implantation.

For emergencies, the Impella 2.5 (supporting peak flows up to 2.5 L/min) or Impella CP (peak flows up to 4.3 L/min) may be selected due to its rapid deployment via the common femoral artery. In semi-urgent cases, the Impella 5.5 (peak flows up to 6 L/min) is preferred when the patient has a suitable target vessel size ($\approx$7 mm in diameter) and is implanted via a chimney Dacron graft anastomosed to the target vessel. Fluoroscopy assists in device placement, while additional echocardiographic imaging can be used for pump positioning and speed titration to achieve the optimal level of hemodynamic support.

16.4.1.3 Practical Considerations for Short-Term VAD Support

Upon initiating LVAD support, inotropic agents should be titrated down appropriately, but not fully discontinued, if the right ventricle requires pharmacologic support. Pulmonary vascular resistance (PVR) can be managed using inhaled nitric oxide, and vasodilators may be necessary to regulate systemic vascular resistance and address hypertension. Typically, patients with severe heart failure present with significantly elevated systemic vascular resistance at the time of cannulation. Once optimal VAD flow and systemic arterial pressure are achieved, systemic perfusion is confirmed through clinical indicators and laboratory parameters. Ventilator settings should also be adjusted to reduce PVR and to maximize right-sided cardiac output, which ultimately determines the filling of the LVAD pump. Temperature control poses a challenge, especially in small children with an open chest, as the short-term VAD circuit does not include a heat exchanger. Overhead radiant heaters or external convective warming devices can be used to address this issue.

Serial evaluation of cardiac function is essential as a guide to weaning MCS. In our experience, 65% (33 of 51) of patients with acute etiologies, such as myocarditis or transplant rejection, were discharged successfully after being weaned from short-term VAD support [17]. Specifically, 73% (16 of 22) of patients with acute myocarditis recovered, compared to a reported 61% recovery rate with ECMO in similar cases. While ECMO may provide adequate, if not optimal, support for most children with acute myocarditis, its limitations in left heart decompression may become critical in managing the most severe cases. The superior outcomes observed with short-term VADs are likely due to their ability to deliver focused and effective left heart decompression, which is essential for addressing the sickest children who may not survive without this targeted intervention.

The use of short-term VAD support in chronic heart failure differs from its application in acute failure, as significant myocardial recovery is generally not achievable in these cases. Instead, short-term VAD support primarily serves as a "rescue" or "salvage" purpose, designed to stabilize the patient by mitigating sustained decompensation and preventing end-organ injury. This stabilization period allows time for recovery and optimization, improving the patient's eligibility for more definitive interventions, such as durable long-term VAD implantation or heart transplantation. A recent study has reported nearly a 90% success rate for short-term VADs in bridging chronic heart failure patients with poor preoperative conditions (e.g., INTERMACS profiles 1 and 2) to long-term VAD support [17]. This bridge-to-bridge strategy has demonstrated improved post-discharge survival rates compared to earlier studies, highlighting the benefits of short-term VAD support in preconditioning patients for long-term VAD therapy and enhancing overall treatment success.

A significant clinical shift accompanying the introduction of catheter-based devices is the earlier initiation of VAD support. Previously, temporary VADs were considered a last-resort option, reserved only for critically ill patients due to the invasive nature requiring a sternotomy for central cannulation. The advent of the Impella, however, has drastically lowered this threshold, enabling rapid deployment as an initial resuscitation strategy. This ease of accessibility is likely a key factor in the improved survival rates observed in these patients [16, 17].

Another noteworthy trend, particularly with Impella use, is the extended duration of temporary support [18]. Our recent experience indicates the feasibility of successful support extending beyond 30 days, enabling patients to be discharged home either after recovery or as a bridge to long-term VAD. This evolving role of catheter-based VADs surpasses their traditional use for durations of less than 2 weeks and is anticipated to expand further with continued advancements in pump technology and next-generation driving consoles. These innovations may enable outpatient management and facilitate a transition toward intermediate- to long-term percutaneous VAD options.

16.4.1.4 Right Heart Short-Term VAD Support

Although short-term VADs are primarily utilized to support systemic circulation, there are specific scenarios where temporary RVAD support is necessary. One such scenario is heart transplantation in patients with elevated PVR. In our experience, the failing RV of a transplanted heart often recovers relatively quickly, allowing RVAD support to be discontinued within a few days. By gradually reducing RVAD flow, clinicians can carefully manipulate the loading condition of the RV, providing a more precise assessment on how much support the RV still needs. In select cases, ECMO may be considered instead of temporary RVAD support. While our preference is to maintain normal physiological circulation using RVAD (i.e., achieving a Qp/Qs ratio of 1:1 with serial circulation), ECMO can offer advantages in situations where the lung parenchyma is the primary issue (e.g., pulmonary hemorrhage), by effectively reducing Qp and providing simultaneous pulmonary support. Another common indication for short-term RVAD support is acute right ventricular failure following the implantation of a long-term LVAD. In cases where the RV dysfunction is deemed transitory, short-term RVAD support can provide an opportunity to evaluate the potential for RV recovery.

For near-adult-sized patients (e.g., teenagers), several percutaneous RVAD options are available. The ProtekDuo® (LivaNova, London, UK) is a right atrium-to-pulmonary artery bypass double-lumen cannula designed for percutaneous, single venous access through the right internal jugular vein. The proximal inflow lumen is positioned in the right atrium, and the distal outflow lumen is positioned in the main pulmonary artery. This device is compatible with multiple MCS pumps and, when equipped with an ECMO circuit, provides oxygenation support, distinguishing it from devices limited to standalone RVAD functionality. The Impella RP Flex™ (Abiomed, Danvers, MA) is another catheter-based device tailored specifically for RVAD support. Similar to other products from the same manufacturer, it utilizes single venous access through the internal jugular vein. One of its most notable advantages is its substantially smaller indwelling catheter size (11 French), which stands in contrast to other percutaneous options, such as ProtekDuo (29 Fr and 31 Fr cannula sizes). The smaller size offers potentially enhanced patient mobility and a reduced risk of vascular complications, making it an appealing choice for appropriate candidates.

16.4.2 Long-Term Ventricular Assist Device

16.4.2.1 Device Options and Configuration

For children with chronic heart disease with relatively stable hemodynamics, long-term VAD implantation should be considered as a primary therapeutic strategy. The selection of an appropriate device is largely determined by the patient's body size. At TCH, the Berlin Heart EXCOR is the preferred option for children with a body surface area of approximately 1.0 m^2 or smaller. In contrast, for larger patients, implantable continuous-flow devices, such as the HeartMate 3, are favored, provided their chest cavity can accommodate the pump without risk of inflow obstruction or compression of adjacent structures. As discussed earlier, the discontinuation of the HeartWare HVAD [7] in June 2021 has had a profound impact on device selection in pediatric patients. This decision, driven by concerns over increased rates of neurological events, pump thrombosis, and mortality, removed a device that was particularly suited to smaller children due to its relatively compact size compared to the HeartMate 3. In the absence of HVAD, the clinical gap in implantable VAD options for smaller children (i.e., body surface area between approximately 0.7 m^2 and 1.3 m^2) has been compensated by increased utilization of the Berlin EXCOR, resulting in greater reliance on this device in recent years [19].

The selection of VAD support configuration, whether isolated LVAD or BiVAD, is a critical decision in the management of pediatric patients with advanced heart failure. Based on our institutional experience, most children can be adequately supported with isolated LVAD implantation, even when echocardiography suggests severe right ventricular dysfunction prior to surgery. Once the LV is decompressed by VAD support, pulmonary artery pressure typically drops, reducing the afterload on the RV. Consequently, RV dysfunction that is secondary to left ventricular failure can often be managed effectively with LVAD support alone.

Nonetheless, there are specific scenarios where BiVAD support may be necessary. These include cases where the RV is intrinsically impaired (e.g., arrhythmogenic right ventricular dysplasia) or when PVR is severely elevated, as seen in restrictive cardiomyopathy. Despite these indications, the use of BiVAD should be approached with caution, as studies consistently report poorer outcomes compared to isolated LVAD support [20]. While some pediatric centers routinely employ BiVAD support, our approach is more selective: unless the RV has intrinsic myocardial dysfunction (e.g., myocardial ischemia in transplant coronary vasculopathy), we prioritize isolated LVAD implantation. If RV function appears insufficient during intraoperative assessment, temporary RV support is used to evaluate recovery potential before committing to durable BiVAD implantation.

For patients with isolated LVAD support, maintaining optimal RV performance is essential for ensuring adequate systemic cardiac output. The LVAD's flow is contingent on the amount of blood received from the RV through the pulmonary circulation, assuming the absence of intracardiac shunting or aortic insufficiency. Key strategies include pharmacological support for the RV, minimizing PVR, and maintaining adequate preload to the right heart. Although echocardiography provides valuable insights into RV function, its findings alone may not always predict clinical outcomes. For instance, in our experience, LVAD filling may remain adequate even when echocardiography suggests severe RV dysfunction.

Direct assessment of the pump's filling status is particularly informative with extracorporeal, pulsatile devices like the Berlin Heart EXCOR, as it provides a straightforward indicator of right heart cardiac output. Additionally, maintaining balanced ventricular function is essential. Excessive LVAD settings can shift the interventricular septum leftward, worsening tricuspid regurgitation and impairing RV performance. Conversely, insufficient LVAD settings can lead to inadequate left heart unloading. In this context, continuous monitoring of left and right atrial pressures is crucial to ensure balanced filling of both ventricles. Septal positioning can also be assessed intermittently via echocardiography, but rapid hemodynamic changes often necessitate real-time atrial pressure monitoring. Careful consideration of these factors allows for a tailored approach that addresses the unique hemodynamic demands of each patient. This ensures that both the device configuration and the management strategy are optimized to support long-term outcomes.

16.4.2.2 Surgical Considerations

Achieving optimal outcomes with pediatric VAD implantation requires meticulous attention to technical details and surgical strategies, particularly given the anatomical and size-related challenges of this patient population. One critical consideration is the "device-patient" size mismatch, which poses unique challenges when implanting adult-sized VADs in children. Devices such as the Berlin Heart EXCOR offer a range of pump and cannula sizes, eliminating this concern for smaller patients. However, implantable continuous-flow devices such as the HeartMate 3, designed primarily for adult populations, inherently introduce size-related complexities in pediatric applications. As clinical efforts push the boundaries of smaller patient sizes, mitigating these challenges has become increasingly important. The accurate placement of the inflow cannula is paramount for successful long-term VAD support, especially in pediatric patients with smaller ventricular chambers. Even adult patients with conditions like restrictive cardiomyopathy, which results in reduced ventricular size, demonstrate limited tolerance for minor misalignments or technical errors [21]. In children, this challenge is further amplified when adult-sized devices are employed, particularly in terms of inflow cannula positioning and intracavitary volume. To prevent complications such as thrombus formation or suction events against the interventricular septum, precise orientation of the inflow cannula is critical. Lessons learned from axial-flow pumps like the HeartMate II highlight that a perpendicular angle relative to the septum is associated with increased rates of pump thrombosis [22]. Ideally, the inflow cannula should align parallel to the septum to facilitate unobstructed flow. While centrifugal pumps such as the HeartWare HVAD and HeartMate 3 differ technologically from axial pumps, this fundamental principle remains relevant.

Although centrifugal pumps have gained widespread adoption in pediatrics due to their compact size [23, 24], these devices often pose unique challenges related to inflow cannula positioning. When implanted intrapericardially, the inflow cannula of centrifugal pumps frequently assumes a perpendicular orientation to the septum (Fig 16.3a), increasing the risk of suction events and suboptimal flow dynamics. To address this issue, some adult cardiac surgeons have modified their techniques, opting to place the inflow cannula through the diaphragmatic surface of the left ventricle rather than the apex [25].

At TCH, a tailored approach is employed to optimize inflow cannula orientation. The cannula is inserted through the left ventricular apex as standard, but the apex is then gently repositioned medially and caudally into a small pocket on the left hemidiaphragm. This maneuver ensures that the inflow cannula lies parallel to the septum, thereby minimizing suction events and promoting efficient flow (Fig. 16.3b). Additionally, this adjustment creates more space for the expansion of the left lower

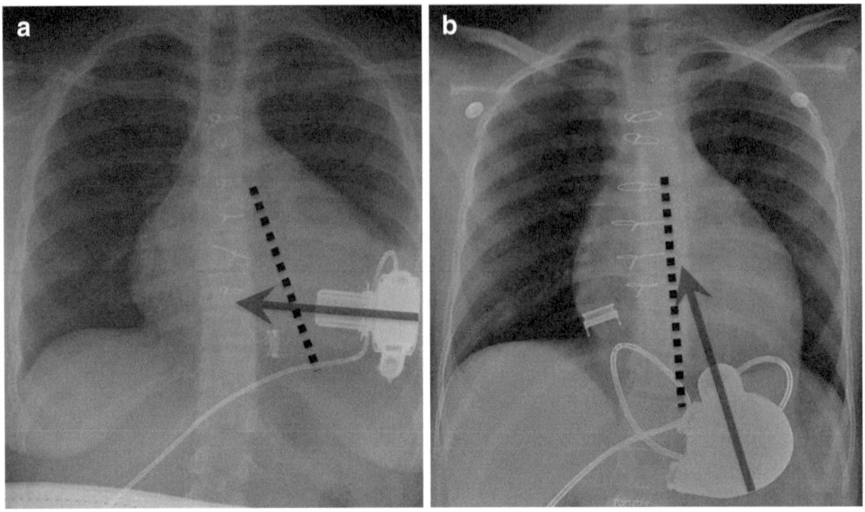

Fig. 16.3 Relationship of the inflow cannula relative to the ventricular septum. Postoperative chest X-rays showing the HeartWare HVAD® implanted with the standard intrapericardial technique (**a**) and with the modified technique at Texas Children's Hospital (**b**). The dotted line represents an imaginary line of the interventricular septum. Note the difference in the relationship of the inflow cannula relative to the ventricular septum. With the modified technique, the inflow cannula lies in a more parallel orientation relative to the ventricular septum. The left lower lobe is well expanded with the modified technique since the device does not occupy the space in the pleural cavity. (Image, courtesy of Texas Children's Hospital 2016)

lung lobe, which is often compromised in patients with severe cardiomegaly, further supporting optimal postoperative physiology. In cases where the left ventricle is unsuitable for cannulation—such as in patients with restrictive or hypertrophic cardiomyopathy, diastolic dysfunction, or chronic cardiac allograft failure with preserved systolic function—left atrial inflow cannulation can serve as an alternative. Although direct left atrial cannulation via Waterston's groove is technically feasible, the use of an "intraatrial" graft has become gradually accepted among surgeons due to its practicality [26, 27] (Fig. 16.4). This approach involves sewing one end of a graft to a surgically created atrial septal defect, with the other end brought out through the right atrial free wall to connect with the pump inflow. The choice of graft size depends on the device: a 20 mm ePTFE ring-supported graft is typically used for the HeartMate 3, while a smaller 10 mm graft may be appropriate for the Berlin EXCOR. To prevent collapse under the negative pressure generated by the pump, using a graft with external support is imperative. While atrial cannulation offers a viable solution in certain cases, it presents unique challenges. First, the intraatrial graft occupies considerable space in the right atrium, which could complicate right-side mechanical support if needed. Second, the shorter outflow graft length required in this configuration can make it more challenging to achieve optimal orientation and flow dynamics. As such, adequate right heart function becomes even more critical in these scenarios than in standard ventricular cannulation.

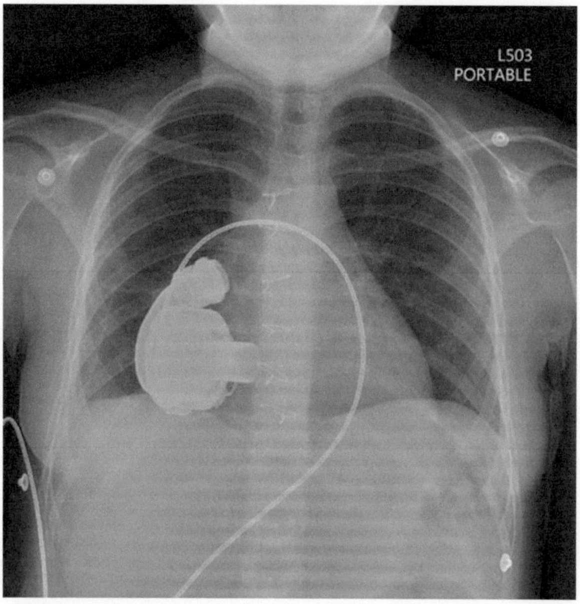

Fig. 16.4 Postimplant chest X-ray demonstrating an alternative cannulation technique utilizing an intraatrial graft with the HeartMate 3™. The graft is sewn to a surgically created atrial septal defect and exits through the right atrial wall. (Image, courtesy of Texas Children's Hospital, 2024)

16.5 VAD Support in Single Ventricle Physiology

As VAD support continues to advance, there has been a growing enthusiasm among clinicians to extend its use to the most challenging patient populations, including those with single ventricle CHD. Data from the second PediMACS report in 2018 indicated that CHD patients made up 21% of pediatric VAD recipients in North America, with 62% of these cases involving single ventricle physiology [28]. By 2022, the proportion of CHD patients receiving VAD support had risen to 25% [29]. Notably, approximately 60% of Berlin EXCOR implants in North America in the same year were placed in patients with CHD, reflecting a clear trend toward expanding the use of VADs in this challenging group [19].

Despite this increased adoption, outcomes for the CHD cohort remain suboptimal compared to their non-CHD counterparts. Mortality rates on support are significantly higher (36% vs. 12%), and the success rate of bridging to transplant is markedly lower (29% vs. 60%) [30]. A key observation from this cohort is the substantial variability in survival rates depending on the stage of single ventricle palliation at the time of VAD implantation. Patients who receive VAD support after Stage 3 palliation (Fontan completion) demonstrate a remarkable 95% survival rate, while survival rates drop to approximately 30% and 40% for Stage 1 and Stage 2 patients, respectively [30]. In Stage 1 patients, it is somewhat predictable that a large proportion (59%) were classified as INTERMACS profile 1, highlighting the critical condition of these individuals. By contrast, fewer than 25% of Stage 2 patients fell under this profile, indicating that the modified hemodynamics of Stage 2 palliation (Glenn physiology) may pose a unique challenge in VAD support.

The challenge of Glenn circulation mainly stems from chronic shunting through veno-venous collaterals between the upper and lower systemic venous systems. The limited decompression achieved by VAD support, which primarily targets venous return from the lower body, can exacerbate the pressure gradient between the upper and lower body. This imbalance may promote the development of collateral vessels that shunt blood away from the pulmonary circulation, further complicating effective hemodynamic support [31]. Although limited data exist on the application of VADs in failing Glenn physiology, transitioning from Stage 2 to Stage 3 (completion of the Fontan procedure) during VAD implantation has been suggested as a strategy to improve cyanosis and exercise capacity [32]. Our experience indicates that concomitant Fontan completion at VAD implantation appears to be a viable option for this exceptionally complex patient population [33]. Unlike VAD support for cardiomyopathy, which is well-established and relatively static, the use of VADs in CHD, particularly in single ventricle physiology, remains a dynamic and evolving field. It is in this area where substantial advancements and outcome improvements are anticipated over the next decade.

16.6 The Future

16.6.1 Devices in Development

The critical need for pediatric-specific VADs, particularly for small children, has been a longstanding concern. To address this, the National Heart, Lung, and Blood Institute (NHLBI) allocated $23 million in 2004 to fund five research groups focused on developing pediatric-specific MCS devices [34]. This initiative set the stage for the Pumps for Kids, Infants, and Neonates (PumpKIN) program, launched in 2010, to advance some of the most promising devices into clinical application [35]. Among these, the Infant Jarvik 2000® (Jarvik Heart, New York, NY) emerged as the sole device carried forward within the program. Extensive modifications and rigorous preclinical testing, both in-vitro and in-vivo, culminated in the development of the Jarvik 2015, a 15 mm VAD specifically designed for pediatric use [36]. The Jarvik 2015 has been tested in the dedicated clinical trial, the so-called "PumpKIN trial" beginning in 2018. However, due to unforeseen circumstances caused by the COVID-19 pandemic, the trial did not proceed as intended. Despite these setbacks, efforts to revive the trial remain active within the pediatric cardiology community, reflecting the continued commitment to advancing this essential technology [37, 38].

Another device on the horizon that may have a significant impact on the pediatric population is the BiVACOR® total artificial heart (TAH) (BiVACOR, Houston, TX; Fig. 16.5). The BiVACOR is the first clinically introduced TAH system based on continuous-flow principles as opposed to the SynCardia TAH (SynCardia Systems, Tucson, AZ), which employs volume displacement with flexible polymer diaphragms. While the SynCardia TAH remains the only FDA-approved TAH in the United States, its role in the pediatric population has been very limited. The

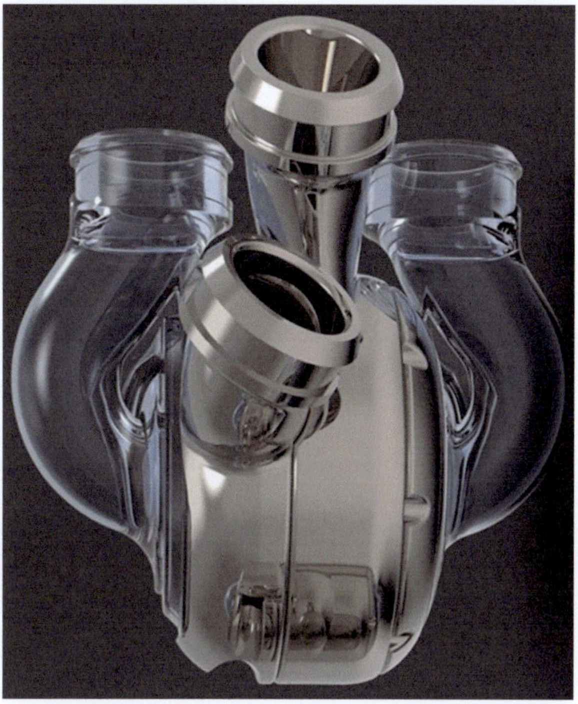

Fig. 16.5 Conceptual illustration of a potential future configuration of the BiVACOR® total artificial heart for pediatric use. (Image, courtesy of BiVACOR, Houston, TX)

BiVACOR TAH represents a major technological advancement, particularly in terms of hemocompatibility and compact design. Currently undergoing a feasibility clinical trial in the United States, the BiVACOR has demonstrated impressively promising initial outcomes [39]. This device holds significant potential in addressing the unmet need for biventricular support, particularly by means of TAH devices. Potential candidates would include those with chronic cardiac allograft failure with severe transplant coronary vasculopathy and a subset of Fontan failure not suitable for isolated systemic VAD support. Despite this need, the use of a TAH in actual practice remains extremely rare. Hesitancy to employ a TAH system, however, may subside once the next-generation devices, such as the BiVACOR TAH, become clinically available. A widespread application of VAD support occurred when continuous-flow technology was first introduced to the clinical arena, and a similar paradigm change may occur with the BiVACOR.

16.6.2 Bridging the Gap in Life Expectancy

The development of the next-generation TAH system offers a glimpse into the future of pediatric MCS. While cardiac transplantation remains the only viable life-saving option for many pediatric patients, ensuring long-term survival remains an unsolved challenge due to the finite durability of donor hearts. This issue is particularly pronounced in children with the most complex CHDs, whose earlier transplant age further widens the gap between "natural" and "transplant-recipient" life expectancy. Despite a 10-year graft survival rate of approximately 70% [40], outcomes after repeat transplantation are significantly worse, with second graft survival dropping to around 30% [41]. These challenges, compounded by persistent organ shortages, highlight the need for alternative strategies [42].

A paradigm shift may lie in integrating long-term MCS with transplantation, redefining the latter as a stepping stone rather than a final solution. Instead of serving solely as an exit strategy for VAD support (i.e., bridge-to-transplant), pediatric heart transplantation could evolve into a bridge-to-permanent VAD support (i.e., reversed-bridge), enabling somatic growth and better anatomical adaptation in younger patients with complex CHD.

Such a paradigm shift is not beyond reach, given the rapid advancements in pediatric VAD technology. Innovations in pump durability, battery technology, and hemocompatibility are set to further improve the feasibility of permanent VAD support. Coupled with growing expertise in outpatient management, these developments promise to revolutionize the management of pediatric heart failure, offering children not only survival but the opportunity to thrive with an extended net life expectancy.

16.7 Summary

The number of children with severe heart failure continues to rise amidst the persistent scarcity of donor hearts for pediatric transplantation. Pediatric MCS will continue to gain clinical importance over time in a true effort to bridge this gap. Ensuring appropriate selection and the optimal application of MCS devices is vital to improving survival outcomes in this vulnerable population. Furthermore, advancements in MCS technology not only address immediate survival needs but also hold the potential to extend net life expectancy, redefining pediatric heart failure management.

References

1. Peng DM, Davies RR, Simpson KE, et al. Seventh annual Society of Thoracic Surgeons Pedimacs report. Ann Thorac Surg. 2024;117(4):690–703.
2. Kirklin JK, Naftel DC, Pagani FD, et al. Seventh INTERMACS annual report: 15,000 patients and counting. J Heart Lung Transplant. 2015;34(12):1495–504.
3. Varshney AS, DeFilippis EM, Cowger JA, et al. Trends and outcomes of left ventricular assist device therapy: JACC focus seminar. J Am Coll Cardiol. 2022;79(11):1092–107.
4. Jorde UP, Saeed O, Koehl D, et al. The Society of Thoracic Surgeons Intermacs 2023 annual report: focus on magnetically levitated devices. Ann Thorac Surg. 2024;117(1):33–44.
5. Birks EJ. The comparative use of ventricular assist devices: differences between Europe and the United States. Tex Heart Inst J. 2010;37(5):565–7.
6. Kirklin JK, Naftel DC, Kormos RL, et al. Fifth INTERMACS annual report: risk factor analysis from more than 6,000 mechanical circulatory support patients. J Heart Lung Transplant. 2013;32(2):141–56.

7. Medtronic press release. 2021. Available at: https://news.medtronic.com/2021-06-03-Medtronic-to-Stop-Distribution-and-Sale-of-HVAD-TM-System. Accessed 1 Nov 2024.
8. Fraser CD Jr, Jaquiss RD, Rosenthal DN, et al. Prospective trial of a pediatric ventricular assist device. N Engl J Med. 2012;367(6):532–41.
9. Adachi I, Fraser CD Jr. Berlin Heart EXCOR Food and Drug Administration investigational device exemption trial. Semin Thorac Cardiovasc Surg. 2013;25(2):100–6.
10. Horton S, d'Udekem Y, Shann F, et al. Extracorporeal membrane oxygenation via sternotomy for circulatory shock. J Thorac Cardiovasc Surg. 2010;139(2):e12–3.
11. MacLaren G, Butt W, Best D, et al. Central extracorporeal membrane oxygenation for refractory pediatric septic shock. Pediatr Crit Care Med. 2011;12(2):133–6.
12. Donker DW, Brodie D, Henriques JPS, et al. Left ventricular unloading during veno-arterial ECMO: a simulation study. ASAIO J. 2019;65(1):11–20.
13. Jiang J, Jain P, Adji A, et al. Afterload pressure and left ventricular contractility synergistically affect left atrial pressure during veno-arterial ECMO. JHLT Open. 2024;3:100044.
14. Puri K, Adachi I. Left heart decompression on extracorporeal membrane oxygenation support and cardiopulmonary bypass. Pediatr Crit Care Med. 2021;22(12):e599–604.
15. Takayama H, Chen JM, Jorde UP, Naka Y. Implantation technique of the CentriMag biventricular assist device allowing ambulatory rehabilitation. Interact Cardiovasc Thorac Surg. 2011;12(2):110–1.
16. Tume SC, Fuentes-Baldemar AA, Anders M, et al. Temporary ventricular assist device support with a catheter-based axial pump: changing the paradigm at a pediatric heart center. J Thorac Cardiovasc Surg. 2023;166(6):1756–63.e2.
17. Cho J, Fuentes-Baldemar AA, Tunuguntla HP, et al. Outcomes of temporary ventricular assist device: a pediatric institutional experience over 25 years. J Thorac Cardiovasc Surg. 2023;166(1):201–11.e2.
18. Lorts A, Eghtesady P, Mehegan M, et al. Outcomes of children supported with devices labeled as "temporary" or short term: a report from the pediatric interagency registry for mechanical circulatory support. J Heart Lung Transplant. 2018;37(1):54–60.
19. Zafar F, Conway J, Bleiweis MS, et al. Berlin Heart EXCOR and ACTION post-approval surveillance study report. J Heart Lung Transplant. 2021;40(4):251–9.
20. Morales DLS, Almond CSD, Jaquiss RDB, et al. Bridging children of all sizes to cardiac transplantation: the initial multicenter North American experience with the Berlin Heart EXCOR ventricular assist device. J Heart Lung Transplant. 2011;30(1):1–8.
21. Kirklin JK, Naftel DC, Kormos RL, et al. Interagency Registry for Mechanically Assisted Circulatory Support (INTERMACS) analysis of pump thrombosis in the HeartMate II left ventricular assist device. J Heart Lung Transplant. 2014;33(1):12–22.
22. Taghavi S, Ward C, Jayarajan SN, et al. Surgical technique influences HeartMate II left ventricular assist device thrombosis. Ann Thorac Surg. 2013;96(4):1259–65.
23. Bansal A, Akhtar F, Zwintscher NP, et al. First pediatric HeartMate 3 implantation: US experience. J Card Surg. 2019;34(11):1383–6.
24. Miera O, Potapov EV, Redlin M, et al. First experiences with the HeartWare ventricular assist system in children. Ann Thorac Surg. 2011;91(4):1256–60.
25. Gregoric ID, Cohn WE, Frazier OH. Diaphragmatic implantation of the HeartWare ventricular assist device. J Heart Lung Transplant. 2011;30(4):467–70.
26. Hoganson DM, Gazit AZ, Boston US, et al. Paracorporeal lung assist devices as a bridge to recovery or lung transplantation in neonates and young children. J Thorac Cardiovasc Surg. 2014;147(1):420–6.
27. Ma M, Yarlagadda VV, Rosenthal DN, et al. A novel inflow cannulation strategy for pediatric mechanical circulatory support in small left ventricles. J Thorac Cardiovasc Surg. 2017;154(3):e47–8.
28. Blume ED, VanderPluym C, Lorts A, et al. Second annual pediatric Interagency Registry for Mechanical Circulatory Support (Pedimacs) report: pre-implant characteristics and outcomes. J Heart Lung Transplant. 2018;37(1):38–45.

29. Adachi I, Peng DM, Hollander SA, et al. Sixth annual Pediatric interagency Registry for Mechanical Circulatory Support (Pedimacs) report: the Society of Thoracic Surgeons Pedimacs annual report. Ann Thorac Surg. 2022;115(5):1098–108.
30. Peng DM, Koehl DA, Cantor RS, et al. Outcomes of children with congenital heart disease implanted with ventricular assist devices: an analysis of the Pediatric Interagency Registry for Mechanical Circulatory Support (Pedimacs). J Heart Lung Transplant. 2018;38:420–30.
31. Adachi I. Ventricular assist device support for complex congenital heart disease: inspiration from history of surgical evolution. J Heart Lung Transplant. 2019;38(4):431–2.
32. Adachi I, Williams E, Jeewa A, et al. Mechanically assisted Fontan completion: a new approach for the failing Glenn circulation due to isolated ventricular dysfunction. J Heart Lung Transplant. 2016;35(11):1380–1.
33. Moon J, Tunuguntla H, Tume S, et al. Ventricular assist device support for failing Glenn circulation: impact of concomitant Fontan completion in select patients. J Heart Lung Transplant. 2023;42(5):637–44.
34. Baldwin JT, Borovetz HS, Duncan BW, et al. The national heart, lung, and blood institute pediatric circulatory support program. Circulation. 2006;113(1):147–55.
35. Baldwin JT, Borovetz HS, Duncan BW, et al. The national heart, lung, and blood institute pediatric circulatory support program: a summary of the 5-year experience. Circulation. 2011;123(11):1233–40.
36. Baldwin JT, Adachi I, Teal J, et al. Closing in on the PumpKIN trial of the Jarvik 2015 ventricular assist device. Semin Thorac Cardiovasc Surg Pediatr Card Surg Annu. 2017;20:9–15.
37. National Library of Medicine (U.S.). Study of [Pumps for Kids, Infants and Neonates (PumpKIN): the Jarvik 2015 pivotal trial (PumpKIN)]. ClinicalTrials.gov. Available at: https://clinicaltrials.gov/study/NCT06348043. Accessed 1 Nov 2024.
38. Almond CS, Davies R, Adachi I, et al. A prospective multicenter feasibility study of a miniaturized implantable continuous flow ventricular assist device in smaller children with heart failure. J Heart Lung Transplant. 2024;43(6):889–900.
39. National Institutes of Health. [The first clinical use of the BiVACOR Total Artificial Heart]. Project No. 10698258. Available at: https://reporter.nih.gov/project-details/10698258. Accessed 1 Nov 2024.
40. Rossano JW, Dipchand AI, Edwards LB, et al. The registry of the international society for heart and lung transplantation: nineteenth pediatric heart transplantation report-2016; focus theme: primary diagnostic indications for transplant. J Heart Lung Transplant. 2016;35:1185–95.
41. Rizvi SA, Luc JGY, Choi JH, et al. Outcomes and survival following heart retransplantation for cardiac allograft failure: a systematic review and meta-analysis. Ann Cardiothorac Surg. 2018;7:12–8.
42. Ubel PA, Arnold RM, Caplan AL. Rationing failure: the ethical lessons of the retransplantation of scarce vital organs. JAMA. 1993;270:2469–74.

Lung Donation After Circulatory Death: Current Challenges and Opportunities in the United States

17

Norihisa Shigemura

Abstract

Since the National Academies of Sciences, Engineering, and Medicine issued a report in 2022 calling for expansion of the supply of transplantable organs, the utilization of lungs acquired through donation after circulatory death (DCD) for transplantation has increased notably in the United States. However, despite collaborative efforts by all stakeholders in the transplant community, the outcomes of DCD lung transplantation have lagged behind the notable successes seen after transplantation of DCD abdominal organs, such as kidneys and livers. To overcome these challenges, the complexities inherent to lung biology and the greater vulnerability of lung tissue to ischemia-reperfusion injury, which make DCD lungs uniquely challenging, need to be understood in depth. The future of DCD lung transplant practices holds promise with evolving strategies potentially capable of bridging this outcome gap. In this review, the potential benefits of transplanting DCD lungs from an organ biology perspective, the evolving role of machines in organ recovery practices, and the role of normothermic regional perfusion in transforming organ recovery will be summarized in light of unique but distinct organ features inherent to lungs.

Keywords

Lung transplantation · DCD · Lung Transplant Collaboratives · Donor pool · Warm ischemic time · DBD · Machine perfusion · NRP · Organ biology

N. Shigemura (✉)
Division of Cardiothoracic Transplantation, University of Pittsburgh, Pittsburgh, PA, USA
e-mail: shigemuran3@upmc.edu

H. Matsuda et al. (eds.), *Heart and Lung Transplantation*,
https://doi.org/10.1007/978-981-96-8810-4_17

17.1 Introduction

A 2022 highly impactful National Academies of Sciences, Engineering, and Medicine(NASEM) report, requested by the United States Congress and sponsored by the National Institutes of Health (NIH), transformed multiple aspects of the clinical practice of organ transplantation [1]. The report strongly advocated equity, accessibility, and improving organ supply across the US transplantation system. One of the significant impacts of this advocacy has been the increased utilization of organs acquired through donation after circulatory death (DCD), which has helped expand the donor pool, particularly in underrepresented populations. DCD donors have been historically underutilized in the entire field of solid organ transplantation [2].

The DCD Lung Transplant Collaborative, organized first in Australia during the early 2010s, has demonstrated the excellent clinical outcomes in DCD lung transplantation during the period of 2006–2011 [3]. In the United States, such activity has launched by Organ Procurement and Transplantation Network (OPTN), ambitiously aimed to improve DCD lung utilization by expanding donor criteria to include lungs from older donors, higher body mass index (BMI) donors, and donors located further from the potential recipient [4]. These adjustments reflect a deliberate broadening of criteria specifically for DCD lungs to address limitations in supply and improve organ availability. This collaborative effort, initiated in late 2022, although bold and challenging, led to a 45% increase in DCD lung transplants across participating centers by mid-2023. The trend of lung transplantation divided by DBD and DCD [6] is shown in Fig. 17.1.

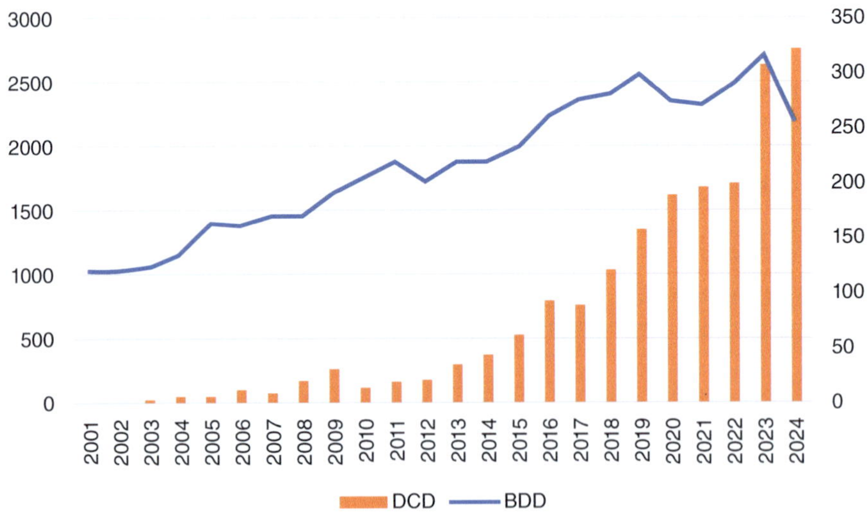

Fig. 17.1 The trend of lung transplantation in the United States, divided by DBD and DCD from 2001 to Nov. 2024. (Data from Ref. [5]. The scale; left: DBD, right: DCD)

For many years, lung transplants in the United States have predominantly used lungs donated by brain-dead donors (DBD). This established a strong bias in favor of transplanting DBD lungs due to their better historical outcomes and predictability. Concerns over lung graft quality stemming from the fear of ischemia-reperfusion injury and associated complications, including primary graft dysfunction (PGD) make many transplant centers cautious about using DCD lungs [6]. Lungs from DCD donors undergo a period of warm ischemia between circulatory arrest and organ procurement, potentially leading to more damage as compared with lungs from DBD donors.

Such biases and concerns about DCD organs, however, have been alleviated with recent, concurrent changes in organ preservation protocols and technologies, evolving roles for machine perfusion (MP), and evolving organ recovery processes, regulations, and logistics [7–9]. In this review, we revisit longstanding questions surrounding the use of lungs from DCD donors and highlight future directions capitalizing on significant opportunities to overcome many of the current challenges in lung transplantation. We will discuss the potential benefits of transplanting DCD lungs from an organ biology perspective, the evolving role of MP in organ recovery practices, and the role of normothermic regional perfusion (NRP) in transforming organ recovery.

17.2 Organ Biology Perspective

From an organ biology and metabolism standpoint, there are several theoretical arguments suggesting that transplanting DCD lungs will likely have advantages over transplanting DBD lungs. Although historically DBD lungs have been preferred due to logistical and clinical factors, there are emerging perspectives that support the potential superiority of DCD lungs in certain respects.

17.2.1 Key Theories Supporting the Use of DCD Lungs

1. **Use of DCD Lungs May Reduce the Catecholamine Storm and Inflammatory Response.**

   In DBD donors, brain death itself triggers a massive sympathetic surge known as the "catecholamine storm". This release of catecholamines (e.g., adrenaline, norepinephrine) leads to systemic vasoconstriction, causing hemodynamic instability, ischemic injury, and inflammatory responses [10]. In the lungs, this can result in increased capillary leakage, alveolar edema, and potential lung injury. This inflammatory environment compromises the lung's structural and functional integrity, making the transplanted lungs more prone to PGD after transplantation [11]. In contrast, DCD donors do not experience brain death, and therefore, this catecholamine surge is avoided. As a result, DCD lungs are less likely to incur the early injury associated with brain death. Theoretically, this should make DCD lungs less inflamed at the time of procurement, potentially preserving their cellular and vascular integrity better as compared with DBD lungs [12].

2. **Shorter Exposure to Mechanical Ventilation.**

   DBD donors are typically maintained on mechanical ventilation for extended periods after the declaration of brain death. Prolonged mechanical ventilation can lead to ventilator-induced lung injury [13], particularly if improper ventilator settings cause overdistension of the alveoli, shear stress, or barotrauma. This mechanical stress is known to injure the alveolar epithelium, contribute to atelectasis, and promote inflammatory processes, all of which may compromise lung function. DCD donors, in contrast, are usually not maintained on mechanical ventilation for extended periods prior to death, in part, because of an expedited process with family-imposed time restrictions [14]. After the withdrawal of life support, the lungs undergo a period of warm ischemia but are less likely to experience the same degree of ventilator-induced lung injury [15]. This may preserve the alveolar architecture and reduce the risk of long-term lung damage.

3. **Metabolic Considerations—Lack of Prolonged Catecholamine and Glucocorticoid Exposure.**

   The catecholamine storm in DBD donors is often accompanied by a surge in stress hormones, such as glucocorticoids. This leads to profound metabolic disturbances including hyperglycemia, insulin resistance, and hypermetabolism. In the lungs, these metabolic disturbances can result in increased oxidative stress, mitochondrial dysfunction, and impaired cellular energy homeostasis [16]. The metabolic derangements can worsen ischemia-reperfusion injury after the lungs are transplanted. Because brain death and its associated metabolic dysregulation are absent in DCD donors, organs recovered from DCD donors maintain more balanced metabolic homeostasis. The absence of excessive hormonal stress could theoretically preserve mitochondrial function, enhance cellular respiration, and reduce oxidative damage, leading to better post-transplant graft recovery [17].

4. **Better Preserved Vascular Endothelium.**

   The inflammatory storm in DBD donors also affects the pulmonary vasculature, causing endothelial dysfunction, increased permeability, and microthrombi formation [18]. This can impair gas exchange and increase the risk of acute lung injury or early graft failure. Lungs from DCD donors may avoid these vascular complications. Without sustained inflammatory and hormonal disruptions, the pulmonary endothelial cells in DCD lungs may remain more intact, preserving normal vasodilatory responses and barrier function. This may contribute to reduced post-transplant edema and better graft function.

5. **Lower Risk of Pulmonary Edema.**

   The combination of inflammation, endothelial damage, and prolonged mechanical ventilation in DBD donors often leads to the development of pulmonary edema in the transplant recipient [19]. This edema makes it harder to oxygenate the lungs, can lead to PGD, and may increase the need for post-transplant intensive care. By avoiding the chain of events that lead to brain death-associated pulmonary edema, DCD lungs might be placed in the recipient in a less edematous state. This could improve the initial function of the lungs, reduce the incidence of PGD, and speed up recovery.

17.3 The Evolving Role of Machine Perfusion in Transformative Organ Recovery Practices

Machine perfusion (MP), whether under moderately hypothermic, subnormothermic, or normothermic conditions, has indeed resulted in significantly better outcomes after kidney or liver transplantation using DCD organs [20]. However, in lungs, this improvement has not yet been consistently demonstrated or clearly appreciated [21].

17.3.1 Key Differences in MP Between DCD Lungs and DCD Kidneys and Livers

1. **Different Roles and Contributions of Ex Vivo Lung Perfusion (EVLP) as MP in Lung Grafts**

   While ex vivo lung perfusion (EVLP) has been instrumental in assessing and improving the quality of marginal donor lungs (both DBD and DCD), the outcomes of transplantation using DCD lungs placed in EVLP have not demonstrated the same dramatic improvements that have been observed after MP of donated kidneys and livers. The reasons for this are multifaceted and include differences in physiology, tolerance for warm ischemia, and the inherent limitations of EVLP. The lungs are highly sensitive to ischemia-reperfusion injury and have complex immune responses due to constant exposure to the external environment [22]. This makes mitigating ischemia-reperfusion injury in the lungs more challenging as compared with mitigation in abdominal organs. Lungs tend to tolerate warm ischemia better than kidneys and livers due to their ability to utilize anaerobic metabolism for longer periods [23]. Therefore, while EVLP is useful for assessing and rehabilitating DCD lungs, the outcomes after transplantation using these lungs have not been significantly better than those observed using DBD lungs [21]. Finally, the degree of recovery post-transplantation, particularly for DCD lungs, remains more limited [24] as compared with the dramatic improvements seen after normothermic perfusion of donated kidneys and livers.
2. **Distinct Features of the Lungs**

   The lungs have different metabolic demands than the kidneys and the liver. While kidneys and livers benefit significantly from metabolic support during perfusion (especially during moderately hypothermic or normothermic perfusion) [25], donated lungs might not derive the same metabolic boost, as their primary function is gas exchange rather than metabolic work. Although EVLP may help in reconditioning donated lungs, reperfusion injury and immune responses in the lungs tend to be more pronounced as compared with abdominal organs, complicating the recovery process even after EVLP [26]. Airway ischemia and reperfusion pose a greater risk for lungs as compared with other organs, and PGD remains a key concern after lung transplantation, particularly in transplanted DCD lungs. The unique structure of the lungs and their reliance on the microvascular circulation may also make recovery more complex, even after EVLP [27]. Moreover, the full potential of EVLP and refinements in lung perfusion technologies are still being realized. While kidney and liver transplantation have benefited rapidly from advancements in perfusion technologies, the lungs may require more targeted strategies. These strategies may include prolonged EVLP with prone positioning or improved perfusion protocols with additives to maximize the benefits of reconditioning [28].

17.4 Transforming Organ Recovery with Normothermic Regional Perfusion in the Lung

The development of normothermic regional perfusion (NRP) had played a pivotal role in the recent notable progress and successful outcomes of DCD transplantation [29]. Indeed, the increase in DCD procedures and the development of NRP have influenced each other, contributing to the growing success of DCD transplantation.

17.4.1 Key Differences Between Lung Transplantation and Transplantation of Other Solid Organs Associated with NRP

1. **The Synergistic Evolution of NRP and DCD Observed in Kidney, Liver, and Heart Transplantation Has Not Been Seen in Lung Transplantation**

   Because NRP continues to show strong results through mitigating the incidences of posttransplant complications associated with organ grafts quality (e.g., biliary complications after liver transplant), it has made DCD donation more attractive to both clinicians and families. Some transplant centers have adopted an aggressive approach, utilizing NRP routinely for DCD donors and thereby increasing the number of transplants performed [30]. The success of NRP has allowed transplant programs to become more confident in accepting and utilizing DCD organs, especially for complex and delicate transplant procedures, such as heart transplant. Without NRP, it was previously unthinkable to transplant hearts from DCD donors [31].

   In lung transplantation, however, the success of NRP remains limited due to multiple factors, largely the distinct physiological characteristics of each organ, lungs versus others, relating to lungs being more vulnerable to edema, making warm ischemia and the reestablishment of perfusion during NRP particularly delicate despite restoring perfusion with controlled pressure and flow (Fig. 17.2).

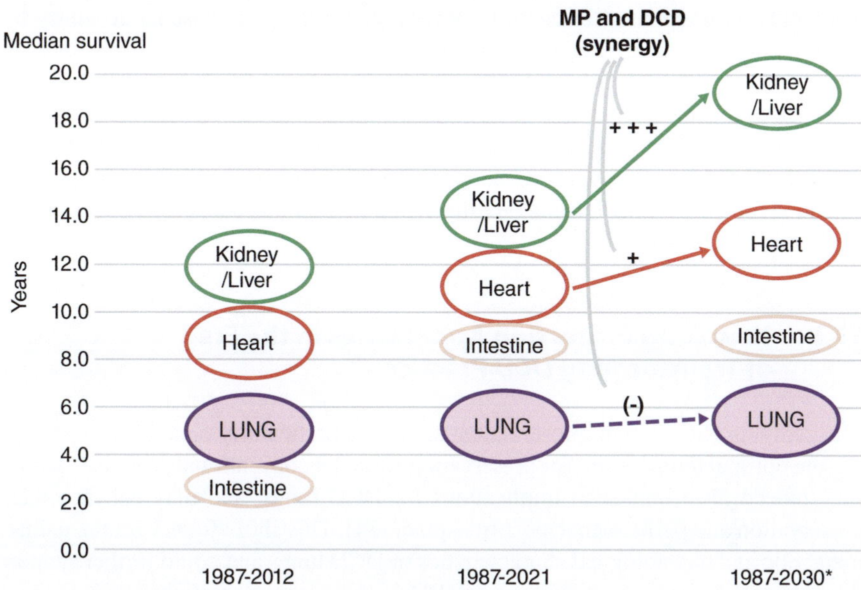

Fig. 17.2 Median survival of solid organ transplants: Where do lungs stand vs. other solid organs in the era of DCD and MP. The past (1987–2012), recent (1987–2021), and potential future (1987–2030) survival outcomes after solid organ transplant for each organ type, and the impact of organ preservation technology with machine perfusion (MP) in the era of increasing donation after circulatory death (DCD). +++ = synergistic, + = additive, and – = minimal benefits

2. **Organ-Specific Physiological Characteristics**

   Organ-specific physiological characteristics likely influence the efficacy of NRP as well. The lungs' unique structure and physiology—thin alveolar walls, the need for continuous ventilation, and susceptibility to pulmonary edema—make maintaining the lung under controlled, optimal conditions during NRP challenging. Reperfusion pressure and flow must be carefully controlled to avoid damaging the fragile pulmonary vasculature. In contrast, kidneys and livers are more tolerant to ischemia than the lungs, making NRP a more feasible strategy for restoring blood flow after DCD. In the liver, for instance, biliary complications and metabolic recovery are closely tied with how well ischemic damage is minimized through techniques like NRP [32].

17.4.2 Key Differences Between NRP and EVLP

NRP and EVLP serve fundamentally different roles and cannot be directly compared, even though both aim to improve outcomes after transplantation, particularly when using organs from DCD donors. While they may overlap in their general purpose for organ preservation and viability assessment, their functions, settings, and contributions differ significantly. NRP occurs in situ and aims to restore perfusion as quickly as possible after death to prevent or reverse warm ischemic injury by using the donor's own vasculature, keeping the organs perfused under physiologic conditions before organ retrieval [33]. EVLP takes place outside the body, and was designed to rehabilitate, assess, and optimize the lungs in a controlled environment. EVLP allows for additional evaluation to determine whether lungs initially deemed to be of marginal quality are suitable for transplantation. EVLP's goal is to provide extended time for evaluation and possible repair of the lung, particularly in marginal quality or DCD lungs.

17.5 New Lung Protection Approaches in the Era of Transforming DCD Practice

The evolving shift in lung preservation strategies, particularly conceptually changing the optimal temperature for preservation from the conventional 4 °C to 8–10 °C, may indeed have important implications for DCD lungs, and may enhance their preservation and performance post-transplant [34]. This shift aligns with the unique metabolic and physiological characteristics of DCD lungs and could further support the potential advantages of DCD over DBD for lung transplantation.

Additionally, in reality, misunderstandings in the lung-transplant community pertaining to DCD transplantation have been present and do not realistically portray newly available EVLP techniques and technology and other organ-preservative strategies [35]. We will further discuss and share these important considerations elsewhere in the near future, as overcoming biases will be an important factor in the widespread adoption of DCD lung transplantation.

17.6 Conclusion

The longstanding biases and concerns over the quality of DCD lungs have been alleviated with recent, concurrent changes in organ preservation protocols and technologies, evolving roles for machine perfusion, and evolving organ recovery process, regulations, and logistics. To capitalize those advantages with DCD lungs, however, deep understanding of distinct organ biology features and robust scientific evidence-based organ preservation techniques inherent to lungs is of paramount importance to move the field in the right directions.

Funding Sources None.

References

1. Realizing the promise of equity in the organ transplantation system. National Academies Press;2022. https://nap.nationalacademies.org/read/26364/chapter/1. Accessed 8 Nov 2024.
2. Morrissey PE, Monaco AP. Donation after circulatory death: current practices, ongoing challenges, and potential improvements. Transplantation. 2014;97(3):258–64.

3. Levvey BJ, Harkess M, Hopkins P, et al. Excellent clinical outcomes from a national donation-after-determination-of-cardiac-death lung transplant collaborative. Am J Transplant. 2012;12:2406–13.
4. https://optn.transplant.hrsa.gov/media/20soedz1/optn-dcd-lung-transplant-collaborative-executive-report.pdf. Accessed 8 Nov 2024.
5. unos.org/news/dcd-lung-transplant-collaborative/. Accessed 8 Nov 2024.
6. Sabashnikov A, Patil NP, Popov A, et al. Long-term results after lung transplantation using organs from circulatory death donors: a propensity score-matched analysis. Eur J Cardiothorac Surg. 2016;49(1):46–53.
7. van Rijn R, Schurink IJ, de Vries Y, van den Berg AP, et al. Hypothermic machine perfusion in liver transplantation – a randomized trial. N Engl J Med. 2021;384(15):1391–401.
8. Abu-Gazala S, Tang H, Abt P, et al. National trends in utilization of normothermic machine perfusion in DCD liver transplantation. Transplant Direct. 2024;10(5):e1596. https://doi.org/10.1097/TXD.0000000000001596.
9. Aburahma K, Davide de Manna N, Kuehn C, et al. Pushing the survival bar higher: two decades of innovation in lung transplantation. J Clin Med. 2024;13(18):5516.
10. Floerchinger B, Oberhuber R, Tullius SG. Effects of brain death on organ quality and transplant outcome. Transplant Rev (Orland). 2012;26(2):54–9.
11. Avlonitis VS, Fisher AJ, Dark JH. Pulmonary transplantation: the role of brain death in donor lung injury. Transplantation. 2003;75(12):1928–33.
12. Ruttens D, Martens A, Ordies S, et al. Short- and long-term outcomes after lung transplantation from circulatory-dead donors: a single-center experience. Transplantation. 2017;101(11):2691–4.
13. Mal H, Santin G, Cantrelle C, et al. Effects of lung-protective ventilation in organ donors on lung procurement and recipient survival. Am J Respir Crit Care Med. 2020;202(2):250–8.
14. Erasmus ME, van Raemdonck D, Akhtar MZ, et al. DCD lung donation: donor criteria, procedural criteria, pulmonary graft function validation, and preservation. Transpl Int. 2016;29(7):790–7.
15. Levvey B, Keshavjee S, Cypel M, et al. Influence of lung donor agonal and warm ischemic times on early mortality: analyses from the ISHLT DCD lung transplant registry. J Heart Lung Transplant. 2019;38(1):26–34.
16. Taylor ME, Jaishankar D, Ho JW, et al. Mitochondrial responses to brain death in solid organ transplant. Front Transplant. 2023;2 https://doi.org/10.3389/frtra.2023.1082227.
17. Tan YB, Pastukh VM, Gorodnya OM, et al. Enhanced mitochondrial DNA repair resuscitates transplantable lungs donated after circulatory death. J Surg Res. 245:273–80.
18. Vieira RF, Breithaupt-Faloppa AC, Matsubara BC, et al. 17 beta-estradiol protects against lung injuries after brain death in male rats. J Heart Lung Transplant. 2018;37(11):1381–7.
19. Wong A, Liu M. Inflammatory responses in lungs from donation after brain death: mechanisms and potential therapeutic targets. J Heart Lung Transplant. 2021;40(9):890–6.
20. Hosgood SA, Callaghan CJ, Wilson CH, et al. Normothermic machine perfusion versus static cold storage in donation after circulatory death kidney transplantation: a randomized controlled trial. Nat Med. 2023;29(6):1511–9.
21. Li SS, Funamoto M, Singh R, et al. Outcomes of donation after circulatory death (DCD) and ex-vivo lung perfusion (EVLP) lung transplantation. J Heart Lung Transplant. 2024;S1053-2498(24):01890–4.
22. Zheng XY, Huang H, Wei ZT, et al. Genetic effect of ischemia-reperfusion injury upon primary graft dysfunction and chronic lung allograft dysfunction in lung transplantation: evidence based on transcriptome data. Transpl Immunol. 2022;71:101556. https://doi.org/10.1016/j.trim.2022.101556.
23. Yu J, Xu C, Lee JS, et al. Rapid postmortem ventilation improves donor lung viability by extending the tolerable warm ischemic time after cardiac death in mice. Am J Physiol Lung Cell Mol Physiol. 2021;321(4):L653–62.

24. Slama A, Schillab L, Barta M, et al. Standard donor lung procurement with normothermic ex vivo lung perfusion: a prospective randomized clinical trial. J Heart Lung Transplant. 2017;36(7):744–53.
25. Raigani S, De Vries RJ, Uygun K, et al. Pumping new life into old ideas: preservation and rehabilitation of the liver using ex situ machine perfusion. Artif Organs. 2020;44(2):123–8.
26. Gouchoe DA, Sanchez P, D'Cunha J, et al. Ex vivo lung perfusion in donation after circulatory death: a post hoc analysis of the normothermic ex vivo lung perfusion as an assessment of extended/marginal donor lungs trial. J Thorac Cardiovasc Surg. 2024;168(3):724–34.
27. Tane S, Noda K, Toyoda Y, et al. Bronchial-arterial-circulation-sparing lung preservation: a new organ protection approach for lung transplantation. Transplantation. 2020;104(3):490–9.
28. Niikawa H, Okamoto T, Ayyat K, et al. Prone ex vivo lung perfusion protects human lungs from reperfusion injury. Artif Organs. 2022;46(11):2226–33.
29. Minambres E, Suberviola B, Dominguez-Gil B, et al. Improving the outcomes of organs obtained from controlled donation after circulatory death donors using abdominal normothermic regional perfusion. Am J Transplant. 2017;17(8):2165–72.
30. Kathawate RG, Abt PL, Bittermann T. Center expansion of liver transplants using donation after circulatory death organs is associated with reduced overall waitlist mortality. Clin Transpl. 2023;37(6):e14960.
31. Siddiqi HK, Trahanas J, Xu N, et al. Outcomes of heart transplant donation after circulatory death. J Am Coll Cardiol. 2023;82(15):1512–20.
32. Gaurav R, Butler AJ, Kosmoliaptsis V, et al. Liver transplantation outcomes from controlled circulatory death donors: SCS vs in situ NRP vs ex situ NMP. Ann Surg. 2022;275(6):1156–64.
33. Hessheimer AJ, Coll E, Torres F, et al. Normothermic regional perfusion vs. super-rapid recovery in controlled donation after circulatory death liver transplantation. J Hepatol. 2019;70(4):658–65.
34. Ali A, Hoetzenecker K, dela Cruz J, et al. Extension of cold static donor lung preservation at 10C. NEJM Evid. 2023;2(6):EVIDoa2300008.
35. Panconesi R, Carvalho MF, Dondossola D, et al. Impact of machine perfusion on the immune response after liver transplantation – a preliminary treatment or just a delivery tool. Front Immunol. 2022;13. https://www.frontiersin.org/journals/immunology/articles/10.3389/fimmu.2022.855263/full

Advancing Donor Lung Preservation and Repair: The Role of Machine Perfusion in Modern Lung Transplantation

18

Takashi Kanou and Yasushi Shintani

Abstract

Lung preservation is crucial for successful transplantation, especially when using marginal donor lungs. Novel organ preservation methods have been developed to improve the quality of donor lungs. Additionally, machine perfusion has been developed and applied clinically for the evaluation of donor lungs. Ex vivo lung perfusion (EVLP) enables normothermic evaluation of donor lungs, assessing parameters like gas exchange and compliance while also allowing therapeutic interventions. Recent studies have explored the use of gene therapy and mesenchymal stem cells (MSCs) during EVLP to reduce ischemia-reperfusion injury and improve graft function. EVLP has proven effective in treating injuries like pneumonia or aspiration damage, offering a promising platform for lung repair. With continued advancements in EVLP, extended preservation and better repair strategies are expected to enhance lung transplantation outcomes.

Keywords

Lung transplantation · DCD · Brain-dead donor · Machine perfusion · Ex vivo lung perfusion · Gene therapy · Cell therapy · Organ preservation · Calpain inhibitor

T. Kanou (✉) · Y. Shintani
Department of General Thoracic Surgery, The University of Osaka Graduate School of Medicine, Suita, Osaka, Japan
e-mail: yshintani@thoracic.med.osaka-u.ac.jp

H. Matsuda et al. (eds.), *Heart and Lung Transplantation*,
https://doi.org/10.1007/978-981-96-8810-4_18

18.1 Introduction

As a countermeasure against donor shortages in brain-dead lung transplantation, the proactive use of marginal donor lungs has been proposed. In Japan, high-quality donor management through the Medical Consultant System has already enabled over 60% of brain-dead donor lungs to be utilized for transplantation [1]. However, some brain-dead donor lungs may suffer from various injuries caused by conditions such as brain-death-related lung injury (e.g., neurogenic pulmonary edema), ventilator-associated lung injury (e.g., barotrauma or infection), blood transfusion, trauma, or aspiration pneumonia. These injuries may exacerbate graft dysfunction, particularly primary graft dysfunction (PGD), which results from ischemia-reperfusion injury following transplantation. In lung transplantation, graft dysfunction remains a leading cause of early post-transplant mortality. The condition of donor organs is a critical factor directly influencing post-transplant outcomes. Therefore, the use of such marginal donor lungs necessitates advanced organ preservation techniques that can accurately evaluate donor lung injury before transplantation and effectively prevent PGD.

In the advancement of organ preservation, machine perfusion (MP) has emerged as an indispensable tool. This chapter provides an overview of the history and evolution of organ preservation in lung transplantation, along with a comprehensive summary of the current state of MP.

18.2 Organ Preservation

Lung preservation is the process of maintaining the lungs removed prior to transplantation in an optimal condition, and it significantly impacts the success of lung transplantation. Research on lung preservation techniques has been a longstanding topic, even before the advent of clinical lung transplantation. From the 1990s to the 2000s, various studies were conducted on preservation solutions, perfusion methods, and techniques for maintaining lung inflation during extraction, leading to the establishment of clinical practices. Meanwhile, research has been conducted on improving organ function and mitigating ischemia-reperfusion injury by adding pharmacological agents to preservation solutions. Traditionally, the cold storage method preserved lungs at near-freezing temperatures, but this approach carries the risk of progressive cellular and tissue damage over time. In recent years, basic and clinical studies on preservation temperatures have regained significant attention.

18.3 Preservation Solution

Compared to kidneys and livers, the lungs have a shorter cold preservation limit and are more susceptible to damage after removal. Consequently, ischemic time being kept within 8 h is considered the top priority in recipient selection criteria for brain-dead lung transplantation. However, improvements in organ preservation solutions and the development of solutions tailored for lung preservation have significantly extended cold preservation times in experimental settings.

Initially, intracellular-type preservation solutions used for kidneys and livers, such as Euro Collins (EC) solution and University of Wisconsin (UW) solution, were employed for lung preservation. In recent years, however, the extracellular-type solution Perfadex has become widely used in major lung transplantation centers in Europe and the United States. Meanwhile, in Japan, ET-Kyoto solution, developed by Kyoto University, is commonly used in many transplantation centers.

ET-Kyoto solution has three key characteristics: (1) its composition resembles extracellular electrolyte solutions, (2) it contains trehalose as a sugar component, and (3) it is stable even at room temperature. While its sodium content is lower and potassium content is higher than standard extracellular solutions, studies have reported that its electrolyte composition offers the highest effectiveness for lung preservation [2]. Trehalose, a non-reducing disaccharide found abundantly in plants and insects that thrive in harsh environments, is widely used in food and cosmetics. It provides protective effects for cell membranes against cold and dehydration and has antioxidant properties.

In recent years, advancements in lung preservation have focused on adding various pharmacological agents to mitigate damage during preservation and after reperfusion. Previous studies have demonstrated that cell death plays a significant role in the pathophysiology of ischemia-reperfusion lung injury following prolonged preservation. This finding has sparked interest in novel strategies targeting cell death to improve graft function. The author has shown that suppressing the activation of RIPK-1 (Receptor Interacting Protein Kinase 1), a key pathway involved in necroptosis, can reduce ischemia-reperfusion lung injury after prolonged preservation [3]. These research findings highlight the importance of inhibiting the activation of necroptosis pathways during preservation, and the author continues to pursue this research theme.

18.4 Preservation Temperature

The optimal preservation temperature for lungs in transplantation has been a subject of repeated discussion. Traditionally, donor lungs have been stored on ice in a cooled container, maintained at 4 °C from procurement to transplantation. However, experimental studies in the 1990s suggested that lung function after transplantation might be better preserved at a higher temperature, prompting a proposal to store lungs at 10 °C. Despite this, practical considerations led to the continued use of ice boxes for preservation.

Recently, a research group in Toronto demonstrated that lung preservation at 10 °C stabilizes mitochondrial function and maintains donor organ viability [4]. Lungs stored at 10 °C were found to have higher levels of metabolites that protect mitochondria—such as itaconate, glutamine, and N-acetylglutamine—compared to those stored at 4 °C. This mechanism reportedly enables prolonged graft function after transplantation. Functional assessments during ex vivo lung perfusion (EVLP) showed that porcine lungs preserved at 10 °C for 36 hours had better compliance and improved gas exchange compared to lungs preserved at 4 °C.

Based on these findings, a multicenter clinical study involving high-volume centers such as Toronto and Vienna was conducted. The study compared outcomes of clinical lung transplantations in which donor lungs were preserved for prolonged periods (12–14 h) at 10 °C with those preserved for less than 8 h at 4 °C [5]. The results demonstrated comparable short- and long-term post-transplant outcomes between the two groups. The 10 °C preservation system is relatively simple, utilizing gel packs arranged inside a traditional cooler to maintain an internal temperature of 10 °C [6]. Future research will focus on introducing this system in Japan.

18.5 Machine Perfusion

To address the shortage of donor lungs in lung transplantation, especially in Japan, the proactive use of marginal donor lungs is crucial. This requires evaluating graft function prior to transplantation to determine their suitability. Internationally, lungs donated after cardiac death (DCD) present additional challenges compared to brain-dead donors, as assessing the extent of injury during the agonal phase and warm ischemia is more difficult.

For the safe utilization of such "injured lungs," it is essential to objectively evaluate the quality of donor lungs prior to transplantation. Currently, ex vivo lung perfusion (EVLP) is gaining international attention, with various clinical trials being conducted, particularly in North America. EVLP preserves donor lungs at normothermic conditions (37 °C) while maintaining ventilation and perfusion. This enables accurate pre-transplant evaluation of lung function and extends the preservation time of donor organs.

18.6 Clinical Implementation of Ex Vivo Lung Perfusion

Currently, three main types of EVLP systems are in use [7]. The Toronto system utilizes a closed-circuit extracorporeal membrane oxygenation (ECMO) type setup, a dome-shaped organ chamber, and specialized pulmonary artery and left atrial cannulas. It employs STEEN Solution (XVIVO Perfusion AB, Göteborg, Sweden), a low-potassium dextran-40 and albumin-containing extracellular fluid, as the perfusate [8]. The Lund system uses the Lund Vivoline LS1 system (Vivoline Medical AB, Lund, Sweden) with STEEN Solution mixed with red blood cells as the perfusate. The third system is the compact, portable Organ Care System (OCS) (TransMedics, Andover, MA, USA), which integrates a ventilator, pulsatile pump, heat exchanger, and monitoring system. The perfusate used in this system consists of OCS-specific solution mixed with red blood cells. A distinctive feature of the OCS is that ventilation and perfusion can begin immediately after donor lung retrieval, allowing graft function to be evaluated during transportation to the transplant center.

The Toronto group conducted the world's first clinical trial using EVLP and reported its favorable outcomes in 2011 [9]. The short-term post-transplant outcomes of 20 lung transplant cases using EVLP with marginal donor lungs (EVLP group) were comparable to those of 116 standard lung transplant cases without EVLP (non-EVLP group). The incidence of PGD grade 2 or 3 at 72 h post-transplant was 15% in the EVLP group compared to 30% in the non-EVLP group. Perioperative mortality rates were 10% in the EVLP group and 5% in the non-EVLP group. More recently, the same group reported favorable long-term outcomes from 230 lung transplants performed using EVLP. The 3-, 5-, and 9-year CLAD-free survival rates were 70%, 56%, and 53%, respectively, in the EVLP group, compared to 72%, 56%, and 36%, respectively, in the non-EVLP group [10].

With the accumulation of clinical cases since its introduction, EVLP is now widely utilized at many transplant centers worldwide.

18.7 Future Perspective of Ex Vivo Lung Perfusion

EVLP not only enables the evaluation of physiological parameters such as gas exchange capacity and compliance prior to transplantation but also allows for the assessment of pulmonary edema over time using bronchoscopy and X-rays. In addition to these parameters obtainable in real-time, the analysis of perfusate holds significant importance. The authors have demonstrated that quantifying cell-free DNA released from injured lungs correlates with the development of PGD [9]. These findings suggest that perfusate analysis is a valuable tool for identifying biomarkers, and recent advancements have explored the use of deep learning to predict post-transplant outcomes more accurately [10].

In recent years, there has been growing attention on utilizing the EVLP system, which enables long-term organ preservation, not merely as a method for evaluating marginal donor lung function but as a platform for pre-transplant treatment and repair of injured lungs. The advantages of treating injured lungs ex vivo include: (1) the ability to perform invasive treatments that are difficult to carry out in multi-organ donors with impaired lung function, (2) the ability to treat and repair the lungs without concern for effects on other organs, and (3) the ability to specifically evaluate the effects of treatment on lung injury.

Brain-dead donor lungs may suffer from various injuries, such as neurogenic pulmonary edema, ventilator-associated lung injury (barotrauma or infection), transfusion-related injuries, trauma, and aspiration pneumonia. During EVLP, individualized treatments tailored to these specific injuries are necessary. Among these, many donor lungs are deemed unsuitable for transplantation due to damage caused by pneumonia. The Toronto group reported that broad-spectrum antibiotic treatment during EVLP improved lung function and significantly reduced bacterial counts in donor lungs, endotoxin levels in the perfusate, and pro-inflammatory cytokines (TNF-α, IL-1β, MIP-1α, MIP-1β) associated with PGD post-transplantation [11]. Similarly, aspiration pneumonia is another major factor contributing to donor lung injury. As a treatment method for donor lungs, administering surfactant intratracheally during EVLP in porcine donor lungs with aspiration pneumonia has been shown to improve both inflammation and graft function.

Additionally, research is advancing on therapeutic interventions involving gene delivery using viral vectors during EVLP perfusion. In studies using lungs deemed unsuitable for clinical transplantation, the intratracheal administration of an adenoviral vector encoding human IL-10 during a 12-h EVLP session improved gas exchange in the graft [12]. Regarding cell-based therapies, treatments using mesenchymal stem cells (MSCs) during EVLP are being developed. Studies have shown that administering MSCs to donor lungs during EVLP improves graft function post-lung transplantation. Furthermore, forcing MSCs to overexpress the anti-inflammatory cytokine IL-10 and administering them has been reported to enhance graft function and reduce inflammation post-transplantation [13]. Thus, EVLP is expected as a platform for treating donor lungs prior to transplantation.

In the future, with further advancements in EVLP technology, it is anticipated that organ preservation for days will become feasible. This could pave the way for organ repair during EVLP through the use of gene therapy and cell therapy with diverse anti-inflammatory and immunomodulatory effects.

18.8 Research in Our Department

The author has demonstrated that inhibiting the activation of RIPK-1 (Receptor Interacting Protein Kinase 1), which is involved in necroptosis, a form of cell death, can mitigate ischemia-reperfusion lung injury after prolonged preservation [3]. These research findings indicate that suppressing the activation of the necroptosis pathway during preservation is crucial, and the author is continuing to investigate this topic. The rat lung transplantation model learned at the University of Toronto was based on the model originally established by Dr. Mizuta, a distinguished senior member of the First Department of Surgery at Osaka University (see Chap. 8 of this book). We also continue to perform research using such animal experiments in our department. The following research projects are being conducted in collaboration with young graduate students, primarily using the rat transplantation model.

18.9 Improvement of Organ Preservation Using Calpain Inhibitors

The regulation of necroptosis involves not only RIPK-1 but also other molecules such as MLKL, as reported in various studies [3, 16, 17]. Among these, we focused on a report demonstrating the suppression of necroptosis using calpain inhibitors [17]. In this study, it was shown that the calpain inhibitor ALLN effectively inhibited cell death, and its underlying mechanism was elucidated. Our experimental verification using an animal model demonstrated a significant protective effect against lung injury, as evidenced by improved gas exchange function and a reduced wet-to-dry weight ratio, a key indicator of pulmonary edema (Fig. 18.1). Notably,

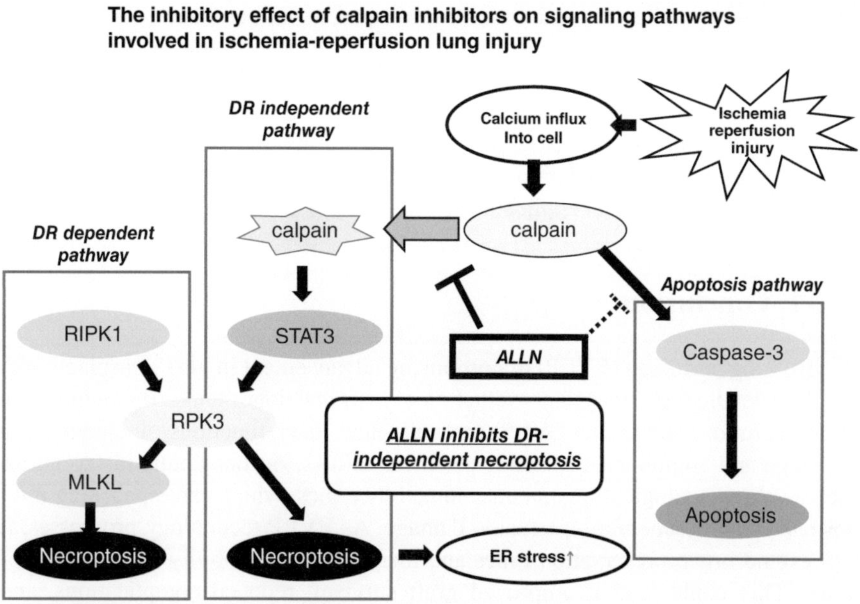

Fig. 18.1 Graphical abstract of the protective effect of calpain inhibition on ischemia-reperfusion lung injury. *DR* Death Receptor, *ER* Endoplasmic Reticulum, *RIPK* Receptor Interacting Protein Kinase. (Courtesy of Dr. Yasushi Shintani)

unlike Nec-1, the addition of the calpain inhibitor solely to the perfusate (administered to the donor only) without recipient administration significantly suppressed organ damage. These findings provide evidence that adding calpain inhibitors to the perfusion preservation solution can inhibit necroptosis and improve graft function in transplanted lungs. However, since this inhibitor is not yet clinically applicable, future research aims to identify clinically applicable drugs with similar effects for potential clinical translation.

18.10 Establishment of a DCD Model and Suppression of Cell Death

The central research question in this study is: "Can we suppress organ dysfunction during the process of DCD lung transplantation to enable safer lung transplantation?" To investigate this question, we are currently developing a rat lung transplantation model simulating controlled DCD, which is the predominant form of DCD in Western countries. Two hours after reperfusion, the animals will be sacrificed, followed by blood gas analysis to evaluate gas exchange function, Western blot analysis to examine necroptosis pathway activation, and histopathological assessment.

To achieve the objectives of this study, we are focusing on two main aspects: (1) analyzing how necroptosis pathways are activated at different time points during the

DCD process by collecting and examining samples at various stages, and (2) evaluating the therapeutic effects of anti-necroptosis drugs (Nec-1 and ALLN as candidates) in mitigating graft dysfunction caused by the DCD process. Through these experimental analyses, we aim to optimize intervention methods (such as perfusate addition and recipient administration), determine effective dosages, and establish a translational research foundation to clarify the therapeutic efficacy of these interventions for future clinical applications.

18.11 Conclusion

Ex vivo lung perfusion (EVLP) is a promising advancement in lung transplantation, enabling detailed pre-transplant evaluation of marginal donor lungs. By maintaining normothermic conditions, EVLP assesses key lung functions, including gas exchange and compliance. Machine perfusion allows for therapeutic interventions such as pharmacological treatments and cell therapies, which can repair lung injuries and reduce ischemia-reperfusion damage. As EVLP technology progresses, it will extend organ preservation times and increase the availability of viable donor lungs. This could lead to improved graft survival, reduced complications, and broader access to lung transplantation.

References

1. Hoshikawa Y, Okada Y, Ashikari J, et al. Medical consultant system for improving lung transplantation opportunities and outcomes in Japan. Transplant Proc. 2015;47:746–50.
2. Wada H, Liu CJ, Hirata T, et al. Effective 30-hour preservation of canine lungs with modified ET-Kyoto solution. Ann Thorac Surg. 1996;61:1099–05.
3. Kanou T, Ohsumi A, Kim H, et al. Inhibition of regulated necrosis attenuates receptor-interacting protein kinase 1-mediated ischemia-reperfusion injury after lung transplantation. J Heart Lung Transplant. 2018;37:1261–70.
4. Ali A, Wang A, Ribeiro R, et al. Static lung storage at 10 °C maintains mitochondrial health and preserves donor organ function. Sci Transl Med. 2021;13(611):abf7601. https://doi.org/10.1126/scitranslmed.abf7601.
5. Ali A, Hoetzenecker K, Luis Campo-Cañaveral de la Cruz J, et al. Extension of cold static donor lung preservation at 10 °C. NEJM Evid. 2023;2(6):EVIDoa2300008. https://doi.org/10.1056/EVIDoa2300008. Epub 2023 Apr 20.
6. Cenik I, Slambrouck JV, Provoost AL, et al. Controlled hypothermic storage for lung preservation: leaving the ice age behind. Gen Thorac Cardiovasc Surg. 2021;69:625–30.
7. Nakajima D, Date H. Ex vivo lung perfusion in lung transplantation. Gen Thorac Cardiovasc Surg. 2021;69:625–30.
8. Watanabe T, Cypel M, Keshavjee S. Ex vivo lung perfusion. J Thorac Dis. 2021;13:6602–17. https://doi.org/10.21037/jtd-2021-23.
9. Cypel M, Yeung JC, Liu M, et al. Normothermic ex vivo lung perfusion in clinical lung transplantation. N Engl J Med. 2011;364:1431–40.
10. Divithotawela C, Cypel M, Martinu T, et al. Long-term outcomes of lung transplant with ex vivo lung perfusion. JAMA Surg. 2019;154:1143–50.

11. Kanou T, Nakahira K, Choi AM, et al. Cell-free DNA in human ex vivo lung perfusate as a potential biomarker to predict the risk of primary graft dysfunction in lung transplantation. J Thorac Cardiovasc Surg. 2021;162:490–9.
12. Sage AT, Donahoe L, Shamandy AA, et al. A machine-learning approach to human ex vivo lung perfusion predicts transplantation outcomes and promotes organ utilization. Nat Commun. 2023;14:4810. https://www.nature.com/articles/s41467-023-40468-7
13. Nakajima D, Cypel M, Bonato R, et al. Ex vivo perfusion treatment of infection in human donor lungs. Am J Transplant. 2016;16:1229–37.
14. Cypel M, Liu M, Rubacha M, et al. Functional repair of human donor lungs by IL-10 gene therapy. Sci Transl Med. 2009;1:4ra9.
15. Nykanen A, Mariscal A, Duong A, et al. Lung transplant immunomodulation with genetically engineered mesenchymal stromal cells-therapeutic window for Interleukin-10. Cells. 2024;13:859. https://doi.org/10.3390/cells13100859.
16. Kim H, Zamel R, Bai XH, et al. Ischemia-reperfusion induces death receptor-independent necroptosis via calpain-STAT3 activation in a lung transplant setting. Am J Physiol Lung Cell Mol Physiol. 2018;315(4):L595–608.
17. Matsui Y, Kanou T, Matsui T, et al. Protective effect of calpain inhibition during cold ischemia on ischemia-reperfusion injury after lung transplantation. Transplantation. 2023;107(9):1945–54.

19 Marginal Donors in Heart Transplantation—Development of a Risk Score Formula for Primary Graft Failure

Yasushi Yoshikawa

Abstract

Heart transplantation in Japan has been developed under severe donor shortage, and aggressive use of marginal donors (MD) seems inevitable. Major concern about the use of MD is the increased risk of primary graft failure (PGF). Therefore, it is crucial to conduct a risk analysis of transplant from marginal donors from the risk of PGF.

Ninety-one cases of heart transplants performed at our institution were examined. Among the overall 10-year cumulative survival rate as 84%, the 10-year survival rate for the PGF(+) group (12 cases, 13%) was 50%, significantly worse than the 92% for the PGF(−) group. Multivariate analysis identified six risk factors for PGF: donor inotropic score, ischemic time, recipient Hb, cardiopulmonary arrest (CPA) time to harvest, donor cardiac function (EF), and donor age.

The PGF risk score derived from these factors is 1.24 + 0.738 log (Donor inotropic score + 1) + 0.014 (Ischemic time) − 0.335 (Recipient Hb) − 0.086 (Time from CPA to Harvest) − 0.073 (Donor EF) + 0.027 (Donor Age), with a c-statistic of 0.785 obtained from the ROC curve.

Keywords

Heart transplantation · Marginal donor · Primary graft failure · Donor shortage · Risk scoring

Y. Yoshikawa (✉)
Division of Cardiovascular Surgery, Tottori University Faculty of Medicine, Yonago, Tottori, Japan
e-mail: yoshikawa@tottori-u.ac.jp

H. Matsuda et al. (eds.), *Heart and Lung Transplantation*,
https://doi.org/10.1007/978-981-96-8810-4_19

19.1 Introduction

The field of heart transplantation in Japan has witnessed remarkable growth since the revision of the organ transplantation law, with the annual number of transplants surpassing 100 cases for the first time in 2023. Moreover, patient outcomes have been exceptional, achieving a 5-year survival rate exceeding 90%. Nonetheless, the persistent and severe shortage of donors remains a pressing issue, with the average waiting time exceeding 5 years and no substantial reduction in waitlist mortality.

Given this unique and challenging environment, every effort must be made to maximize the utilization of available donor hearts, including marginal donors (MDs). MDs are defined as donors whose organ characteristics are on the borderline of acceptability for transplantation. Utilizing MD hearts carries a heightened risk of acute graft failure, potentially leading to poor transplant outcomes.

When transplant surgeons elect to proceed with transplantation using marginal donor hearts, such decisions are typically based on a meticulous evaluation of the recipient's prognosis while on the waiting list versus the anticipated risks and complications post-transplantation. In Japan, risk scoring has been implemented in lung transplantation through the lung allocation score (LAS). Similarly, efforts to develop risk scoring systems for heart transplantation have been made in Western countries [1]. However, the donor shortage in Japan is far more severe compared to Western nations, underscoring the necessity for a risk scoring system uniquely tailored to Japan's specific circumstances.

The evaluation of MDs is intrinsically linked to the organ allocation system, which, except for adjustments in pediatric donor policies, has remained unchanged for over two decades in Japan. The revision of this allocation system can be approached from two perspectives: optimizing the use of MDs and evaluating the risk of waitlist mortality. The latter approach is particularly relevant for conditions such as failed Fontan procedures, adult congenital heart disease, and restrictive cardiomyopathy.

The following study outlines an investigation conducted at Osaka University, aimed at addressing these challenges.

19.2 Objective

Despite an increase in heart transplants following the revised organ transplantation law, the severe scarcity of donors compels Japan to adopt a more proactive approach to utilizing MD hearts compared to other nations. To enhance the outcomes of heart transplantation in Japan, we analyzed donor and recipient factors from cases at our institution to construct a risk scoring model for primary graft failure (PGF).

19.3 Methods

1. Study Population:

   The study analyzed 91 heart transplant cases performed at Cardiovascular Surgery of Osaka University between January 1999 and December 2017. The cohort consisted of 63 male and 28 female recipients, with a mean age of 38 ± 14 years. The mean Status 1 waiting period was 923 ± 305 days.
2. Definition of Marginal Donors:

   Internationally recognized criteria for defining MDs are summarized in Table 19.1 [2, 3]. When applied to the 91 cases in this study, at least one MD factor was identified in 71 cases as 77% (Fig. 19.1), and the prevalence of key MD factors, including cardiac arrest (51%), donor age over 50 years (27%), and high-dose inotropic support (21%), respectively.

PGF, a leading cause of mortality following heart transplantation, occurs in approximately 40% of cases [4, 5]. Both donor and recipient factors are associated with PGF. Identifying and mitigating these risk factors are essential for improving transplant outcomes. The definition of PGF was based on the criteria proposed by Kobashigawa and his colleagues in 2014 (Table 19.2) [6].

Table 19.1 General definitions of marginal donors

Age	Donors aged 50 years or older
Cardiac arrest	History of cardiac arrest
Inotropic support	Requirement for high-dose inotropic agents (e.g., ≥10 μg/kg/min of dopamine or dobutamine, or use of adrenaline or noradrenaline)
EF	EF < 55%
LVDd	LVDd <36 mm
Gender mismatch	Female donor to male recipient
Cardiac hypertrophy	Left ventricular posterior wall thickness > 13 mm or evidence of left ventricular hypertrophy pattern on ECG
Size mismatch	Donor-to-recipient body weight ratio < 0.8

EF Ejection fraction, *LVDd* Left ventricular diastolic dimension

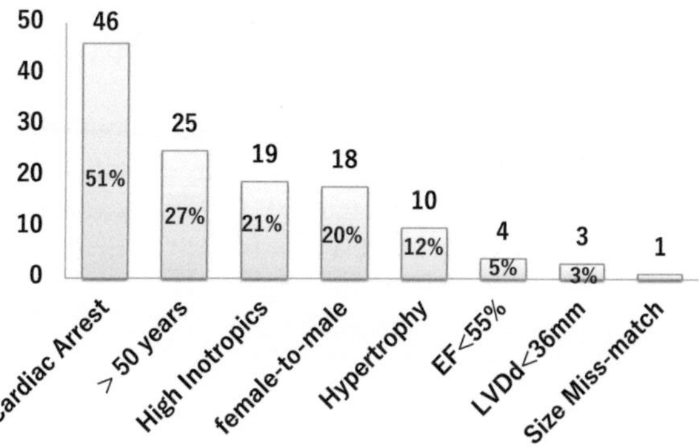

Fig. 19.1 Frequency of marginal donor factors leading to heart transplantation in our cohort of 91 patients. *EF* Ejection fraction, LVDd: Left ventricular diastolic dimension

Table 19.2 Definition of primary graft failure

Moderate PGF:
PGF is classified as moderate if both of the following conditions (I and II) are met:
I. Hemodynamic dysfunction:
LVEF ≤40%
Or CVP > 15 mmHg combined with:
PCWP >20 mmHg
CI < 2.0 L/min/m^2
II. High-dose inotropic support or mechanical support:
Inotropic score > 10
Or use of an IABP
Severe PGF:
PGF is classified as severe if mechanical circulatory support is required, including:
ECMO
LVAD
BiVAD

Inotrope score = dopamine (x1) + dobutamine (x1) + amrinone (x1) + milrinone (x15) + epinephrine (x100) + norepinephrine (x100) with each drug dosed in µg/kg/min)
PGF Primary graft failure, *LVEF* Left ventricular ejection fraction, *CVP* Central venous pressure, *PCWP* Pulmonary capillary wedge pressure, *CI* Cardiac Index, *IABP* intra-aortic balloon pump, *ECMO* Extracorporeal membrane oxygenation, *LVAD* Left ventricular assist device, *BiVAD* Biventricular assist device

19.4 Results

1. Incidence and Outcomes of PGF:
   Moderate PGF occurred in five cases (5.5%), while severe PGF was observed in seven cases (7.7%). The cumulative survival rate was significantly worse in recipients who experienced PGF compared to those who did not. At 10 years post-transplantation, the cumulative survival rate was 92% in the non-PGF group, compared to 50% in the PGF group (Fig. 19.2).
2. Risk Factors for PGF
   Univariate analysis identified hemoglobin levels ($P = 0.0176$) and pulmonary vascular resistance ($P = 0.08$) as significant recipient-related risk factors (Fig. 19.3). Donor-related risk factors included inotropic score ($P = 0.00005$), time from CPA to harvest ($P = 0.00205$), EF ($P = 0.0144$), age ($P = 0.0639$), and ischemic time ($P = 0.118$) (Fig. 19.4).

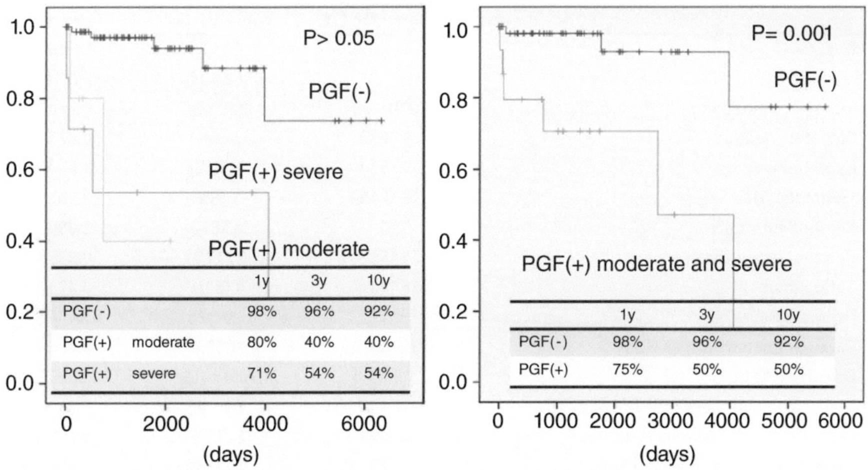

Fig. 19.2 Kaplan-Meier curves for overall survival, stratified by the severity of PGF. Left: comparison among 3 groups of PGF (no, moderate, severe). Right: comparison between two groups of PGF (no, moderate, and severe)

	Without PGF (79)	With PGF (12)	p-value
Male	56	7	
Female	23	5	0.503
Age (year)	38±14	37±16	0.805
DM	2 (3%)	1 (8%)	0.439
Amiodarone	14 (18%)	5 (42%)	0.119
RVAD	6 (8%)	3 (25%)	0.0939
Driveline infection	26 (33%)	5 (42%)	0.534
Inotropic support	9 (11%)	1 (8%)	0.577
Ventilator	0	1 (8%)	0.132
Mean PA pressure	21± 10	19±7	0.517
PVR	2.3±1.2	1.7±0.5	0.080
Hb	12.0±1.8	10.7±1.7	0.0176
Na	137±3	136±3	0.113
BUN	16.8±7.5	21.0±11.4	0.102
Creatinine	0.86±0.31	1.00±.047	0.183
Total bilirubin	0.84±0.72	0.64±0.35	0.353
CRP	0.66±1.06	0.61±0.80	0.889

Fig. 19.3 Recipient risk factors for PGF by univariate analysis. *RVAD* Right ventricular assist device, *PA* Pulmonary artery, *PVR* Pulmonary vascular resistance, *Hb* Hemoglobin, *Na* Natrium, *BUN* Blood Urea Nitrogen, *CRP* C-reactive protein

	Without PGF (79)	With PGF (12)	P-value
Age (year)	41 ± 12	48 ± 14	0.0639
Ejection fraction (%)	67 ± 6	62 ± 12	0.0144
Ischemic time (min.)	210 ± 39	229 ± 38	0.118
Diabetes mellitus	9 (8%)	1 (8%)	0.577
Hypertension	9 (8%)	1(12%)	1.000
Traumatic brain injury	19 (24%)	1 (8%)	0.289
Cerebral infarction	0	1 (8%)	1.000
Cerebral hemorrhage	7 (9%)	2 (17%)	0.338
Suffocation	16 (20%)	4 (33%)	0.453
Inotropic Score	6 ± 8	20 ± 23	0.00005
Cardiopulmonary arrest (CPA)	39 (49%)	7(58%)	0.758
Days from CPA to Harvest	7.9 ± 4.5	4.0 ± 1.3	0.00205
Left ventricular mass index (cm^3/m^2)	89 ± 27	98 ± 45	0.360
Left ventricular diastolic dimension < 36mm	3 (4%)	2 (17%)	0.141
Female donor to male recipient	15 (19%)	3 (25%)	0.699
Weight difference (Donor/Recipient)	1.20 ± 0.32	1.27 ± 0.42	0.493
BSA ((Donor/Recipient)	1.08 ± 0.14	1.14 ± 0.26	0.231

Fig. 19.4 Donor risk factors for PGF by univariate analysis. *BSA* Body surface area

Through cross-validation using C-statistics and Brier scores, six key risk factors were identified: inotropic score, ischemic time, hemoglobin levels, time from CPA to harvest, donor age, and donor EF (C-statistic 0.785, Brier Score 0.102). These factors formed the basis for constructing the following risk score formula (Fig. 19.5).

$$\text{Risk score} = 1.24 + 0.738^{*} \log(\text{donor} - \text{inotropic score} + 1) \\ + 0.014^{*} \text{ ischemic time} - 0.335^{*} \text{ Hb} - 0.086^{*} \text{ time from CPA} \\ \text{to harvest} - 0.073^{*} \text{ donor EF} + 0.027^{*} \text{ age}$$

The frequency of PGF across six risk score strata is illustrated with Strata 6 exhibiting the highest PGF incidence (Fig. 19.6).

Parameters in the final scoring model for PGF

Variable	AOR	95% CI	p-value
log (Donor Inotropic score + 1)	2.09	(0.97 - 4.49)	0.059
Ischemia duration (min)	1.01	(1.00 - 1.03)	0.131
Hb	0.72	(0.45 - 1.14)	0.161
Time from CPA to Harvest (days)	0.92	(0.76 - 1.11)	0.380
Donor EF	0.93	(0.84 - 1.03)	0.159
Donor Age	1.03	(0.96 - 1.10)	0.413

AOR, addjusted odds ratio; CI, confidence interval.

risk score = 1.24 + 0.738*log(d_inotrope score + 1) + 0.014*Ischemic time – 0.335*Hb – 0.086*Time from CPA to Harvest – 0.073*Donor EF + 0.027*Age

Fig. 19.5 The final model of risk scoring formula for PGF. *CPA* Cardiopulmonary arrest, *EF* Ejection fraction, *CPA* Cardiopulmonary arrest

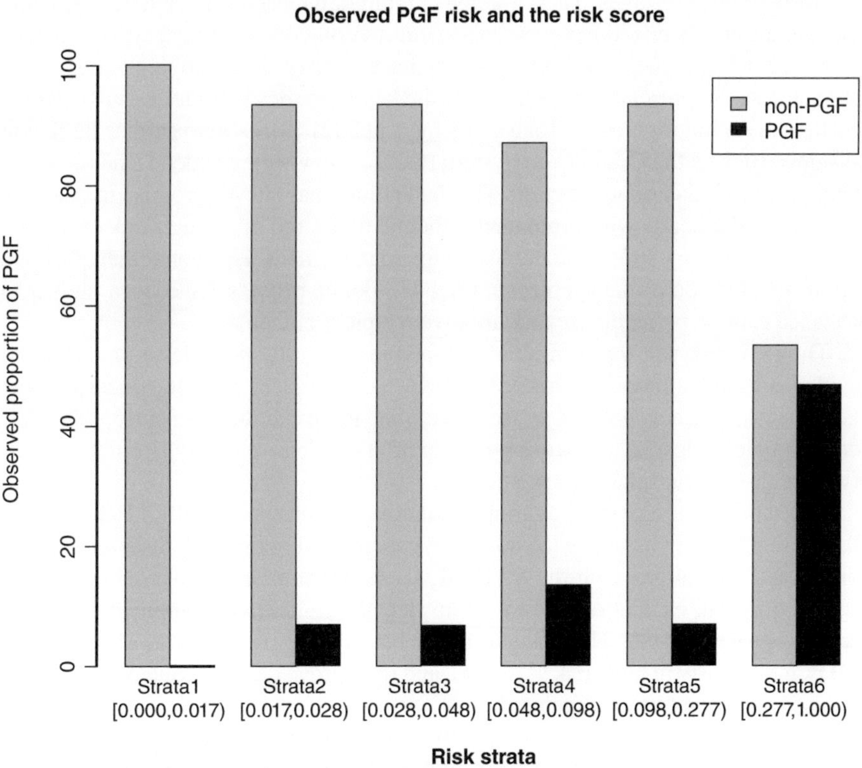

Fig. 19.6 The frequency of PGF across six risk score strata. Strata 1 (0.000–0.017), Strata 2 (0.017–0.028), Strata 3 (0.048–0.098), Strata 4 (0.048–0.098), Strata 5 (0.098–0.277), and Strata 6 (0.277–1.000)

19.5 Discussion

Heart transplantation in Japan faces the persistent challenge of a severe donor shortage. The average waiting time for transplantation is approximately 5 years [7], with over 90% of candidates reliant on left ventricular assist devices (LVADs) [3, 8]. This limited donor pool necessitates the frequent use of MDs. In our study, 77% of transplanted donor hearts met the criteria for marginal donors, a rate that is consistent with the high dependence on MDs observed across Japan.

MDs are characterized by factors such as advanced age, high-dose inotropic support, prolonged ischemic time, or reduced left ventricular ejection fraction. Despite the increased risks associated with MDs, such as PGF, careful donor selection and recipient management have demonstrated the potential for favorable long-term outcomes [9].

In our study, PGF was observed in 13% of cases, with the 10-year survival rate for PGF cases notably lower at 50% compared to 92% in non-PGF cases. This underscores the critical importance of effective risk assessment and donor selection strategies, especially in contexts like Japan, where MDs are frequently utilized due to severe donor shortages. These findings highlight the need for accurate prediction models and advanced clinical protocols to improve outcomes for high-risk recipients.

Recent advancements in MD utilization have focused on improving donor evaluation and organ preservation [9]. One of the key strategies includes ex vivo cardiac perfusion. As highlighted by Tong and Khush in 2021 [9], ex vivo cardiac perfusion systems, such as the Organ Care System (OCS), allow for extended ischemic times while preserving cardiac function. This technology has shown promise in enabling the use of MD hearts with prolonged ischemic times and other high-risk characteristics. Another key strategy includes donor Management. Hormonal therapies and optimized inotropic management during the donor process have been shown to enhance cardiac performance and improve recipient outcomes.

The PGF risk scoring formula developed in our study provides a practical and evidence-based approach to assessing donor and recipient risks. By incorporating key variables such as donor age, ischemic time, inotropic requirements, and recipient hemoglobin levels, this scoring system offers a robust predictive tool for identifying high-risk transplant cases.

The model demonstrated a strong predictive performance, with a C-statistic of 0.785, highlighting its utility in stratifying patients and optimizing decision-making processes. This aligns with the RADIAL score and similar international efforts to standardize risk evaluation in heart transplantation [1, 9]. The application of this scoring system enables clinicians to better balance the risks and benefits of using MDs, particularly in high-risk scenarios, and to improve recipient outcomes through tailored perioperative management.

While the model's initial validation demonstrates its utility, future efforts should focus on expanding the dataset to include multi-center and nationwide data. This will ensure the generalizability of the scoring system across diverse clinical settings. Additionally, incorporating data from regions with varying donor profiles and medical practices will further strengthen the robustness and applicability of the model.

19.6 Conclusion

The developed PGF risk scoring formula has been validated as robust and effective. Its application is critical for the appropriate selection of marginal donors (MDs), facilitating PGF risk analysis and improving transplant outcomes.

The findings indicate that this scoring model holds significant potential to enhance the accuracy and efficiency of risk evaluation in heart transplantation. Moving forward, the development of a risk scoring formula based on nationwide, all-Japan data is anticipated to further refine risk assessment and improve clinical decision-making.

These results also highlight the potential utility of this risk scoring system in addressing challenges associated with the current heart allocation framework, paving the way for its practical application and integration.

References

1. Segovia J, Cosio MD, Barcelo JM, et al. RADIAL: a novel primary graft failure risk score in heart transplantation. J Heart Lung Transplant. 2011;30(6):644–51.
2. Amarelli C, De Santo LS, Marra C, et al. Early graft failure after heart transplant: risk factors and implications for improved donor-recipient matching. Interact Cardiovasc Thorac Surg. 2012;15(1):57–62.
3. Fujita T, Toda K, Yanase M, et al. Risk factors for post-transplant low output syndrome. Eur J Cardiothorac Surg. 2012;42(3):551–6.
4. D'Alessandro C, Golmard JL, Barreda E, et al. Predictive risk factors for primary graft failure requiring temporary extra-corporeal membrane oxygenation support after cardiac transplantation in adults. Eur J Cardiothorac Surg. 2011;40(4):962–9.
5. Rhee Y, Kim HJ, Kim JJ, et al. Primary graft dysfunction after isolated heart transplantation—incidence, risk factors, and clinical implications based on a single-center experience. Circ J. 2021;85(9):1451–9.
6. Kobashigawa J, Zuckermann A, Macdonald P, et al. Report from a consensus conference on primary graft dysfunction after cardiac transplantation. J Heart Lung Transplant. 2014;33(4):327–40.
7. The registry report of Japanese heart transplantation-2023. Jpn J Transplant. 2023;58(3):179–80.
8. Seguchi O, Fujita T, Murata Y, et al. Incidence, etiology, and outcome of primary graft dysfunction in adult heart transplant recipients: a single-center experience in Japan. Heart Vessel. 2016;31(4):555–62.
9. Tong CKW, Khush KK. New approaches to donor selection and preparation in heart transplantation. Curr Treat Options Cardiovasc Med. 2021;23(5):28.

20 Exploring Advancements in DCD Heart Transplantation: Preservation Techniques, Ethical Challenges, and Clinical Outcomes

Masafumi Shibata and Yasuhiro Shudo

Abstract

Donation after circulatory death (DCD) has emerged as a viable strategy to expand the donor pool for heart transplantation. Initially limited by technical, ethical, and logistical challenges, advancements in preservation and evaluation methods—such as normothermic regional perfusion (NRP) and ex situ machine perfusion—have renewed interest in this approach. Historically, DCD heart transplantation lagged behind liver and kidney transplantation due to the concerns about ischemia-reperfusion injury. However, recent innovations have shown that the outcomes of DCD heart transplantation are comparable to those of donation after brain death.

This manuscript reviews the evolution of DCD heart transplantation, highlighting key breakthroughs in donor heart preservation, assessment techniques, and the implementation of NRP and ex situ machine perfusion systems. Despite ongoing clinical challenges, including ethical considerations surrounding NRP protocols and the economic burden of ex-situ machine perfusion systems, DCD heart transplantation has proven effective in reducing transplant waiting times and improving access for patients with end-stage heart failure.

M. Shibata · Y. Shudo (✉)
Department of Cardiothoracic Surgery, Stanford University, Stanford, CA, USA
e-mail: ymiyamoto@otemae.gr.jp

H. Matsuda et al. (eds.), *Heart and Lung Transplantation*,
https://doi.org/10.1007/978-981-96-8810-4_20

Keywords

Heart transplantation · Donation after circulatory death · Machine perfusion · Normothermic regional perfusion · Warm ischemic time · Ischemic reperfusion injury · Primary graft dysfunction

20.1 Introduction

Heart transplantation remains the gold standard for treating end-stage heart failure. However, with over 3300 candidates on the waiting list, according to the United Network for Organ Sharing (UNOS), the demand for donor hearts far exceeds supply. To address this disparity, donation after circulatory death (DCD) has gained renewed global attention. Around 2015, Australia [1] and the United Kingdom [2] became early adopters of DCD heart transplantation, reporting promising outcomes. In the United States (U.S.), DCD donor hearts have been utilized for transplantation since 2019 [3]. Studies suggest that expanding the use of DCD hearts could increase the number of heart transplants by up to 30% [4]. By 2024, DCD heart transplantation has grown rapidly, with approximately 730 procedures performed annually [5] (Fig. 20.1). This review provides clinicians with an overview of the current state of DCD heart transplantation. It examines the historical background, technical advancements, retrieval and preservation strategies, clinical outcomes compared to donation after brain death (DBD) transplants, and the ethical considerations influencing this evolving field.

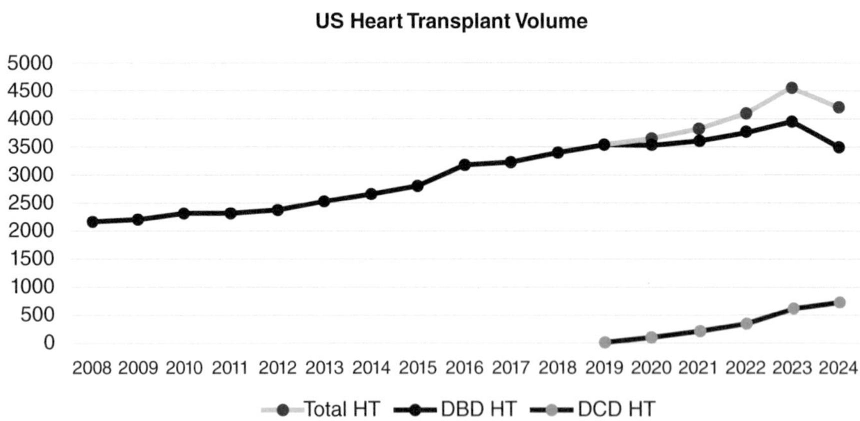

Fig. 20.1 Trends in heart transplantation in the United States. (Source; https://www.acc.org/Latest-in-Cardiology/Articles/2022/11/21/13/31/Emerging-Frontier-in-Heart-Transplantation. *HT* heart transplantation, *DBD* donation after brain death, *DCD* donation after circulatory death)

20.2 Historical Background of DCD

The evolution of heart transplantation has been closely tied to advancements in medical science, ethical principles, and technological innovation. The world's first heart transplant was performed by Christiaan Barnard in Cape Town, South Africa, on December 3, 1967 [6]. The donor was a 25-year-old woman who sustained a head injury in a car accident. After cardiac arrest was confirmed following extubation, the donor heart was removed under hypothermic regional perfusion (16 °C) using cardiopulmonary bypass (CPB) and transplanted into a 53-year-old man with chronic heart failure. Barnard performed a second heart transplant on January 2, 1968, in a similar manner.

Norman E. Shumway performed the first adult heart transplant in the United States at Stanford University in California on January 6, 1968. The donor in this case was a brain-dead patient on a ventilator, and the donor's heart was removed and transplanted under hypothermic conditions after cardiac arrest was confirmed in a manner similar to earlier procedures [7]. In the early days of heart transplantation, donor hearts were not removed directly from brain-dead patients, as is standard practice today, but rather after cardiac arrest, a process now referred to as Donation after Circulatory Death (DCD). That same year, the 30th heart transplant worldwide—and the first in Japan—was performed by Professor Juro Wada and his colleagues at Sapporo Medical University in Hokkaido. Over subsequent years, more than 100 institutions began performing heart transplants. However, at that time, the definition of brain death had not been universally established, leading to ongoing ethical debates and criticism regarding the use of patients with clinically confirmed cessation of cerebral function as donors.

In September 1968, the diagnosis of brain death—defined as the cessation of brainstem activity—was introduced to the medical community by the Harvard Brain Death Committee [8]. Heart transplants continued to be performed in various parts of the United States at the discretion of transplant physicians until 1979 when the Natural Death Act was enacted in California. This was followed by a 1981 federal court ruling that formally recognized brain death as legal death.

After 1981, heart transplantation using donation after brain death (DBD) became the standard practice. The introduction and widespread use of cyclosporine, further advanced transplantation outcomes, leading to a rapid increase in the number of heart transplants [8, 9]. In 1993, the University of Pittsburgh issued a policy for DCD transplantation [10] that included the stipulation that surgeons must not participate in the declaration of death. This policy, originally intended for DCD transplantation, was developed in parallel with an increase in DCD liver transplants led by pioneers such as Thomas Starzl and his colleagues. It remains a foundational guideline for DCD organ donation today. Despite these developments, DCD heart transplantation faced major delays compared to liver and kidney transplantation. Challenges included the complexity of heart retrieval methods, storage limitations, and ethical concerns surrounding the practice.

20.3 Advancing DCD Heart Transplantation

Efforts to advance DCD heart transplantation in the United States focus on addressing technical, institutional, and ethical challenges. On the technical side, new evaluation criteria and techniques are being developed to assess the viability of DCD hearts. Marked progress has been made in heart reperfusion, proper preservation methods, and transplantation techniques aimed at improving the safety and success rates of DCD heart transplantation. On the institutional side, guidelines and regulations governing programs involving DCD donors have been established. Enhanced data sharing and collaboration among transplant centers and medical institutions further support the effective implementation and monitoring of DCD heart transplant procedures. Ethical efforts prioritize transparent consent processes for patients and their families. Comprehensive explanations are provided, decision-making support is offered, and ethical concerns and values are carefully addressed to ensure an informed and respectful approach.

These collective efforts have contributed to maintaining high success rates in DCD heart transplantation. Studies have reported comparable outcomes in patient survival and quality of life between DCD and DBD heart transplants, along with shorter transplant waiting times [11, 12]. Continued advancements in long-term outcomes, organ preservation techniques, and systems compared to brain death transplantation are anticipated to enhance the field of DCD heart transplantation further.

20.3.1 Defining and Optimizing DCD Heart Donation

Following the University of Pittsburgh's foundational policy statement in 1993, the definition and categorization of DCD were further refined during the 1995 Maastricht meeting. The updated Maastricht criteria classify DCD donors into specific categories [13, 14] (Table 20.1). For heart transplantation, DCD donors typically fall within Maastricht category III, representing controlled DCD donation. A Maastricht III donor is generally an individual who has suffered irreversible neurological injury and is not expected to achieve meaningful neurological recovery but does not meet the strict criteria for brain death. According to the World Health Organization's pathways for organ donation, potential controlled DCD donors include individuals who do not meet the criteria for DBD, are reliant on life-sustaining therapies due to irreversible illness or injury, and are expected to experience imminent death following the planned withdrawal of life support [15, 16].

The total warm ischemic time (WIT) and functional warm ischemic time (fWIT) are critical metrics in the process of withdrawal of life-sustaining therapy (WLST) leading to circulatory arrest. WIT is defined as the time elapsed from the initiation of WLST to organ reperfusion, while fWIT refers to the period from the onset of hypoperfusion and/or hypoxia to the restoration of coronary blood flow. In the OCS DCD Heart trial, the onset of organ ischemia was marked by peripheral blood oxygen saturation dropping below 70% or systolic blood pressure falling below

Table 20.1 Modified Maastricht criteria for organ donation after cardiac death

Modified Maastricht Criteria		
Category I	IA: Found dead out of hospital	Unexpected cardiac arrest without attempted resuscitation
Uncontrolled	IB: Found dead in hospital	
Uncontrolled	IIB: Witnessed in hospital arrest	
Category III	Withdrawal of life-sustaining therapy	Planned withdrawal of life support.
Controlled		
Category IV	Cardiac arrest after brain death	Cardiac arrest after brain death diagnosis during donor
Controlled or uncontrolled		Management, but prior to organ recovery

Data from Ref. [13, 14]

50 mmHg [17]. This phase is commonly known as the "agonal phase". Most institutions currently define the onset of the agonal phase as the moment when systolic blood pressure drops below 50 mmHg. Given the potential unreliability of oxygen saturation measurements under hypotensive conditions, many centers rely exclusively on blood pressure monitoring to determine the onset of this critical phase.

Preclinical studies suggest that an fWIT of less than 30 min is optimal for complete graft recovery [18]. Institutional policies and the implant surgeon's discretion may vary, but organs are often excluded if the fWIT exceeds this threshold. If pulseless electrical activity (PEA) does not occur within this window, or if cardioplegia infusion is not completed in time, the organ may be deemed unusable—a scenario commonly referred to as a "dry run".

Many centers enforce a "stand-off" period, typically 5 min, between circulatory arrest and the declaration of death. However, some institutions have reduced this interval to 2 min, aligning with the Pittsburgh Protocol and the 2013 joint statement issued by the American Thoracic Society (ATS), International Society for Heart and Lung Transplantation (ISHLT), Society of Critical Care Medicine (SCCM), Association of Organ Procurement Organizations (AOPO), and United Network for Organ Sharing (UNOS).

Clinical factors associated with rapid progression to cardiac death after WLST include younger age, a high inspired oxygen fraction, and the use of nonspontaneous ventilation modes [19]. Risk scoring systems, such as the University of Wisconsin donation after cardiac death evaluation tool and the UNOS scoring system, have been developed to identify patients likely to experience circulatory collapse within a timeframe suitable for DCD donation [20]. According to the UNOS consensus committee criteria, over half the patients meeting at least one predictor for rapid progression to circulatory arrest (Table 20.2) experienced circulatory death within 1 h of WLST [21]. The probability increased with the number of criteria met: 65% of patients meeting two criteria and 82% of those meeting three criteria died within 60 min.

Table 20.2 UNOS DCD consensus committee criteria

UNOS DCD consensus committee criteria
Apnea
Respiratory rate < 8
Respiratory rate > 30
Left ventricular assist device
Right ventricular assist device
Venoarterial extracorporeal membrane oxygenation
Pacemaker-unassisted heart rate < 30
PEEP ≧ 10 and ≦ SaO2 92%
FiO2 ≧ 0.5 and ≦ SaO2 92%
Venovenous extracorporeal membrane oxygenation
Norepinephrine or phenylephrine ≧ 0.2
Dopamine ≧ 15
Intra-aortic balloon pump 1:1
-or-
Dobutamine or dopamine ≧ 10 and cardiac index ≦ 2.2 L/min/m2
Intraaortic balloon pump 1:1 and cardiac index ≦ 1.5 L/min/m2

Data from Ref. [22]

20.3.2 Heart Evaluation and Perfusion Methods

In DCD heart transplantation protocols, the donor heart is exposed to hypotension and hypoxia for an extended period, often several tens of minutes, and remains without circulation for several minutes after the onset of PEA. As a result, both ventricles and atria dilate, increasing the heart's susceptibility to ischemia and reperfusion injury compared with that after conventional brain death donation. Given these risks, it is essential to evaluate the feasibility of transplantation by reanimating the donor heart to assess its functionality.

Current evaluation methods involve reanimating the donor heart either in situ or ex situ. These techniques are essential for determining the viability of the donor heart. As of 2024, transplant surgeons employ one of two primary methods for DCD organ procurement and preservation based on the recipient hospital's institutional policies and logistical considerations. Direct procurement perfusion (DPP) or normothermic regional perfusion (NRP) are the methods of choice for DCD heart transplantation, and they are described in the following text.

20.3.3 DCD-DPP(DCD-OCS)Method

The DPP method involves excising the donor heart and resuscitating it using an ex-situ machine perfusion (MP) system. This approach is based on the Langendorff perfusion model, which focuses on perfusion of the coronary arteries. Building on this concept, the commercial normothermic ex-situ heart perfusion system, the

TransMedics (Andover, MA, USA) Organ Care System (OCS), was developed and has received approval from the US Food and Drug Agency following multiple clinical trials [22] (Fig. 20.2). The OCS is a portable device featuring a wireless display

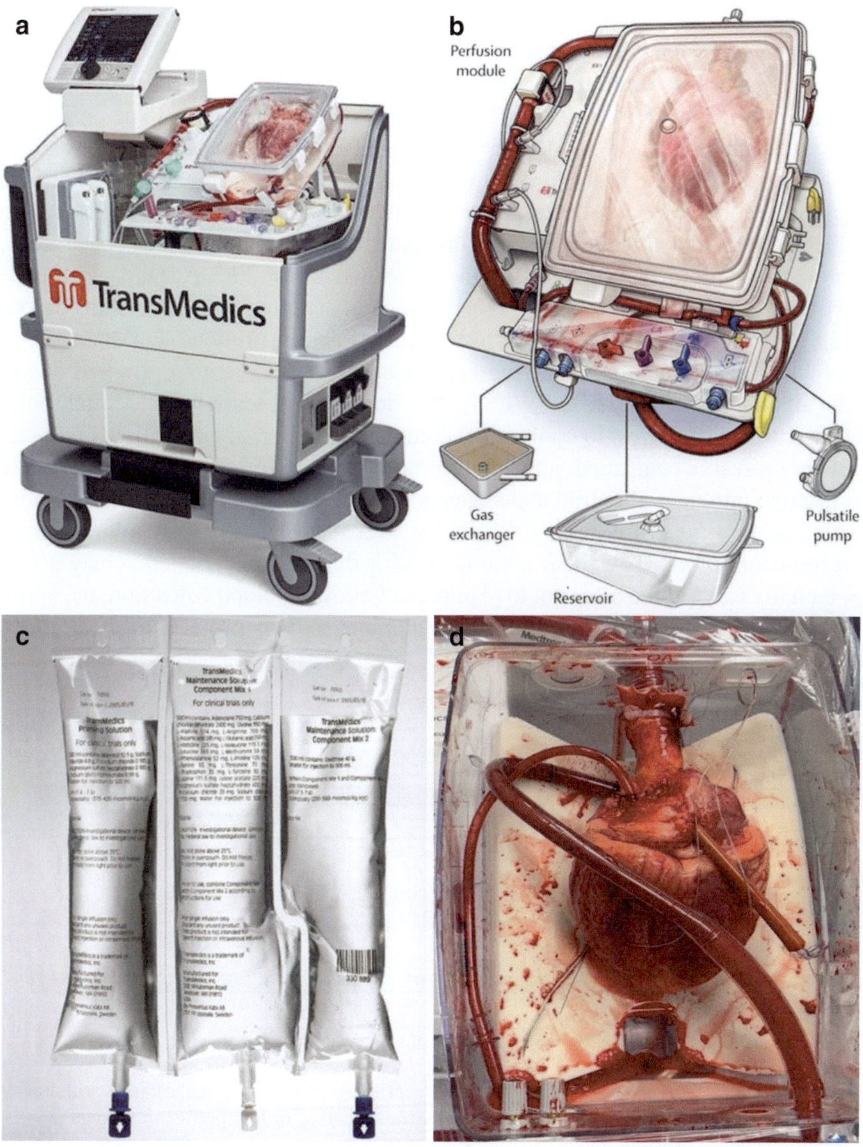

Fig. 20.2 Ex-situ heart preservation. Normothermic ex-situ heart preservation, organ care system (OCS), is composed of a portable heart console (**a**), heart perfusion module (**b**), and heart solution set (**c**). The ascending aorta and pulmonary artery are cannulated. The left ventricular vent is placed and secured at the left atrium. The superior vena cava, inferior vena cava, right atrial incision, and left atrial appendage are securely closed. The heart is actively beating inside the box (**d**). (Source: Ardehali et al. [22])

monitor and a perfusion system comprising a pulsatile pump, gas exchanger, and heater. Together, these components deliver oxygenated blood, nutrient solutions, and supplements to the heart, which is connected to the perfusion module. During ex-situ machine perfusion, the donor heart's function and condition are evaluated through its beating activity and laboratory analysis. To assess the condition of the donor heart, physiological parameters are monitored. Changes in electrolyte levels and enzyme activity in both heart tissue and blood are observed to detect potential damage and evaluate functionality. If the donor heart is determined to be unsuitable for transplantation based on these assessments, it is referred to as a "turn down".

Before starting the procedure, all necessary surgical instruments and materials, including donor blood collection bags, should be prepared on a designated side table for the surgical team. The OCS instrumentation kit is set up on a back table. The standard protocol of the DPP method is shown in Fig. 20.3. A standard practice involves administering 30,000 IU of heparin approximately 5 min before WLST. However, practices vary across countries and institutions. For example, in the United Kingdom, administering heparin before WLST is not permitted due to ethical considerations. After WLST, the donor is observed for 5 min post-electromechanical arrest to confirm the complete cessation of circulation. Once circulatory arrest is confirmed, a median sternotomy is performed. A venous cannula is inserted into the right atrial appendage to collect 1200–1400 mL of donor blood, which is used for priming the OCS. If the liver team inadvertently administers a preservation solution (e.g., UW solution) during this step, hyperkalemia may occur, potentially causing the heart not to reanimate. Following blood collection, the aortic cross-clamp is applied. Cardioplegia is administered to protect the heart from

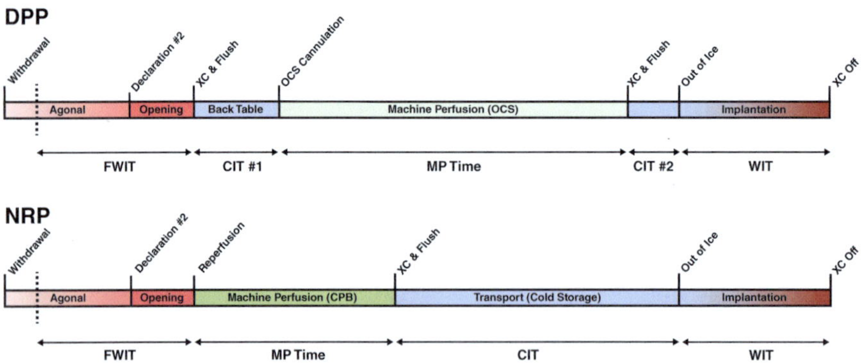

Fig. 20.3 Time sequences in DCD heart procurement. With DCD donation, the care is withdrawn, and the donor is allowed to expire. The donor reaches a period of low perfusion (agonal phase), typically defined as systolic blood pressure < 50 mmHg and oxygen saturation < 70%. The time from when the agonal phase begins to cold organ flushing (in DPP) or machine perfusion (NRP) is the functional warm ischemic time (f-WIT). Source: https://www.acc.org/Latest-in-Cardiology/Articles/2022/11/21/13/31/Emerging-Frontier-in-Heart-Transplantation. *DPP* direct procurement and machine perfusion, *NRP* normothermic regional perfusion, *f-WIT* functional warm ischemic time, *XC* aortic cross-clamp, *MP* machine perfusion, *CIT* cold ischemic time, *WIT* warm ischemic time

ischemic damage. Both chambers of the heart are vented. Topical cooling is achieved using ice slush or cold saline. The heart is explanted using techniques similar to those employed in DBD procedures [23]. The donor heart is transferred to the back table for OCS instrumentation. The OCS circuit is primed with donor blood mixed with TransMedics priming solution, which contains mannitol and electrolytes. Antibiotics, steroids, albumin, and supplements are added to the circuit, along with epinephrine, levothyroxine, and the TransMedics maintenance solution, which includes multivitamins, electrolytes, dextrose, insulin, and adenosine.

The heart is inspected for anatomical defects such as a patent foramen ovale (PFO) or septal defects, which are repaired if present. Any incisions made in the right and/or left atrial appendages for donor blood collection or left-sided heart venting are also repaired. The superior and inferior vena cavae are closed. The pulmonary artery and ascending aorta are cannulated. A left ventricular (LV) vent is inserted via left atriotomy. Once the aortic cannula is connected to the circuit and de-aired, oxygenated blood is perfused at 34 °C through the coronary arteries. This blood returns to the coronary sinus at the right atrium, enters the right ventricle through the tricuspid valve, and drains across the pulmonary valve into the pulmonary artery cannula [24]. After gentle cardiac massage is performed to decompress the heart, it typically begins to beat. If ventricular fibrillation (Vf) occurs, it is treated with defibrillation. Biventricular pacing wires are placed, and the ventricular pacing rate is set for VVI at 80 beats per minute. Once sinus rhythm is established, the pulmonary artery cannula is connected to its port [24]. During transportation, the aortic pressure is adjusted to 65–90 mmHg, and the coronary flow is maintained at 650–900 mL/min using a combination of epinephrine infusion, pump flow adjustments, and maintenance solution infusion to ensure optimal heart condition. Serial arterial and venous blood gases and lactate levels are monitored to assess myocardial lactate extraction, with levels below 5 mmol/L indicating adequate function [25].

When the recipient is ready for implantation, the OCS pump is turned off, and cold cardioplegia is administered to achieve rapid electromechanical arrest. The heart is disconnected from the OCS and transferred to the recipient's surgical field [25]. In March 2023, the Stanford team introduced an innovative technique to reduce ischemic reperfusion injury during the transplantation process. The unique feature of this method is that the heart is transplanted while it is still beating and avoids a second cardioplegic arrest by maintaining coronary perfusion. The donor heart is connected to the recipient's cardiopulmonary bypass circuit before being disconnected from the OCS circuit [26].

20.3.4 DCD-NRP Method

The standard protocol of the NRP method is shown in Fig. 20.3. In the NRP method, after the donor is pronounced dead, the chest is opened immediately, and the three branches of the aortic arch are clamped. CPB, or extracorporeal membrane oxygenation (ECMO), is initiated to restore oxygenated blood perfusion, enabling cardiac resuscitation. The hospital blood bank prepares four units of washed-packed red blood cells for priming the NRP circuit. The technique closely resembles the method used in the first heart transplant pioneered by Christiaan Barnard. Once the cardiac function is assessed and deemed suitable for transplantation, the donor heart is excised. The heart can be cooled and transported in a manner similar to DBD or transported using the OCS. NRP protocols may vary based on the specific organs being recovered.

1. **Thoracoabdominal normothermic regional perfusion (TA-NRP)**

TA-NRP is used when the heart, lungs, and/or abdominal organs are being recovered (Fig. 20.4). Perfusion is reestablished using veno-arterial extracorporeal membrane oxygenation (VA-ECMO) or CPB with central cannulation of the ascending aorta and right atrium [27]. Before perfusion is restored, the three cephalic vessels (innominate, left common carotid artery, and left subclavian arteries) are clamped to exclude cerebral circulation. This step is critical to prevent inadvertent cerebral perfusion, which raises ethical issues.

TA-NRP is initiated with a targeted flow of 5 L/min. The heart typically begins to beat within 2–3 min of perfusion restoration. If Vf occurs, internal defibrillation at 10 J is performed. Initial cardiac function is assessed visually and supported with inotropes or vasopressors to maintain a mean arterial blood pressure (MAP) > 50 mmHg. Functional assessment is performed using transesophageal echocardiography (TEE) and pulmonary artery catheter monitoring. The donor is reintubated and ventilated using a low tidal volume strategy to prevent atelectasis and reduce pulmonary vascular resistance. As cardiac function improves, inotropes and vasopressors are gradually weaned off. Arterial blood gas (ABG) analysis and

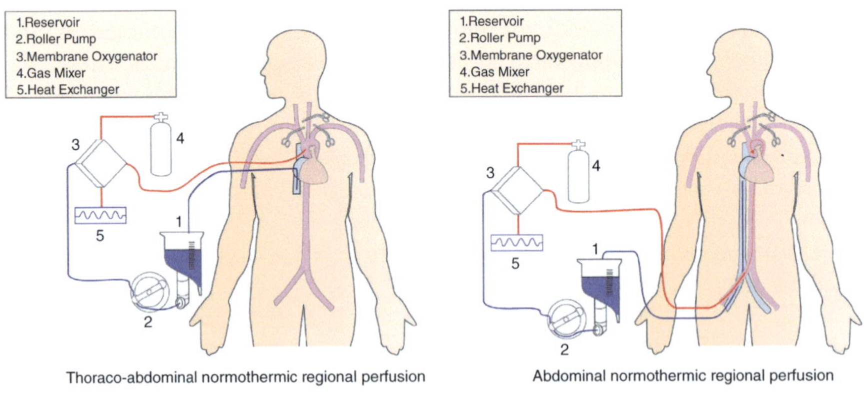

Fig. 20.4 Schematic of normothermic regional perfusion. Left: Thoracoabdominal normothermic regional perfusion (TA-NRP). The ascending aorta and right atrium are cannulated. The innominate artery, the left common carotid artery, and the left subclavian artery are clamped. Right: Abdominal normothermic regional perfusion (A-NRP). The femoral artery and femoral vein are cannulated. Veno-arterial ECMO circuit is similar for both Thoracoabdominal NRP and abdominal NRP. (Source: Alamouti-Fard et al. [31])

lactate levels are monitored to confirm adequate organ perfusion. NRP typically continues for 45–90 min, depending on the improvement in cardiac contractility [28]. After this period, the donor is weaned off the NRP circuit to evaluate unsupported cardiac function. The following criteria must be met to accept the donor heart for transplantation: left ventricular ejection fraction (LVEF) ≥50% (assessed by TEE); cardiac index (CI) ≥ 2.5 L/min/m^2; central venous pressure ≤ 12 mmHg; and pulmonary capillary wedge pressure (PCWP) ≤ 12 mmHg [27]. If the donor heart meets the acceptance criteria, cold cardioplegia is administered to achieve cardiac arrest [29]. The excision process mirrors that of DBD heart procurement. The donor heart can be transported using static cold storage (e.g., SherpaPak) or OCS [28, 30].

Using the OCS after NRP could minimize cold ischemic time compared to static cold storage. Moreover, for recipients undergoing complicated redo-sternotomy requiring extended mediastinal dissection, OCS provides additional time to allow for meticulous dissection after the donor heart has arrived in the operating room [31].

TA-NRP facilitates earlier, continuous warm blood perfusion, restoring cardiac function while simultaneously perfusing other organs. This approach can reduce costs associated with OCS by enabling multiple organ recovery under physiological conditions. When combined with static cold storage, TA-NRP is less expensive than using the OCS alone [32]. Despite its advantages, ethical concerns surrounding NRP persist in certain regions of the United States. These concerns include the risk of inadvertent cerebral reperfusion, which may still occur despite the clamping of cephalic vessels [29, 32, 33].

2. **Abdominal Normothermic Regional Perfusion (A-NRP)**

A-NRP was initially developed for the recovery of abdominal organs (Fig. 20.4). Recently, it has been adapted for combined use in abdominal organ recovery and DCD heart and/or lung procurement using the OCS. Arterial cannulation is performed via the femoral artery or abdominal aorta, and venous cannulation is conducted through the femoral vein or IVC, depending on the protocol. To prevent cerebral and thoracic recirculation, the abdominal aorta is clamped below the diaphragm, or an endovascular balloon occluder is inserted via the abdominal aorta, advanced to the thoracic aorta and inflated. The IVC is clamped to block thoracic recirculation [31]. For additional security, an aortic clamp may be applied to the thoracic descending aorta, just above the balloon occlusion. In some protocols, the three cephalic vessels from the aortic arch are clamped or ligated to ensure complete exclusion of cerebral perfusion. Increased blood flow to thoracic veins may result in generalized bleeding within the chest cavity. To mitigate this, bleeding veins should be ligated one by one using clips to prevent excessive blood loss. The theoretical and practical advantages and disadvantages of DPP and NRP are shown in Table 20.3.

Table 20.3 The theoretical and practical advantages and disadvantages of DPP and NRP

	Advantages	Disadvantages
DCD-DPP	The viability of the organ can be repeatedly assessed during the ex vivo perfusion Ex situ machine perfusion is less likely to face ethical opposition Longer travel time accepted	Ex situ machine perfusion is required for all procured organs to assess their viability before transplantation It is significantly more expensive compared to NRP
DCD-NRP	The time to reperfusion is shorter compared to DCD-OCS Cardiac function can be evaluated in vivo before organ procurement It is markedly more cost-effective compared to DCD-OCS	The donor heart is exposed to high levels of catecholamines present in the donor's blood during reperfusion There is a risk of cerebral reperfusion if cerebral circulation is not properly isolated before reperfusion Ethical objections exist in certain countries and regions The assessment takes time

20.3.5 Transport Methods in the DCD-NRP Procedure

In the DCD-NRP procedure, three primary methods are utilized for transporting the donor heart.

1. **Paragonix SherpaPak Cardiac Transport System**

   The Paragonix SherpaPak Cardiac Transport System is an advanced alternative to the traditional icebox for transportation (Fig. 20.5). It maintains a consistent storage temperature between 4 °C and 8 °C, effectively reducing the risk of myocardial damage caused by supercooling—a known limitation of conventional icebox storage [34]. Studies have shown promising outcomes in both DBD heart transplantation and DCD-NRP procedures. A multicenter study in the United States demonstrated reduced rates of severe primary graft dysfunction and lower post-transplant ECMO usage compared to traditional icebox storage [35]. Urban et al. reported on 12 DCD-NRP cases using the SherpaPak with a median storage time of 158 min (range: 37–224 min). Among these cases, one death (8%) occurred due to graft dysfunction [36].
2. **Organ Care System (OCS)**

   The second method for transporting the donor heart after NRP procurement involves using the OCS. This approach focuses on improving outcomes by minimizing cold ischemic time. A report from Royal Papworth Hospital in the United Kingdom evaluated 19 cases of DCD-NRP followed by OCS. The study demonstrated shorter ventilator time, lower postoperative hemofiltration rates, and reduced hospital stay compared to the DCD-DPP method that used OCS alone [37]. Despite its clinical benefits, the combined use of NRP and OCS causes higher costs and requires additional procedure time, which should be carefully weighed in clinical decision-making.

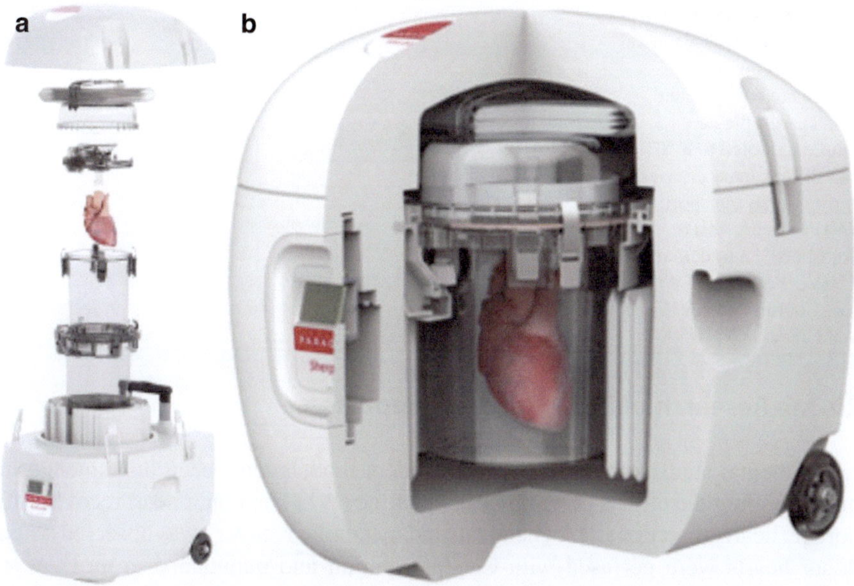

Fig. 20.5 Paragonix SherpaPak Cardiac Transport System. (**a**) Exploded view of the device, demonstrating its components and assembly process. (**b**) Cross-sectional view of the assembled device, showing a preserved heart within the system. This novel device can maintain the heart in the cold static status between 4 and 8 °C. Courtesy of Paragonix Technologies, Inc. Massachusetts, USA

3. **XVIVO Heart Assist Transport system**
   The XVIVO Heart Assist Transport system offers a novel approach to organ transport and preservation. Unlike the OCS, which operates at room temperature, the XVIVO system continuously perfuses the coronary arteries with oxygenated cardioplegic solution cooled to 8 °C during transport (Fig. 20.6). A study demonstrated a significantly lower incidence of severe primary graft dysfunction in the XVIVO group compared with that in the conventional icebox group (28% vs. 11%) [38]. The XVIVO system is currently being evaluated in the PRESERVE trial in the United States for extended criteria donor case hearts. Eligibility for the trial requires at least one of the following conditions: an estimated cross-clamp time of 4 h or more or a cross-clamp time of 2 h or more in combination with one or more additional risk factors. Additional risk factors included donor age of 50 years or older; left ventricular ejection fraction (LVEF) of 40–50% at the time of provisional acceptance; a downtime of 20 min or longer; evidence of left ventricular hypertrophy with a septal thickness between 12 mm and 16 mm; or angiographic findings of luminal irregularities without significant coronary artery disease (CAD).

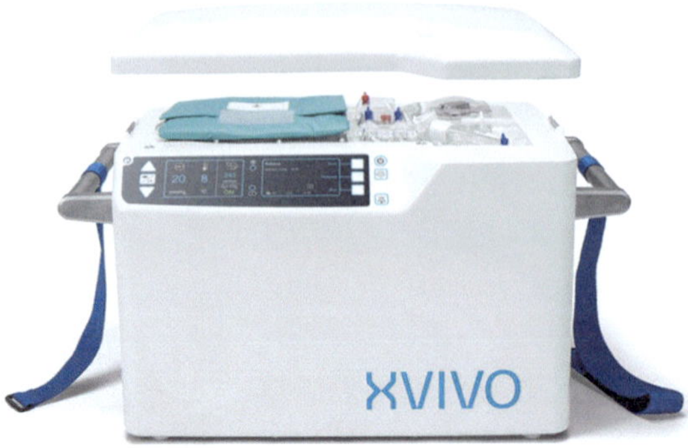

Fig. 20.6 XVIVO Heart Assist Transport This novel device continuously recirculates oxygenated blood cardioplegic solution, cooled to 8 °C, into the coronary arteries during organ transport. XVIVO Heart Assist Transport™ a trademark of XVIVO Perfusion AB. Courtesy of XVIVO Inc. Golden, CO. USA

20.3.6 Research of DCD: Outcome Reports

Experimental studies using porcine and rodent models have been instrumental in understanding the effects of warm ischemic time (WIT) on donor heart recovery. In porcine hearts, functional, biochemical, and metabolic recovery was observed when donor hearts were perfused with Celsior solution and maintained in an ex vivo device, provided the WIT was limited to 20 min [39]. Similarly, in rat models, contractile parameters such as end-systolic elastance (Ees) and dp/dt max were reduced after 15 min of WIT during reperfusion with ECMO. Despite this, cardiac output was preserved [36]. In a recent human study, myocardial biopsies were obtained at WLST, circulatory arrest, and every 2 min thereafter in 16 DCD donors. The findings demonstrated that cellular function and viability remained stable for up to 10 min post-circulatory arrest. Significant declines in myocardial contractility and cell viability were observed beyond 10 min, with severe impairment occurring thereafter [40, 41]. These studies establish a critical threshold for warm ischemia at approximately 10 min following circulatory cessation.

Since 2015, clinical outcomes of DCD heart transplantation have been reported from multiple single-center studies, consistently demonstrating results comparable to DBD heart transplantation [17, 42, 43]. St. Vincent's Hospital reported the first three successful DCD heart transplants in 2015, with all hearts supported by OCS for over 4 h [1]. A subsequent report between the years 2014 and 2018 detailed 45 potential DCD donors, of whom 23 underwent transplantation, 9 recipients required ECMO, and one died on postoperative day 6. The mortality rate was 4.4% over 4 years. All surviving patients maintained normal cardiac function without acute rejection [39]. In a 2020 report, of the 49 patients who had undergone DCD-DPP, 32 (65%) underwent heart transplantation, and temporary VA-ECMO was required in 31%, with survival rates of 96%, 94%, and 94% at 1, 3, and 5 years, respectively [44]. Outcomes were comparable to DBD transplantation. The Royal Papworth Hospital in the United Kingdom reported 26 DCD heart transplants, showing no significant survival differences compared to DBD transplantation. The 90-day survival rates were 92% for DCD and 96% for DBD ($p = 1.0$), while 1-year survival rates were 86% and 88% ($p = 0.98$) [2]. In the subsequent 5-year report, the number of DCD donors increased to 164, but there were no significant differences in 30-day survival (DCD group 97% vs. DBD group 99%, $P = 1.00$) or 1-year survival (DCD group 91% vs. DBD group 89%, $P = 0.72$) [45]. The adoption of DCD heart transplantation in the United States began in 2019 at Duke University Hospital. Since then, the frequency of DCD heart transplants has increased from 0.2% (7 cases) in 2019 to 8.8% (288 cases) in 2022 [46]. According to the UNOS (United Network for Organ Sharing) database, of the 288 DCD heart transplants performed in 2022, 110 cases (38%) utilized the DCD-NRP method, while the remaining 178 (62%) cases used DPP. Between 2020 and 2023, Vanderbilt University performed 122 DCD heart transplants, with 83% utilizing the DCD-NRP method. The outcomes were comparable to 263 DBD heart transplants performed at the same institution during the same period. Specifically, 1-year survival rates showed no significant differences. Rejection rates and readmission rates were also similar between the two groups [44].

In June 2023, a randomized controlled trial confirmed that the 6-month survival rate for DCD hearts preserved with OCS was equivalent to that of DBD hearts preserved in cold storage [17]. However, it is important to note that the DCD patient group had a significantly lower preoperative listing priority, suggesting a less severe condition compared to that in the DBD group. Despite these encouraging results, DCD heart utilization remains low. A UNOS registry study conducted between January 2020 and February 2021 reported that only 136 out of 3611 DCD donors (3.8%) were used for heart transplantation [47]. The DCD donor hearts selected for transplantation exhibited the following characteristics: younger age (median 29 years [IQR: 23–36] vs. 47 years [IQR: 36–56]) for unused donors; male predominance (90%); blood type O (79%); and lower prevalence of comorbidities, including diabetes (2.21% vs. 12.86%), hypertension (12.50% vs. 41.49%), and coronary artery disease (CAD) (0% vs. 7.78%) [47].

20.3.7 Issues in DCD

Currently, the choice of method depends on institutional policies and regional organ network consensus. However, a comprehensive evaluation of ethical considerations, cost-effectiveness, and transplant outcomes is crucial to determining the most appropriate approach.

1. **Ethical Considerations**

One of the primary ethical debates surrounding NRP is the potential for cerebral blood flow restoration. In DCD, the heart is excised only after cardiac death is confirmed, strictly adhering to the definition of death. However, in NRP, blood flow is mechanically restored to all organs while they remain in the body, raising questions about whether this practice conflicts with the cardiac death criteria. Proponents argue that clamping the cephalic vessels (originating from the aortic arch) ensures conditions equivalent to brain death. Critics, however, raise concerns about potential collateral blood flow from the descending aorta, which could perfuse the posterior cranial fossa, leading to incomplete cerebral blood flow cessation. In 2021, the American College of Physicians recommended against the use of NRP, citing unresolved ethical and medical concerns regarding its compatibility with the definition of death [43]. On the contrary, transcranial Doppler studies have shown no evidence of cerebral blood flow during NRP in isolated case reports, suggesting that further research is needed to clarify these concerns [48]. This debate regarding the use of NRP remains unresolved. Decisions about its implementation are left to the discretion of the ethical committees of individual institutions and regional organ networks. For A-NRP, cerebral blood flow is avoided by clamping the descending aorta at the diaphragm, ensuring that perfusion is limited to abdominal organs. Since the heart is not perfused during A-NRP, it is procured separately using the DPP technique [49].

2. **Cost-effectiveness**

The OCS is a technologically advanced method for organ preservation and transport, but its use is associated with high costs. The per-use cost is approximately $80,000 to $100,000. In comparison, the NRP method is relatively more cost-effective. Additionally, donor hearts assessed via OCS may ultimately be deemed unsuitable for transplantation, compounding the economic burden by incurring high costs without clinical benefit. Logistical challenges also arise when DCD candidates fail to progress to cardiac death after extubation, resulting in major time and resource burdens for procurement teams.

20.4 Conclusions

DCD heart transplantation, already well-established in Europe and Australia, is now being conducted on a large scale in the United States. However, achieving a global consensus on the optimal methods for organ perfusion and transport remains a challenge, with key considerations spanning ethical, economic, and long-term prognostic aspects. In Japan, the development of a cost-effective and safe DCD heart transplantation system will require close observation of ongoing research and clinical outcomes from other countries. Additionally, much progress is needed in fostering a broad understanding of the detailed definitions and processes involved in ventilator withdrawal, extubation, and the determination of cardiac death. These efforts are essential for ensuring the consistent and ethical implementation of DCD heart transplantation across diverse healthcare systems. By integrating insights obtained from international advancements and addressing ethical challenges while standardizing the best practices, DCD could become a universally accepted method to solve the donor shortage in heart transplantation.

References

1. Dhital KK, Iyer A, Connellan M, et al. Adult heart transplantation with distant procurement and ex-vivo preservation of donor hearts after circulatory death: a case series. Lancet. 2015;385(9987):2585–91.
2. Messer S, Page A, Axell R, et al. Outcome after heart transplantation from donation after circulatory-determined death donors. J Heart Lung Transplant. 2017;36(12):1311–8.
3. Abbasi J. Donation after circulatory death heart transplant is a US first. JAMA. 2020;323(2):111.
4. Jawitz OK, Raman V, DeVore AD, et al. Increasing the United States heart transplant donor pool with donation after circulatory death. J Thorac Cardiovasc Surg. 2020;159(5):e307–e9.
5. Fiedler A, Miller PN, Smith JW. Expanding the donation after circulatory death transplant Pool in the United States. Ann Thorac Surg. 2023;116(6):1121–3.
6. Barnard CN. A human cardiac transplant: an interim report of a successful operation performed at Groote Schuur hospital. Cape Town South African Med J. 1967;41:1271–4.
7. Baumgartner WA, Reitz BA, Gott VL, et al. Norman E. Shumway, MD, PhD: visionary, innovator, humorist. J Thorac Cardiovasc Surg 2009;137(2):269–277.
8. Beecher HK. A definition of irreversible coma. Report of the ad hoc Committee of the Harvard Medical School to examine the definition of brain death. JAMA. 1968;205:337–40.
9. Modry DL, Oyer PE, Jamieson SW, et al. Cyclosporine in heart and heart-lung transplantation. Can J Surg 1985;28(3):274–80, 82.
10. Casavilla A, Ramirez C, Shapiro R, Nghiem D, et al. Experience with liver and kidney allografts from non-heart-beating donors. Transplantation. 1995;59(2):197–203.
11. Gernhofer YK, Bui QM, Powell JJ, et al. Heart transplantation from donation after circulatory death: impact on waitlist time and transplant rate. Am J Transplant. 2023;23(8):1241–55.
12. Page A, Messer S, Large SR. Heart transplantation from donation after circulatory determined death. Ann Cardiothorac Surg. 2018;7(1):75–81.
13. Hann A, Osei-Bordom DC, Neil DAH, et al. The human immune response to cadaveric and living donor liver allografts. Front Immunol. 2020;11:1227.
14. Laurie J, Morrison CS, Grunau B, et al. Organ donation after out-of-hospital cardiac arrest: a scientific statement from the international liaison committee on resuscitation. Circulation. 2023;148(10):e120–46. https://doi.org/10.1161/CIR.0000000000001125. Epub 2023 Aug 8.
15. Dominguez-Gil B, Delmonico FL, Shaheen FA, et al. The critical pathway for deceased donation: reportable uniformity in the approach to deceased donation. Transpl Int. 2011;24(4):373–8.
16. Morrissey PE, Monaco AP. Donation after circulatory death: current practices, ongoing challenges, and potential improvements. Transplantation. 2014;97(3):258–64.
17. Schroder JN, Patel CB, DeVore AD, et al. Transplantation outcomes with donor hearts after circulatory death. N Engl J Med. 2023;388(23):2121–31.
18. White CW, Ambrose E, Muller A, et al. Assessment of donor heart viability during ex vivo heart perfusion. Can J Physiol Pharmacol. 2015;93(10):893–901.
19. Suntharalingam C, Sharples L, Dudley C, et al. Time to cardiac death after withdrawal of life-sustaining treatment in potential organ donors. Am J Transplant. 2009;9(9):2157–65.
20. Lewis JPJ, Nelson H, Snyder W, et al. Development of the University of Wisconsin donation after cardiac death evaluation tool. Prog Transplant. 2003;13:265–73.
21. Kotloff RM, Blosser S, Fulda GJ, et al. Management of the Potential Organ Donor in the ICU: Society of Critical Care Medicine/American College of Chest Physicians/Association of Organ Procurement Organizations Consensus Statement. Crit Care Med. 2015;43(6):1291–325.
22. Ardehali A, Esmailian F, Deng M, et al. Ex-vivo perfusion of donor hearts for human heart transplantation (PROCEED II): a prospective, open-label, multicentre, randomised non-inferiority trial. Lancet. 2015;385(9987):2577–84.
23. Shudo Y, Hiesinger W, Oyer PE, et al. Operative technique and pitfalls in donor heart procurement. Asian Cardiovasc Thorac Ann. 2017;25(1):80–2.

24. Kasinpila P, Ruaengsri C, Koyano T, et al. Case report: heart retransplant from a donor after circulatory death and extended transport period with normothermic perfusion. Front Cardiovasc Med. 2023;10:1212886.
25. Alomari M, Garg P, Yazji JH, et al. Is the organ care system (OCS) still the first choice with emerging new strategies for donation after circulatory death (DCD) in heart transplant? Cureus. 2022;14(6):e26281.
26. Krishnan A, Kasinpila P, Wang H, et al. First-in-human beating-heart transplant JTCVS Tech. 2023;19:80–5.
27. Beuth J, Falter F, Pinto Ribeiro RV, et al. New strategies to expand and optimize heart donor pool: ex vivo heart perfusion and donation after circulatory death: a review of current research and future trends. Anesth Analg. 2019;128(3):406–13.
28. Copeland H, Hayanga JWA, Neyrinck A, et al. Donor heart and lung procurement: a consensus statement. J Heart Lung Transplant. 2020;39(6):501–17.
29. Fiedler AG, DeVries S, Czekajlo C, et al. Normothermic regional perfusion surgical technique for the procurement of cardiac donors after circulatory death. JTCVS Tech. 2022;12:113–5.
30. Monteagudo Vela M, Garcia Saez D, Simon AR. Current approaches in retrieval and heart preservation. Ann Cardiothorac Surg. 2018;7(1):67–74.
31. Alamouti-Fard E, Garg P, Wadiwala IJ, et al. Normothermic regional perfusion is an emerging cost-effective alternative in donation after circulatory death (DCD) in heart transplantation. Cureus. 2022;14(6):e26437.
32. Hess NR, Ziegler LA, Kaczorowski DJ. Heart donation and preservation: historical perspectives, current technologies, and future directions. J Clin Med. 2022;11(19)
33. Truby LK, Casalinova S, Patel CB, et al. Donation after circulatory death in heart transplantation: history, outcomes, clinical challenges, and opportunities to expand the donor pool. J Card Fail. 2022;28(9):1456–63.
34. Messer S, Cernic S, Page A, et al. A 5-year single-center early experience of heart transplantation from donation after circulatory-determined death donors. J Heart Lung Transplant. 2020;39(12):1463–75.
35. Shudo Y, Leacche M, Copeland H, et al. A paradigm shift in heart preservation: improved post-transplant outcomes in recipients of donor hearts preserved with the SherpaPak system. ASAIO J. 2023;69(11):993–1000.
36. Urban M, Castleberry AW, Siddique A, et al. Utilization of Paragonix Sherpapak cardiac transport system for the preservation of donor hearts after circulatory death. Transplant Proc. 2023;55(9):1997–2002.
37. Kaliyev R, Bekbossynov S, Nurmykhametova Z. Sixteen-hour ex vivo donor heart perfusion during long-distance transportation for heart transplantation. Artif Organs. 2019;43(3):319–20.
38. Rega F, Lebreton G, Para M, et al. Hypothermic oxygenated perfusion of the donor heart in heart transplantation: the short-term outcome from a randomised, controlled, open-label, multicentre clinical trial. Lancet. 2024;404(10453):670–82.
39. Ayyaz A, Ali PD, Singh G, Qi W, et al. Rat model of veno-arterial extracorporeal membrane oxygenation. J Transl Med. 2014;12:37.
40. Sanchez-Camara S, Asensio-Lopez MC, Royo-Villanova M, et al. Critical warm ischemia time point for cardiac donation after circulatory death. Am J Transplant. 2022;22(5):1321–8.
41. Iyer A, Gao L, Doyle A, et al. Increasing the tolerance of DCD hearts to warm ischemia by pharmacological postconditioning. Am J Transplant. 2014;14(8):1744–52.
42. Madan S, Saeed O, Forest SJ, et al. Feasibility and potential impact of heart transplantation from adult donors after circulatory death. J Am Coll Cardiol. 2022;79(2):148–62.
43. Siddiqi HK, Trahanas J, Xu M, et al. Outcomes of heart transplant donation after circulatory death. J Am Coll Cardiol. 2023;82(15):1512–20.
44. Dhital K, Ludhani P, Scheuer S, et al. DCD donations and outcomes of heart transplantation: the Australian experience. Ind J Thorac Cardiovasc Surg. 2020;36(Suppl 2):224–32.
45. Messer S, Ardehali A, Tsui S. Normothermic donor heart perfusion: current clinical experience and the future. Transpl Int. 2015;28(6):634–42.

46. Chew HC, Iyer A, Connellan M, et al. Outcomes of donation after circulatory death heart transplantation in Australia. J Am Coll Cardiol. 2019;73(12):1447–59.
47. Shivank Madan OS, Forest SJ, Daniel J, et al. Feasibility and potential impact of heart transplantation from adult donors after circulatory death. J Am Coll Cardiol. 2022;79(2):148–62.
48. Perez Redondo M, Alcantara Carmona S, Villar Garcia S, et al. Transplantation of a heart donated after circulatory death via thoraco-abdominal normothermic regional perfusion and results from the first Spanish case. J Cardiothorac Surg. 2020;15(1):333.
49. Parent B, Caplan A, Moazami N, et al. Response to American College of Physician's statement on the ethics of transplant after normothermic regional perfusion. Am J Transplant. 2022;22(5):1307–10.

Multi-organ Transplantation in the United States

21

Alice V. Vinogradsky, Yoshifumi Naka, and Koji Takeda

Abstract

Multi-organ transplantation involves the simultaneous or sequential transplantation of more than one organ into a single recipient and may be offered to patients with end-stage organ failure affecting multiple organs due to a variety of underlying conditions. This chapter details the history and current landscape of multi-organ transplantation in the United States, discusses modern-day organ allocation policies, and provides an overview of the heart-liver, heart-kidney, and triple-organ transplantation experience. We highlight how ethical considerations regarding the just and equitable distribution of limited resources pose similar, albeit more nuanced, challenges to multi-organ transplantation as they do to single-organ transplantation and describe how careful candidate selection and ongoing refinements in surgical technique and medical management have allowed increasingly more patients, including those with irreversible, multisystem organ failure, to benefit from organ transplantation.

Keywords

Multi-organ transplant · Heart-liver transplant · Heart-kidney transplant · Combined transplant · Continuous distribution system · Organ allocation · Fontan operation · FALD

A. V. Vinogradsky · K. Takeda (✉)
Department of Cardiothoracic Surgery, Columbia University Irving Medical Center, New York, NY, USA
e-mail: avv2113@cumc.columbia.edu; kt2485@cumc.columbia.edu

Y. Naka
Department of Cardiothoracic Surgery, Cornell University Medical Center, New York City, New York, USA
e-mail: yn33@cumc.columbia.edu

H. Matsuda et al. (eds.), *Heart and Lung Transplantation*,
https://doi.org/10.1007/978-981-96-8810-4_21

21.1 Introduction

The development of organ transplantation in the world to date has been remarkable and has brought many lives and healthy life to many patients. On the other hand, the shortage of donors has limited the opportunities for patients to receive organs, and in the case of combined transplantation, there have been restrictions on the priority allocation of donor organs from the viewpoint of fair allocation. However, this institutional constraint has been improved by the recent increase in the donation from the donors, and the number of actual multiple organ transplants has been increasing.

There are several challenges associated with such combined organ transplantation: equitable mechanisms for organ allocation, demanding transplantation procedures, differences in transplantation immunologic responses of different organs, evaluation of organ failure for transplantation, and indications for retransplantation. This paper presents the current status of multi-organ transplantation in the United States based on the authors' experience at Columbia University at New York and discusses some of the controversial issues.

21.2 The United States Organ Allocation System

Demand for organs for transplantation far exceeds the available supply. To promote just and medically utile transplantation, the Organ Procurement and Transplantation Network (OPTN), a unique private-public partnership managed by the United Network for Organ Sharing (UNOS), links all US professionals involved in deceased-donor organ transplantation. Individual organ procurement organizations (OPOs), of which there are currently 58, are responsible for procurements in each region and are all members of the OPTN [1].

Prior to 2018, a classification-based system of organ allocation was utilized. Waitlist candidates were grouped together with others who had similar characteristics to a given donor. Following grouping, candidates were placed into classifications sorted by unique factors—including medical need, distance from donor hospital, biological makeup, and life expectancy—which were reviewed in a specific order. Given the prioritization of certain factors over others, candidates would often encounter hard boundaries that would prevent them from being ranked highly when a list of potential recipients for a given organ was generated. In 2018, the OPTN initiated a major overhaul of all US deceased-donor organ allocation policies with the goal of creating a more efficient, equitable, and inclusive system by instituting a continuous distribution system [2]. In this framework, no single factor determines a candidate's placement on the waitlist. Instead, one's score is a composite of medical urgency, predicted post-transplant survival, biology, and access, among other metrics.

This continuous distribution system has been introduced to provide the following patients' benefits [2]:

Table 21.1 The continuous distribution attributes in heart transplantation by OPTN Heart Transplantation Committee

	Medical urgency	Reducing biological disadvantages	Patient access	Placement efficiency	Post-transplant survival
Attributes	Adult statuses Pediatric statuses Waiting time on LVAD	Blood type Sensitization	Priority for pediatric candidates Priority for prior living donors Waiting time	Distance between transplant and donor hospital	NA

Source: Ref. [3]

- It's a more fair and flexible system, because multiple factors will be considered at the same time.
- Equity is predicted to increase among potential recipients.
- Patients can provide their feedback earlier in the policy development process.
- It's a single distribution framework that can be adapted to all organ types.

Allocation of each organ type (lung, kidney and pancreas, liver and intestine, or heart) depends on a set of attributes specific to that organ that collectively contribute to a patient's overall rank. Candidates receive points from multiple attributes, and the score is unique to each organ offer. In heart transplantation, the OPTN Heart Transplantation Committee identified the attributes in 2024 (Table 21.1) [3].

Specific allocation policies are in place to address the growing need for multi-organ transplantation. These generally require OPOs to allocate multiple organs from the same donor to patients who meet proper criteria and are updated as single-organ policies continue to evolve [4]. Still, given organ scarcity, allocating more than one organ to a single patient poses certain ethical dilemmas. To address this issue, in 2021, the OPTN established the Ad Hoc Multi-Organ Transplantation Committee. This group's primary charge is to develop and propose equitable organ allocation policies that address multiple organ groups. The Committee further works to ensure that all proposed multi-organ policies are in alignment with federal regulations governing the OPTN and a continuous distribution framework [4].

21.3 Multi-organ Transplantation

Patients who have several organs that have failed or are likely to fail may be in need of a multi-organ transplant, though it is also possible that organ function will recover after single-organ transplantation alone. In the case of simultaneous multi-organ transplantation, organs from the same donor are often transplanted, as doing so is believed to reduce the recipient's immune response and lower the risk of rejection. If a patient has more than one failing organ but only one is transplanted, should the failing organ not regain function, the patient may receive special priority for

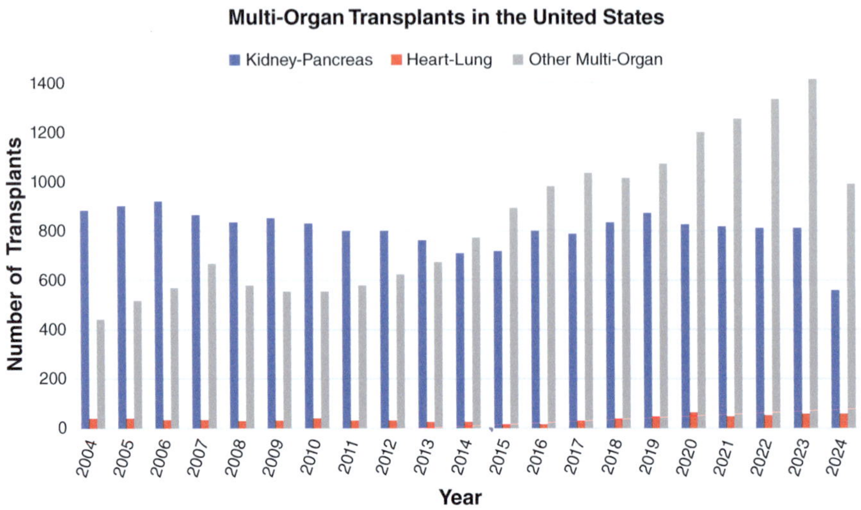

Fig. 21.1 Bar graph of the number of multi-organ transplants performed in the United States between 2004 and 2024. (Source: Ref. [6])

transplant of the second organ under a safety net multi-organ policy [5]. In either case, multi-organ transplants are rare, accounting for about 5% of all deceased donor organ transplants in the United States in the past 20 years [6].

The most frequent combination of transplanted organs—kidney-pancreas—comprises ~40% of all multi-organ transplants [7], and up to 90% of multi-organ transplants include a kidney [8]. While the combinations of pancreas-kidney and heart-lung have specific, policy-defined listing criteria and OPTN waitlists, others have no specified criteria, and a second organ is often allocated together with the primarily allocated organ [7]. To date, over 28,000 pancreas-kidney, 1500 heart-lung transplants, and 20,000 multi-organ transplants of various other combinations have been performed (Fig. 21.1). Heart-kidney transplantation is particularly common, with over 3500 to date, and heart-liver transplants, while relatively rare, are growing in number [6].

21.4 Multi-organ Transplantation at Columbia University Irving Medical Center

Thousands of transplants are done every year at Columbia University Irving Medical Center, including unique multi-organ procedures. The first heart transplant at Columbia was performed in 1977. Since then, Columbia's heart transplant program has grown to perform over 80 transplants annually, with more than 3000 to date, making it one of the largest in the United States by volume. The adult heart transplant volume at Columbia in the past 5 years, as well as the number of dual-organ transplants, involves the heart and either lung, kidney, or liver (Fig. 21.2). Note the

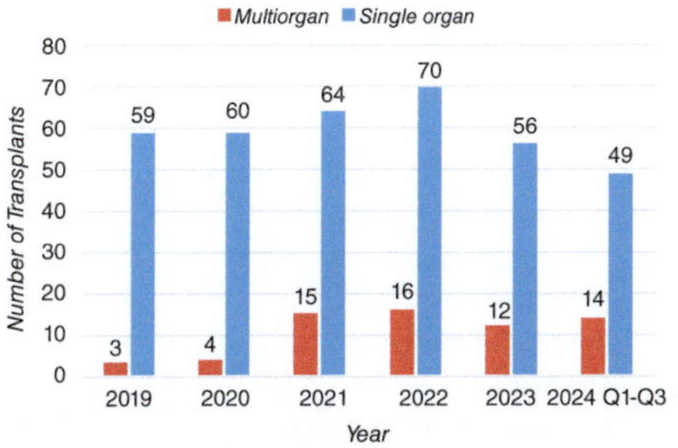

	2019	2020	2021	2022	2023	2024 Q1-Q3
Heart/Kidney	0	2	9	10	7	7
Heart/Liver	2	1	3	5	3	3
Heart/Lung	1	1	3	1	2	4
Overall %	**5%**	**7%**	**23%**	**23%**	**22%**	**28%**

Fig. 21.2 Adult heart transplant volume at Columbia University Irving Medical Center between 2019 and 2024. Bar graph (left) shows the number of isolated heart transplants (blue) as well as number of heart transplants performed in combination with at least one kidney, liver, or lung. Chart (right) demonstrates the number and percent of all heart transplants in a given year that were performed as part of a heart-kidney, heart-liver, or heart-lung transplant

significant increase in the percent of heart transplants done as part of a multi-organ operation, from 5% in 2019 to 28% in the first three quarters of 2024. As of June 2024, the adult heart transplant program is proud to report the highest three-year survival outcomes in the country, and our mechanical circulatory support program has expanded options for the sickest of patients, including those with multisystem organ failure. Such favorable outcomes in extremely sick patients have supported us in making the decision to list patients for multi-organ transplant, though we maintain that close interdisciplinary collaboration and judicious candidate selection are the foundation of any successful program.

21.5 Heart-Liver Transplantation

Combined heart and liver transplantation (CHLT) may be indicated for select patients with coexisting end-stage heart and liver disease. First described in 1984 by Starzl and colleagues [9], CHLT has become an internationally accepted strategy when the pathophysiology of the disease process underlying dual organ failure is a contraindication to single organ transplantation [10]. The various indications for CHLT and associated underlying diseases are shown in Table 21.2. Regardless of indication, outcomes are relatively favorable; in a recent UNOS database analysis of 364 CHLT recipients between 1987 and 2020, patient survival at 1, 3, and 5 years was found to be 87%, 80%, and 78%, respectively (Fig. 21.3) [11].

Although CHLT remains a rare operation largely due to donor organ scarcity and allocation protocols, it has gained increasing popularity in recent years [11]. In the United States, over 600 cases have been performed since 1992, with 350 in the past 5 years (Fig. 21.4) [6]. The leading indication for CHLT had long been familial amyloidosis involving both the heart and liver, though congenital heart disease (CHD) predominates in the modern era. Indeed, more adults with CHD have undergone CHLT between 2018 and 2020 than in the previous 18 years [11–13].

Table 21.2 Various indications and associated underlying diseases for combined heart-liver transplantation

Etiology of organ failure	Underlying disease
Abnormal amyloid deposition	Familial amyloid polyneuropathy
Primary liver disease and concurrent end-stage cardiac disease	Alcohol use disorder Cirrhotic cardiomyopathy Drug toxicity Familial hypercholesterolemia Hepatitis C Hepatocellular carcinoma Hereditary hemochromatosis Metabolic syndrome, nonalcoholic steatohepatitis
End-stage cardiac disease and secondary liver disease	Congenital heart disease Fontan-associated liver disease

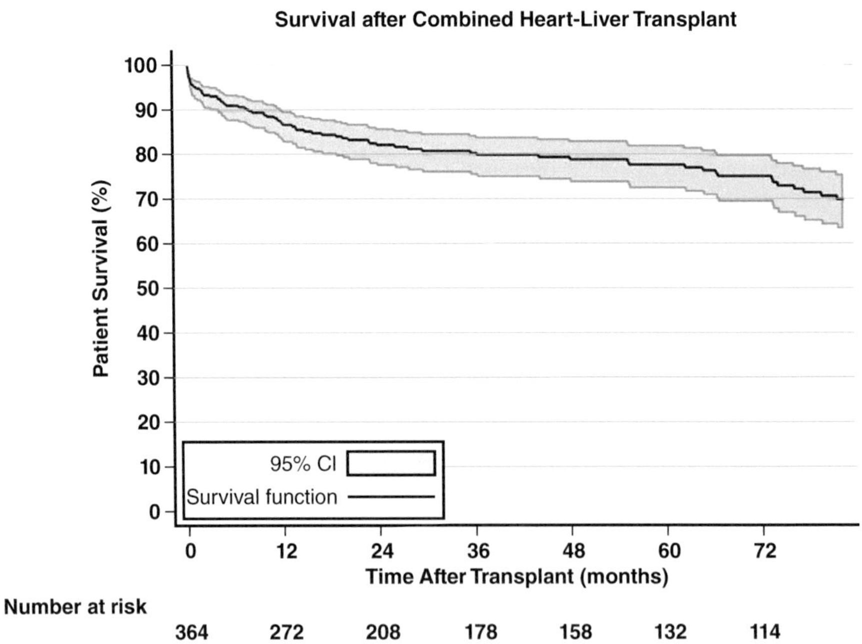

Fig. 21.3 Long-term survivals of combined heart-liver transplantation. Kaplan-Meier survival curve demonstrating 3-year survival among 364 adults undergoing combined heart-liver transplantation between December 1989 and August 2020 in the United States. (Source: Ref. [11] (open access))

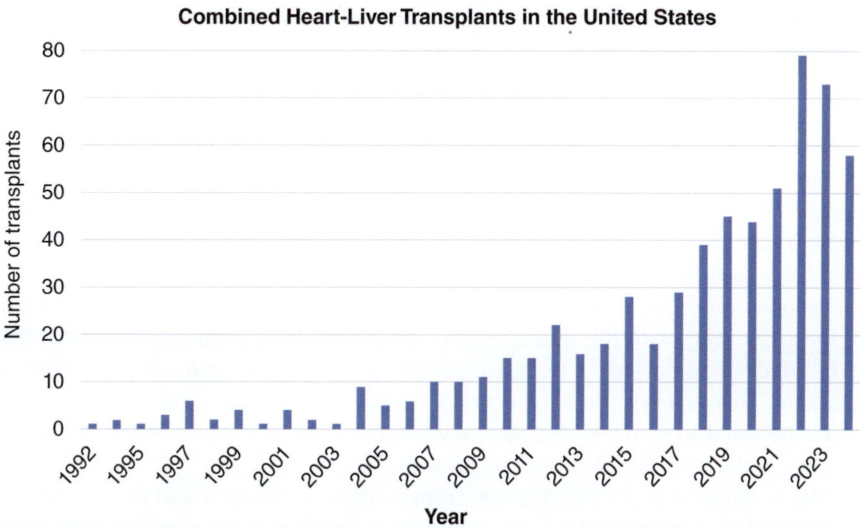

Fig. 21.4 Number of combined heart-liver transplants performed in the United States. (Data from Ref. [6])

Nowadays, nearly 95% of children with CHD survive to adulthood, though a substantial number go on to develop heart failure and hepatic cirrhosis secondary to elevated right-sided pressures associated with either the original intracardiac pathology, surgical repair, or biventricular dysfunction. A recent OPTN analysis found that 8% of all adults with CHD undergoing heart transplantation undergo CHLT[12]. Authors reported highly favorable 30-day and 1-year survival rates of 90% and 81%, which largely parallel those of mixed cohorts with various indications for CHLT. Furthermore, survival outcomes between CHD patients undergoing isolated heart transplant and CHLT were similar, with stable survival across the decades despite the boom in case volume. Similarly, a 2023 multicenter analysis of adult Fontan patients undergoing either isolated heart transplant or CHLT revealed significantly improved post-transplant survival in the years after 2010 (1-year: 76% vs. 46%; 5-year: 87% vs. 59%) [14]. These works highlight the feasibility and promise of CHLT as a strategy for patients with complex CHD and life-threatening complications of failing Fontan circulation. As there remain no explicit indications for CHLT in the Fontan population complicated by liver dysfunction, known as FALD [15] (Fontan-associated liver disease), further work to delineate factors associated with early hepatic dysfunction will be essential to identifying CHD patients who would benefit from CHLT [12].

Surgical approaches to heart-liver transplantation vary widely across transplant centers and include (1) staged transplantation during separate operations, (2) sequential implantation, and (3) en bloc dual-organ transplantation [16]. Of these, sequential, heart-first implantation is the most common [17]. In such cases, liver transplantation, particularly the anhepatic phase, may cause dramatic hemodynamic instability in a patient with a newly transplanted heart with temporarily reduced function. Various strategies for intraoperative hemodynamic support may be employed, including the continuation of cardiopulmonary bypass or transition to veno-arterial extracorporeal membrane oxygenation (V-A ECMO) or veno-venous bypass (VVB) [13, 18]. VVB is used to shunt blood from the inferior vena cava and mesenteric system to the right ventricle to maintain adequate preload while the cava and portal vein are clamped. However, there is concern that VVB may not provide enough support to accommodate the acute, large-volume fluid shifts that occur once the liver is reperfused, and V-A ECMO may instead be considered [19]. Alternatively, the en bloc technique, first described in 2012, allows both organs to be transplanted at the same time, with the inferior vena cava maintaining connection between the two, which may provide a technical advantage in patients with aberrant venous anatomy. This strategy also allows for a reduced ischemic time of the liver allograft and is believed to confer tighter hemodynamic control, decreased bleeding/coagulopathy, and improved early graft function [17].

Much enthusiasm for CHLT stems from evidence to suggest that the simultaneous transplantation of both organs may be immunoprotective, with the liver graft enhancing tolerance of the cardiac allograft [20]. In a large single-center series, Alturi and his colleagues were among the first to highlight a considerably lower-than-anticipated rate of rejection in CHLT recipients [21]. Most recently, Bakhtiyar and colleagues similarly saw a lower incidence of rejection episodes in patients with congenital heart disease who undergo CHLT compared to isolated heart transplant recipients [12]. Though the mechanisms underlying this phenomenon remain unclear, some have attributed it to shedding of soluble human leukocyte antigens by the liver, which acts as an "antigen sink" [22]. A review by Cannon and his colleagues also revealed a lower incidence of acute liver rejection among patients with graft survival greater than 1 year in the CHLT group compared to those undergoing liver transplant alone (5.2% vs. 12.2%) [20]. That CHLT patients have previously been successfully maintained on lower doses of immunosuppression compared to patients who undergo isolated heart transplantation further speaks to this immunoprotective effect [23].

Recently, a scientific statement has been released from the American Heart Association proposing the decision-making algorithm for CHLT [24]. And the concept consists of the parameters including regular liver function test, biochemical assays, and MEDL-XI Score (The Model of End-Stage Liver Disease Excluding INR), and abdominal ultrasound/CT. The final decision for CHLT is proposed as the presence of approved hepatic cirrhosis and MELD-X Soce over 11 points.

21.6 Heart-Kidney Transplantation

Given the close physiological interdependence of the cardiac and renal systems, kidney dysfunction is common in patients with end-stage heart failure. Dysfunction of one organ can affect the other—cardiogenic shock may cause renal hypoperfusion, volume overload may lead to overaction of the renal-angiotensin-aldosterone system, and neurohormonal disturbances may affect both the heart and kidneys [25]. Renal injury may also occur after cardiac transplantation, in part due to the necessity of cardiopulmonary bypass and the use of nephrotoxic immunosuppressive medications postoperatively [26, 27]. In either case, renal impairment—before or after heart transplantation—is associated with poor outcomes and increased post-transplant mortality [28].

First reported in 1978 by Norman and colleagues [29], combined heart-kidney transplantation (CHKT) has become a widely recognized treatment modality for patients with comorbid end-stage heart and renal failure. In the past 15 years, the number of CHKT performed has risen nearly fivefold, now to >300 annually [30] (Fig. 21.5), as studies have shown a survival advantage, less rejection, and less cardiac allograft vasculopathy in patients undergoing CHKT compared to heart-alone transplantation [6, 24, 31].

Like other multi-organ transplants, heart-kidney transplantation may be performed in a simultaneous (either as simultaneous procedures or sequentially within 24 h of one another) or staged fashion, the latter of which offers the benefits of hemodynamic optimization and stabilization and may decrease surgical complexity [31]. Some patients may also recover renal function after heart-alone transplantation, making appropriate patient selection for these scarce resources a challenge. UNOS policy holds that candidates must meet specific medical criteria for either chronic kidney disease or sustained acute kidney injury to be eligible for a required kidney share on a heart match. Safety net policies are also in place for kidney-after-heart allocation, and priority classifications are available for thoracic organ transplant recipients who are later listed for kidney transplant [31]. Kidney-after-heart transplantation may be indicated for patients with pretransplant kidney dysfunction

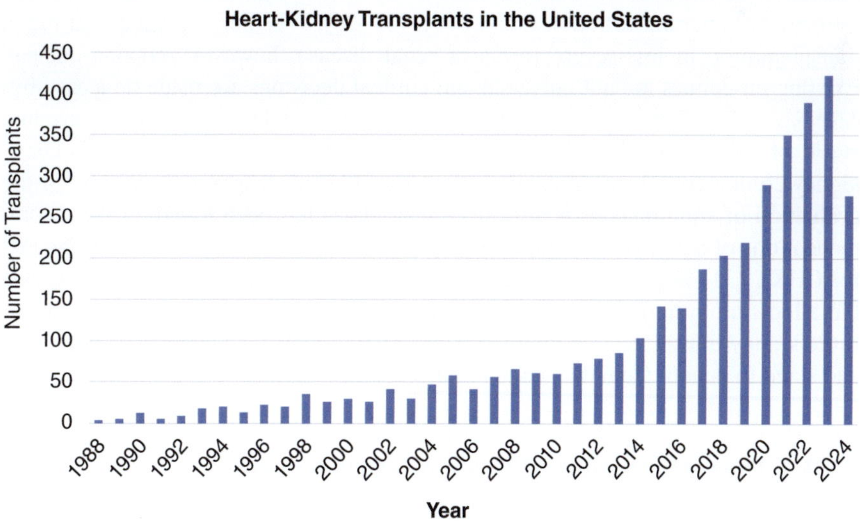

Fig. 21.5 Number of heart-kidney transplants performed in the United States. (Data from Ref. [30])

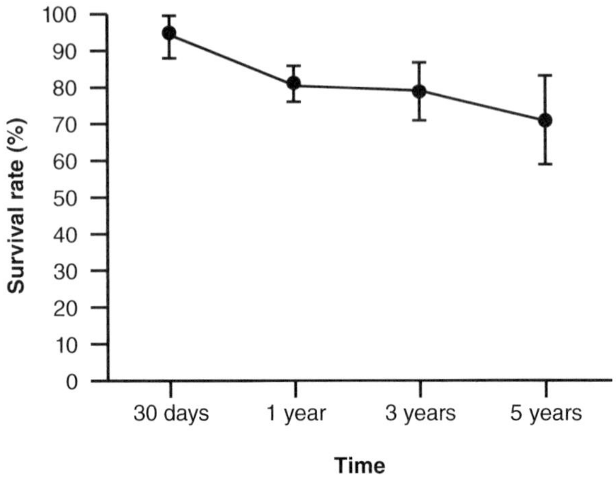

Fig. 21.6 Long-term survivals of heart-kidney transplantation. Kaplan-Meier survival curve showing a 30-day, 1-, 3-, and 5-year survival of 95% (95% CI: 88–100%), 81% (95% CI: 76–86%), 79% (95% CI: 71–87%), and 71% (95% CI: 59–83%), respectively, in a meta-analysis of 376 patients who underwent combined heart-kidney transplantation between 1996 and 2019 at 15 transplantation centers across the globe. (Source: Ref. [32] (open access))

or unanticipated severe kidney injury post-transplant; such patients will often undergo kidney transplantation before the initiation of dialysis and frequently receive living-donor grafts [31].

Retrospective studies have consistently demonstrated favorable survival after CHKT [32] (Fig. 21.6) as well as improved survival compared to heart-alone transplantation in dialysis-dependent candidates or those with a significantly reduced estimated glomerular filtration rate (eGFR) [33–36]. Whether to pursue dual-organ transplantation in less-severe forms of renal disease, however, remains unclear. Existing guidelines are not universal and clinical decisions are made on a case-by-case basis, though recent work suggests that heart candidates with a pre-transplant eGFR of <45 mL/min/1.73 m^2 have superior outcomes after simultaneous heart-kidney compared to heart-alone transplantation [37]. A proposed algorithm for the evaluation of simultaneous heart-kidney candidates has been based on the recommendations of a 2019 consensus conference seeking to establish national standards for CHKT [31, 38]. Ultimately, additional investigations are necessary to improve the allocation system for heart and kidney transplantation to avoid premature or futile kidney transplantation while also accurately identifying candidates who need and stand to benefit from dual-organ transplantation.

21.7 Transplantation of Three or More Organs

Transplantation of three or more organs is rare, though may be the only option for certain patients with multi-organ dysfunction. In advanced heart failure, congestion and hypoperfusion may precipitate congestive hepatopathy, hepatic cirrhosis, and cardiorenal syndrome. Meanwhile, end-stage liver disease may cause alterations in splanchnic vasodilation, leading to renal malperfusion, irreversible end-organ damage, hepatorenal and/or hepatopulmonary syndromes, and hepatopulmonary hypertension [39]. At present, multivisceral transplantation of the liver, intestine, and pancreas is the most common triple-organ transplant, with over 1200 to date, followed far behind by the four-organ combination of liver-kidney-intestine-pancreas (n = 134). Among transplants that include at least one thoracic organ, liver-heart-kidney is the most common, with nearly 70 to date, and the proportion that each ≥3 organ combination contributes to all multi-organ transplants [9] (Fig. 21.7).

While dual-organ transplantation has become a well-established strategy for patients with concomitant organ damage [38, 40, 41], the question of whether to allocate three or more organs, and to whom, requires careful evaluation of outcomes and what makes for the equitable and effective distribution of a limited resource. Few have published robust outcomes studies on the subject, with the available literature largely limited to case reports and small series. The largest retrospective analysis of the UNOS/OPTN database investigating the United States experience with triple organ transplantation was published in 2024; Adjei and his colleagues looked at the triple organ combinations of heart-kidney-lung (n = 12) and heart-kidney-liver (n = 37) and compared their survival with that of dual-organ transplants. Authors showed that patients undergoing triple organ transplant had similar 10-year survival to their corresponding dual-organ cohorts (45% for heart-lung-kidney group, 49% for heart-liver-kidney) (Fig. 21.8) [39]. Similarly, in a recent

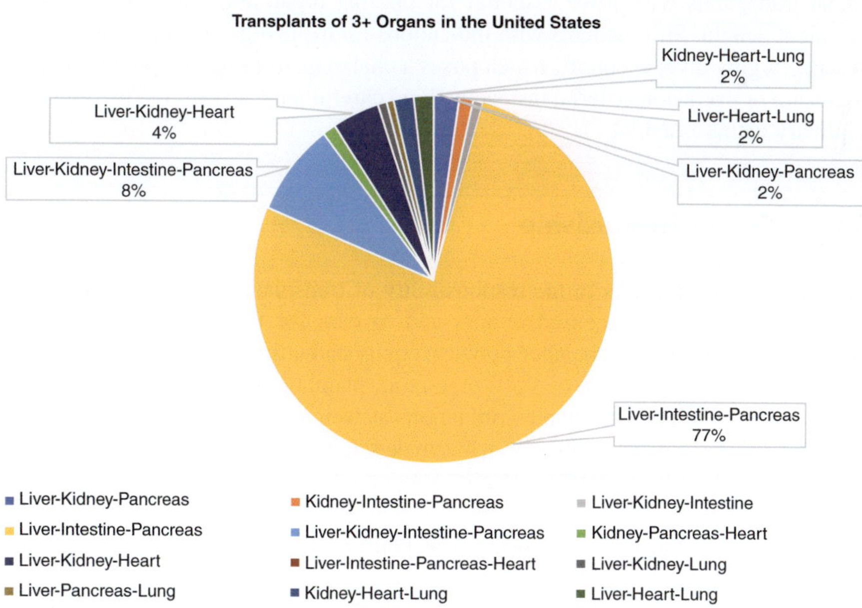

Fig. 21.7 Chart demonstrating the makeup of all transplants of 3+ organs in the United States. (Data from Ref. [6])

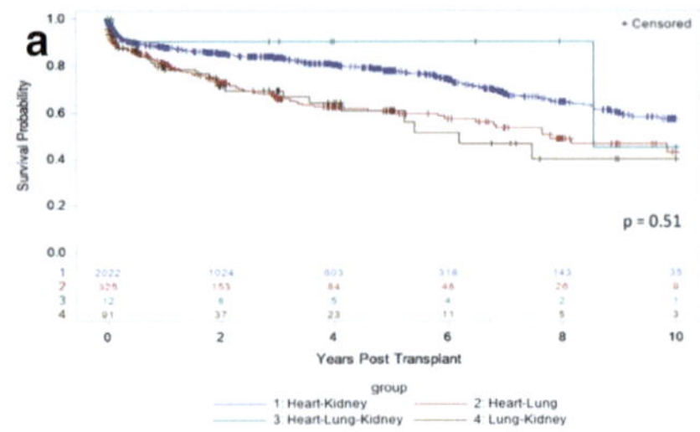

Years	Heart-Lung-Kidney		Heart-Kidney		Heart-Lung		Kidney-Lung	
	N at risk	Survival %	N at risk	Survival %	N at risk	Survival %	N at risk	Survival %
0	12	100	2022	100	325	100	91	100
1	8	90.0	1313	87.9	214	80.5	53	79.6
3	7	90.0	796	83.4	114	65.7	29	69.4
5	4	90.0	453	77.6	64	60.7	16	60.7
10	1	45.0	35	57.4	9	42.8	3	40.0

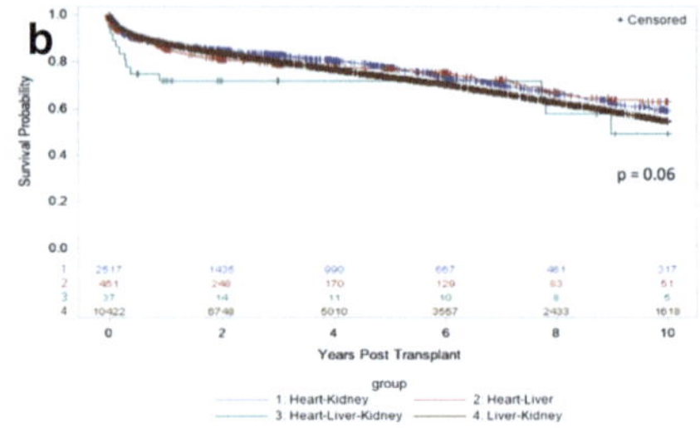

Years	Heart-Liver-Kidney		Heart-Kidney		Heart-Liver		Liver-Kidney	
	N at risk	Survival %	N at risk	Survival %	N at risk	Survival %	N at risk	Survival %
0	37	100	2517	100	451	100	10422	100
1	20	72.0	1741	87.6	307	85.0	7897	87.6
3	11	72.0	1193	82.9	203	78.7	5832	80.0
5	11	72.0	821	77.2	153	76.9	4252	73.2
10	5	49.4	317	58.9	51	62.6	1618	54.5

Fig. 21.8 Estimates of 10-year survival and number at risk of multiorgan transplantation in the United States between 1987 and 2022. (**a**) heart-lung-kidney, heart-kidney, lung-kidney, and heart-lung transplants. (**b**) heart–liver–kidney, heart–kidney, liver–kidney, and heart–liver transplants. (Source; Ref. [39] with permission)

UNOS study of triple organ heart transplants (heart-kidney-liver, heart-lung-kidney, heart-kidney-pancreas, and heart-lung-liver) between January 1989 and June 2023, authors reported a median survival of 81.5% (73.1–90.7%) at 1 year, and 69.9% (59.7–81.8%) at 5 years as well as a trend towards improved survival in recent years [42]. Taken together, these works suggest that triple organ transplants represent a reasonable allocation option in properly selected patients [39]. Given constraints on the donor pool, additional evaluation of outcomes data from simultaneous triple organ transplants will prove essential for optimal organ allocation and maximal recipient benefit. Still, patients with indications for triple organ transplantation represent a highly diverse cohort, which poses a challenge to the development of strict inclusion or exclusion criteria, instead making careful patient selection by multidisciplinary teams essential.

21.8 Organ Stewardship

Organ stewardship refers to the responsibility of transplant professionals to fairly allocate organs from deceased donors and to care for living donors. Doing so requires striking a careful balance between equity and utility, which may be particularly challenging in the field of multi-organ transplantation. Given the heterogeneity in patient population and organ combinations as well as the recency of the practice, data driving our understanding of what makes for good multi-organ stewardship remain limited. Still, the OPTN strongly supports the practice of multi-organ transplantation, as it is a life-saving therapy for patients who have no other options. In select situations, however, multiorgan transplantation may be less defensible, such as when the expected survival of the recipient is poor or when the need for a second organ is unclear. Per the OPTN public comment, proposal on the ethical implications of multi-organ transplants are as follows [43]:

- When the chance of survival is low, a transplant center should not proceed with multiorgan transplant.
- When the need for the second organ is unclear, a transplant center should only proceed after a thorough review of the candidate's condition and available data, and only if there is a reasonable chance that the second organ is necessary.

21.9 Conclusions and Future Perspectives

Ultimately, growing enthusiasm for multi-organ transplantation in recent years highlights the reality that many patients deemed inappropriate candidates for single-organ transplantation may not only be considered for, but also enjoy favorable outcomes after multi-organ transplant. With a meticulous approach to patient selection in the face of this rapid upstroke in case volume, increasingly more patients, including those with irreversible, multisystem organ failure, may benefit from transplantation. Extensive and unified efforts across organ transplant programs are necessary to coordinate care and continue to optimize outcomes for this challenging population of patients with multi-organ failure.

References

1. Organ Procurement and Transplantation Network (OPTN). About the OPTN. Health Resources and Services Administration (HRSA) https://optn.transplant.hrsa.gov/about/. Accessed 4 Jan 2025.
2. Organ Procurement and Transplantation Network (OPTN). A closer look at continuous distribution. Health Resources and Services Administration (HRSA) https://optn.transplant.hrsa.gov/policies-bylaws/a-closer-look/continuous-distribution/. Accessed 4 Jan 2025.
3. Organ Procurement and Transplantation Network (OPTN). Public Comment. Continuous Distribution of Hearts Update, Summer 2024. https://optn.transplant.hrsa.gov/media/vch-h1kty/pcsummer2024_edvideo_heart_cd-update.pdf
4. Organ Procurement and Transplantation Network (OPTN). A closer look at multi-organ transplantation. Health Resources and Services Administration (HRSA). https://optn.transplant.hrsa.gov/policies-bylaws/a-closer-look/multi-organ-transplantation/. Accessed 13 Nov 2024.
5. Organ Procurement and Transplantation Network (OPTN). Establish eligibility criteria and safety net for heart-kidney and lung-kidney allocation. https://optn.transplant.hrsa.gov/policies-bylaws/public-comment/establish-eligibility-criteria-and-safety-net-for-heart-kidney-and-lung-kidney-allocation/ Accessed 13 Nov 2024.
6. Organ Procurement and Transplantation Network (OPTN). OPTN data: National reports. Health Resources and Services Administration (HRSA). https://optn.transplant.hrsa.gov/data/. Accessed 13 Nov 2024.
7. Aeder M, Andreoni KA. Multi-organ allocation: medical and ethical considerations. Curr Transplant Rep. 2022;9:5–11.
8. Westphal SG, Langewisch ED, Robinson AM, et al. The impact of multi-organ transplant allocation priority on waitlisted kidney transplant candidates. Am J Transplant. 2021;21(6):2161–74.
9. Starzl TE, Bilheimer DW, Bahnson HT, et al. Heart-liver transplantation in a patient with familial hypercholesterolaemia. Lancet. 1984;1(8391):1382–3.
10. Zhao K, Mclean RC, Hoteit MA, et al. Combined heart and liver transplant: indication, patient selection, and allocation policy. Clin Liver Dis (Hoboken). 2019;13(6):170–5.

11. Alexopoulos SP, Wu WK, Ziogas IA, et al. Adult combined heart-liver transplantation: the United States experience. Transpl Int. 2022;35:10036.
12. Bakhtiyar SS, Sakowitz S, Ali K, et al. Combined heart-liver vs isolated heart transplantation in adults with congenital heart disease. Ann Thorac Surg. 2023;S0003-4975(23):00371–5.
13. Tracy KM, Matsuoka LK, Alexopoulos SP. Update on combined heart and liver transplantation: evolving patient selection, improving outcomes, and outstanding questions. Curr Opin Organ Transplant. 2023;28(2):104–9.
14. Lewis MJ, Reardon LC, Aboulhosn J, et al. Morbidity and mortality in adult Fontan patients after heart or combined heart-liver transplantation. J Am Coll Cardiol. 2023;81(22):2161–71.
15. Emamaullee J, Zaidi AN, Schiano T, et al. Fontan-associated liver disease; screening, management, and transplant consideration. Circulation. 2020;142:591–604.
16. Rauchfuss F, Breuer M, Dittmar Y, et al. Implantation of the liver during reperfusion of the heart in combined heart-liver transplantation: own experience and review of the literature. Transplant Proc. 2011;43(7):2707–13.
17. Mullis DM, Garrison A, Heng E, et al. Heart-liver transplantation using the en bloc technique: a single-center experience over two decades. J Thorac Cardiovasc Surg. 2024;S0022-5223(24):00765–7.
18. Lapisatepun W, Lapisatepun W, Agopian V, et al. Veno-venous bypass during liver transplantation: a new look at an old technique. Transplant Proc. 2020;52(4):905–9.
19. Smeltz AM, Kumar PA, Arora H. Anesthesia for combined heart and liver transplantation. J Cardiothorac Vasc Anesth. 2021;35(9):3350–61.
20. Cannon RM, Hughes MG, Jones CM, et al. A review of the United States experience with combined heart-liver transplantation. Transpl Int. 2012;25(12):1223–8.
21. Atluri P, Gaffey A, Howard J, et al. Combined heart and liver transplantation can be safely performed with excellent short- and long-term results. Ann Thorac Surg. 2014;98(3):858–62.
22. McMillan RW, Gelder FB, Zibari GB, et al. Soluble fraction of class I human histocompatibility leukocyte antigens in the serum of liver transplant recipients. Clin Transpl. 1997;11(2):98–103.
23. Hollander SA, Reinhartz O, Maeda K, et al. Intermediate-term outcomes after combined heart-liver transplantation in children with a univentricular heart. J Heart Lung Transplant. 2013;32(3):368–70.
24. Kittleson MM, Sharma K, Brennan DC, et al. Dual-organ transplantation: indications, evaluation, and outcomes for heart-kidney and heart-liver transplantation: a scientific statement from the American Heart Association. Circulation. 2023;148(7):622–36.
25. Rangaswami J, Bhalla V, Blair JEA, et al. Cardiorenal syndrome: classification, pathophysiology, diagnosis, and treatment strategies: a scientific statement from the American Heart Association. Circulation. 2019;139:e840–78.
26. Fortrie G, Manintveld OC, Caliskan K, et al. Acute kidney injury as a complication of cardiac transplantation. Transplantation. 2016;100:1740–9.
27. Sikma MA, Hunault CC, Kirkels JH, et al. Association of whole blood tacrolimus concentrations with kidney injury in heart transplantation patients. Eur J Drug Metab Pharmacokinet. 2018;43:311–20.
28. Itagaki S, Toyoda N, Moss N, et al. Outcomes of simultaneous heart and kidney transplantation. JACC. 2023;81(8):729–40.
29. Norman JC, Brook MI, Cooley DA, et al. Total support of the circulation of a patient with post-cardiotomy stone-heart syndrome by a partial artificial heart (ALVAD) for 5 days followed by heart and kidney transplantation. Lancet. 1978;1:1125–7.
30. United Network for Organ Sharing (UNOS). New data fields available June 29 to prepare for simultaneous heart-kidney and lung-kidney allocation. UNOS. Published June 29, 2024. Available from: https://unos.org/news/policy-changes/new-data-fields-available-june-29-shk-sluk/
31. Karamlou T, Welke KF, McMullan DM, et al. Combined heart-kidney transplant improves post-transplant survival compared with isolated heart transplant in recipients with reduced glomerular filtration rate: analysis of 593 combined heart-kidney transplants from the united network organ sharing database. J Thorac Cardiovasc Surg. 2014;147(1):456–61.e1.

32. Sampaio NZ, Faleiro MD, Vieira LVDS, et al. Simultaneous heart and kidney transplantation: a systematic review and proportional meta-analysis of its characteristics and long-term variables. Transpl Int. 2024;37:12750.
33. Schaffer JM, Chiu P, Singh SK, et al. Heart and combined heart-kidney transplantation in patients with concomitant renal insufficiency and end-stage heart failure. Am J Transplant. 2014;14:384–96.
34. Kilic A, Grimm JC, Whitman GJR, et al. The survival benefit of simultaneous heart-kidney transplantation extends beyond dialysis-dependent patients. Ann Thorac Surg. 2015;99:1321–7.
35. Karamlou T, Welke KF, McMullan DM, et al. Combined heart-kidney transplant improves post-transplant survival compared with isolated heart transplant in recipients with reduced glomerular filtration rate: analysis of 593 combined heart-kidney transplants from the united network organ sharing database. J Thorac Cardiovasc Surg. 2014;147:456–61.
36. Gill J, Shah T, Hristea I, et al. Outcomes of simultaneous heart-kidney transplant in the US: a retrospective analysis using OPTN/UNOS data. Am J Transplant. 2009;9:844–52.
37. Feng I, Wang AS, Takeda K, et al. Simultaneous heart-kidney transplant compared with heart transplant alone in patients with borderline renal function who are not dialysis dependent. J Thorac Cardiovasc Surg. 2024;168(1):149–60.e15.
38. Kobashigawa J, Dadhania DM, Farr M, et al. Consensus conference on heart-kidney transplantation. Am J Transplant. 2021;21:2459–67.
39. Adjei MA, Wisel SA, Steggerda JA, et al. Incidence and outcomes of simultaneous thoracoabdominal triple organ transplantation in the United States. Transplant Proc. 2024;56(1):161–8.
40. Rucker AJ, Anderson KL, Mulvihill MS, et al. Simultaneous versus sequential heart-liver transplantation: ideal strategies for organ allocation. Transplant Direct. 2019;5(1):e415.
41. Engen R, Shepherd D, Bradford MC, et al. Impact of multiorgan and kidney–pancreas allocation policies on pediatric kidney-alone transplant candidates in the United States. Pediatr Transplant. 2022;26(8):e14394.
42. Dunbar EG, Ambrosio M, Tchoukina IF, et al. Combined triple-organ transplantation: review of survival outcomes. Abstract only. J Heart Lung Transplant. 2024;43(4):Supplement S22.
43. OPTN/UNOS Ethics Committee. Public comment proposal: ethical implications of multi-organ transplants. Published June 2019. Available from: https://optn.transplant.hrsa.gov/.

Transplantation Immunology in Lung

22

Tomoyuki Nakagiri

Abstract

Transplantation immunology is a unique field that studies its immune response which occurs artificially after organ transplantation; Although it is a basic medical science, but a field in which the clinical department must be involved. In the case of lung transplantation, although the organ is connected to the outside environment, it requires a large dose of immunosuppressive drugs due to its own strong defense mechanism. However, the prognosis for lung transplantation is much poorer than for other solid organ transplants due to chronic lung allograft dysfunction (CLAD), which still occurs in more than 50% of transplant recipients. Prevention of CLAD without immunosuppressive drugs is urgently needed, and it is important to study its immunological pathogenesis. In this chapter, as the basis of lung transplantation immunology, it was described the unique defense mechanisms, the basic of immunology, risk factors for CLAD and their immunological mechanisms, and for the study of CLAD, biomarkers are mentioned from the clinical side and animal models from the experimental transplantation immunology.

Keywords

Transplantation immunology · Lung transplantation · Acute cellular rejection (ACR) · Chronic lung allograft dysfunction (CLAD) · Risk factors · Innate immunity · Acquired immunity · Antibody-mediated rejection (AMR) · Animal models

T. Nakagiri (✉)
Department of Cardiothoracic, Transplantation and Vascular Surgery, Hannover Medical School, Hannover, Germany
e-mail: Nakagiri.Tomoyuki@mh-hannover.de

H. Matsuda et al. (eds.), *Heart and Lung Transplantation*,
https://doi.org/10.1007/978-981-96-8810-4_22

22.1 Introduction

As for organ transplantation, immunological rejection of the foreign organs is the primary problem. The transplantation immunity is an immune state, as a reaction that occurs after the surgical therapeutic intervention. In other words, it is a special basic science field that requires the involvement of surgeons. Conversely, because of the operative involvement, it is still a poorly recognized area in the field of basic immunology.

In terms of transplantation immunity, especially regarding solid organ transplantation, relatively advanced research has been made on kidney, liver, pancreas, and heart transplantations, while research results that will lead to clinical practice have not yet been produced on lungs. Clinically the median survival for kidney, liver, pancreas, and heart transplantation is 14.76, 14.59, 16.10, and 11.73 years, respectively, while the median survival after lung transplantation is only 5.58 years [1]. This is due to the dilemma of the lung being an organ in contact with the outside environments and having its own defense mechanisms, and because of that, requiring strong immunosuppression after transplantation. However, too much immunosuppression increases the risk of side effects, such as infection, kidney damage, and development of malignant diseases. The major leading cause of death after lung transplantation is chronic lung allograft dysfunction (CLAD) [2], the mechanism of which is still unknown and animal models for research are insufficient. Currently, the gold standard for diagnosis of acute rejection is bronchoscopic biopsy, and there are also no non-invasive or minimally invasive biomarkers needed to diagnose early CLAD [3]. Furthermore, cellular immunity has been the focus of attention as a mechanism of rejection, but in the last two decades, it has become clear that antibody-mediated rejection (AMR) is also involved in the development of CLAD and has entered as a new factor of transplantation immunity that needs to be clarified [4, 5]. In addition, the intermediating mechanisms between the risk factors for CLAD, including acute rejection, and the development of CLAD remain unclear and continue to be investigated.

22.2 Unique Defense Mechanisms

22.2.1 Anatomical Physiology

The lung is an organ that is connected to the outside environment, therefore has an extensive vascular bed. Because of that, it is susceptible to damage from the destruction of donor and/or recipient erythrocytes and damage to the epithelium, which release various inflammatory agents, to ischemia-reperfusion injury (IRI) due to non-infectious inflammation [6]. In addition, goblet cells found from the trachea to the bronchioles and Clara cells found after the bronchioles produce antimicrobial peptides as well as mucins. Normally, the mucin-entrapped pathogens are expelled by epithelial ciliary movement and cough reflex. However, after transplantation, the nerves for the cough reflex are disconnected and inadequate, making the patient more susceptible to pneumonia. In deeper respiratory bronchi, they lack cartilage for structural maintenance, and collapse is prevented by a surfactant secreted by the type II alveolar epithelium.

22.2.2 Innate Immunity

When pathogens cross the epithelial barrier and invade, first, the complement accessory pathway (second pathway) is activated on the bacterial surface, and then surfactant proteins activate the lectin pathway [7, 8]. Thus, post-transplantation, the cells are susceptible to complement-mediated damage. In addition, the activated fragments of complement, C3a and C5a, cause histamine release from tissue mast cells and increase vascular permeability (Fig. 22.1) [8, 9]. This leads to the recruitment of neutrophils, macrophages, and tissue NK cells to the graft, and to the activation of tissue-resident lymphocytes, especially innate immune T cells (γδ-T cells) earlier than after other solid organ transplantations (Fig. 22.2) [10–13]. These tissue-resident immune cells remain in the tissue for several years after transplantation and are a major contributor to the strong post-transplant rejection response.

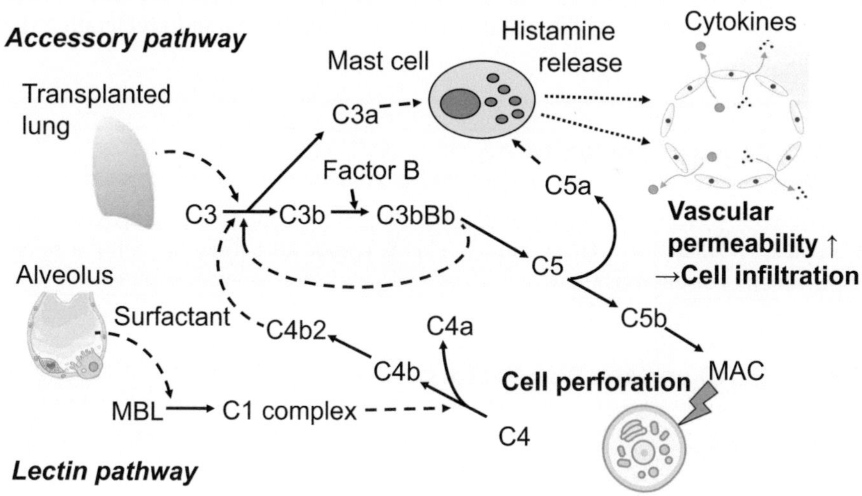

Fig. 22.1 Complement pathways in lung transplantation. Unlike the classical pathway (not shown), the accessory pathway does not require immune complexes. Complement 3 (C3) is cloven into C3a and C3b upon graft stimulation. The C3b binds to Factor B in the blood (C3bBb). This complex further activates C3 (broken lines: stimulation). The C3bBb binds to the graft cell, leading to a cascade of complement activity that cleaves down C5 into C5a and C5b. The C5b forms a membrane-attack complex (MAC), which disrupts the graft cell membrane. In addition, C3a and C5a stimulate mast cells, which release histamine, resulting in increased permeability of the vessel wall, cytokine influx, and inflammatory cell infiltration. In the lectin pathway, mannose-binding lectin (MBL) is activated by alveolar surfactant and forms C1 complex. This activates C4, forming C4b2, which activates the accessory pathway

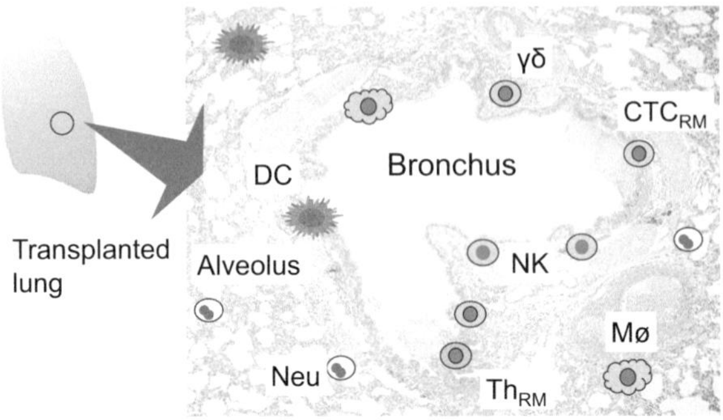

Fig. 22.2 Tissue-resident immune cells. A variety of immune cells are resident in the lungs, bronchi, and alveoli. In addition to dendritic cells (DCs), natural killer cells (NKs), and macrophages (Mø), the bronchioles contain numerous lymphocytes (Th_{RM}: Tissue-resident helper memory cells, CTC_{RM}: Tissue-resident cytotoxic memory cells, γδ: γδ T cells, and B-resident memory cells). DCs, Mø, resident memory lymphocytes, and neutrophils (Neu) are also present in the alveoli

Furthermore, epithelial cells and macrophages recognize cells, produce inflammatory cytokines, increase vascular permeability, and allow further phagocytic invasion into the tissue [14, 15]. This is also a major factor in posttransplant rejection. The transplanted lung epithelium and tissue macrophages themselves are foreign bodies to the recipient, which can cause chronic stimulation and accelerating the immune response [16].

22.2.3 Acquired Immunity

The immune system that is activated after antigen presentation, primarily by lymphocytes, is called acquired immunity. This is responsible for acute cellular rejection, which is discussed below.

22.3 CLAD and the Risk Factors

22.3.1 CLAD

CLAD is the main cause of death after lung transplantation, and is now classified into two types, bronchiolitis obliterans syndrome (BOS) and restrictive allograft syndrome (RAS) [2, 17]. See other chapters for descriptions of these. In this section, only historical trends relevant to the study of transplantation immunity will be discussed.

First, chronic rejection was defined as irreversible fibrotic obstructions of the bronchioles after lung transplantation, bronchiolitis obliterans (BO) [18]. In other words, the histological diagnosis of lung tissue that had undergone irreversible pathological changes was defined as chronic rejection, so the mechanism of its

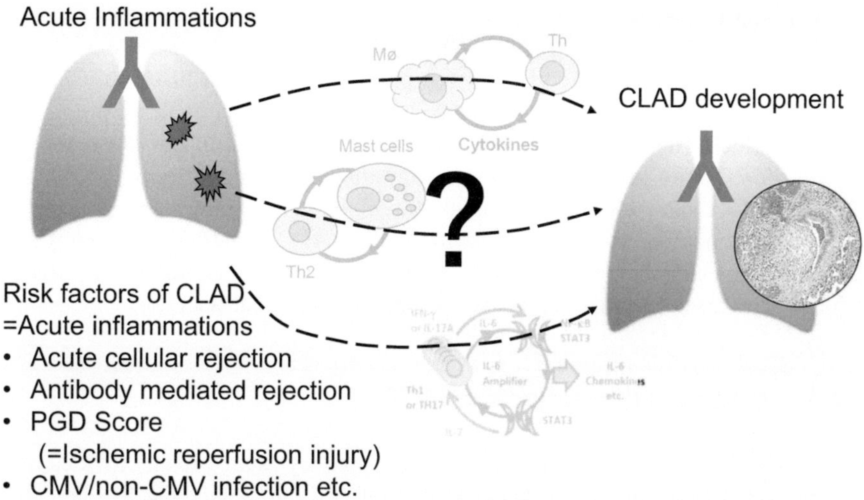

Fig. 22.3 Risk factors of chronic lung allograft dysfunction (CLAD) development. Risk factors of CLAD include the intensity and frequency of acute rejection, high primary graft dysfunction (PGD) scores, cytomegalovirus (CMV) infection or other pneumonia, etc.

development was unknown. Bronchoscopic tissue biopsy was essential for this diagnosis, but it was difficult to perform such an invasive bronchoscopy for patients with respiratory failure. Therefore, BOS was defined as a clinical diagnosis as an alternative without invasive examinations [19–21]. In this entity, a group of patients with rapid deterioration was classified and defined as a clinical diagnosis of RAS [2, 17]. The histopathology of RAS differs from that of BO and it is characterized by fibrosis of the alveolar interstitium and visceral pleura. However, the pathogenesis of both CLAD is still not well known. We know only clinical risk factors including the frequency and severity of acute rejection, acute lung inflammation such as primary graft dysfunction (PGD), cytomegalovirus pneumonia or other pneumonias, and gastroesophageal reflux disease [2, 17] (Fig. 22.3). Except for acute rejection, the other risk factors can have different inflammatory mechanisms from rejection, and we also study these.

22.3.2 Ischemic Reperfusion Injury (IRI)

Clinically, it is considered the most common cause of high score of primary graft dysfunction (PGD). At the reperfusion, aseptic inflammation, increasing vascular wall permeability, and infiltration of inflammatory cells can be caused [22]. In addition, the activation of complement causes vascular wall damage, activation of immune cells in the tissues, and formation of intravascular thrombi, all of which contribute to decreased permeability of chest radiographs and hypoxia [23].

22.3.3 Acute Rejection

Self and nonself are identified by polymorphisms of the major histocompatibility complex (MHC, also called human leukocyte antigen: HLA in humans) present on the cell surface. There are two classes: Class I is expressed on all types of cells, and presents foreign substances such as viruses invading the body and waste products on the cell surface and passes the information to immune cells (NK cells, etc.), while class II is expressed on antigen-presenting cells (APC: dendritic cells, etc.) and presents antigens to helper T cells (see below). This initiates an immune response, which in the case of transplantation results mainly in cellular rejection.

22.4 Acute Cellular Rejection (ACR)

As a systemic acquired immune mechanism, lymphocytes are broadly divided into T cells and B cells, the former being further divided into helper T cells (Th-cells: CD4 positive T cells) and cytotoxic T cells (CTCs: CD8 positive T cells, killer T cells). Undifferentiated dendritic cells phagocytose foreign substances (grafts) to become mature dendritic cells and simultaneously present antigens bound to MHC class II on the cell surface as antigen-presenting cells (APCs) [24]. Th-cells recognize this MHC class II-bound antigen. This leads to the production of various cytokines, which promote the activation of immune cells. CTCs recognize antigens bound to MHC class I that are expressed on the surface of phagocytes, especially macrophages and mature dendritic cells as APC. There are three pathways (combinations) between the MHC classes and T cell subtypes, direct pathway, semi-direct pathway, and indirect/late pathway (Fig. 22.4) [25]. B cells encounter the antigen and produce IgM. B cells then receive approval from Th-cells to transform into plasma cells and produce IgG antibodies (discussed below in the AMR section).

Th-cells can be further classified into effector Th-cells and regulatory T cells (Tregs). Effector Th-cells can be further classified into Th1, Th2, and Th17 cells. In addition, Th9, Th22, and Tfh cells are nowadays also known, but these are omitted here. In general, Th1 cells have a fraction in the natural state to regulate the attack against intracellular viruses. Their differentiation is mediated by the transcription factor T-bet. Th1 cells produce IFN-γ, TNF-α and β, and activate macrophages and NK cells. Th2 cells promote the differentiation of the B cells and are originally responsible for attacks against parasites. GATA3 is important as a transcription factor, and the surface markers CCR4 and CXCR4, as well as IL-4 by intracellular staining, are used for identification. It is known that not only DCs but also macrophages, B cells, and eosinophils (EOS) present antigens. Recently, it has been reported that eosinophils are responsible for Th2 induction [26].

One subset of Th2 cells is known to cause chronic airway inflammation in mice [27], and animal studies have shown eosinophil infiltration of grafts and the presence of IL-5 [29], although its role in transplantation immunity remains not well known clinically. Th17 is a subset which has become known in the last two decades and has an interesting relationship with Tregs. Th17 cells produce IL-17A and

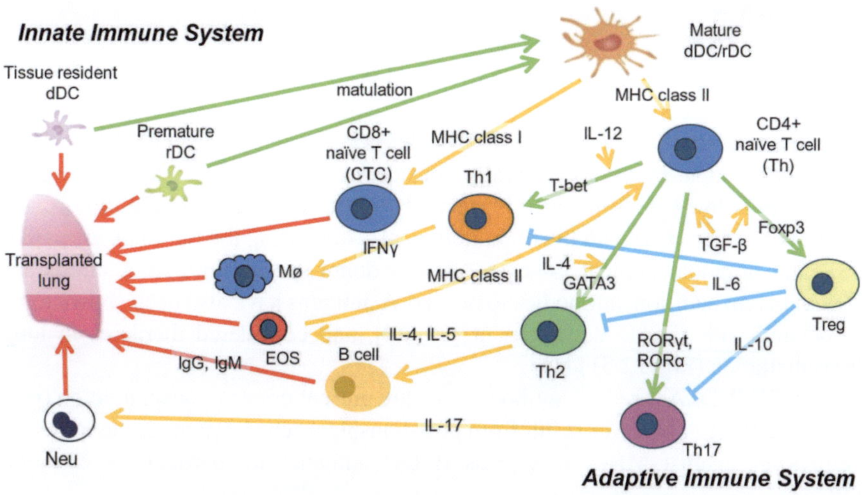

Fig. 22.4 Innate and adaptive immune systems. In addition to the text, graft is first rejected by the innate immune system. At this event, resident dendritic cells in the lung, i.e., donor-derived dendritic cells (dDCs), are also recruited and subsequently mature and work as antigen-presenting cells (APCs). Antigen presentation to recipient naïve lymphocytes is mediated via major histocompatibility complex (MHC) class I for cytotoxic T cells (CTCs) and MHC class II for helper T cells (Ths). This dDC-mediated pathway is called the direct/early pathway. Later, recipient DCs (rDCs) also phagocytose the donor graft and present antigens to Ths. This is called the indirect/late pathway. Recently, antigen presentation by rDC mediated by donor-derived MHC I/II has been reported and classified as a semi-direct pathway. *Treg* regulatory T cell, *EOS* eosinophils

IL-17F, and induce G-CSF and chemokines, which collect neutrophils and fibroblasts [24]. Th17 cells are mainly responsible for bacterial attack in early phase. TGFβ and IL-6 are required for differentiation, and RORγt and RORα are important transcription factors. This subset is identified by the surface marker CCR6 and the intracellular stains IL-17A and IL-17F. They have been reported to contribute to acute rejection and CLAD formation [24, 28]. Unlike the effector Th-cells as described above, Tregs are a subgroup of lymphocytes that suppress immune responses.

Mechanisms include the expression of IL-10 and CTLA4. Classical Tregs have FoxP3 as their master transcription factor. Interestingly, TGF-β is required for Treg differentiation, as is Th17; however, the additional presence of IL-6 induces RORγt and naive T cells differentiate into Th17, whereas the absence of IL-6 induces FoxP3, and Treg differentiation [28]. Tregs are still functional during acute rejection, but the effects of effector Th-cells and drug therapy seem to be stronger than Treg effect [30]. However, the percentage of Tregs in lymphocytes in the early postoperative period affects the chronic phase [31]. Several studies have shown that patients with CLAD have significantly less Tregs than stable resilient in the chronic phase [32, 33], and already early after lung transplantation [31, 34].

22.5 AMR

AMR is a syndrome defined by graft dysfunction and the presence of antibodies [2], but currently no consensus diagnostic criteria exist [35]. It is generally considered to have a poorer prognosis than ACR. The detection of complement C4d deposition by bronchoscopic biopsy is generally considered the pathologic standard, but its specificity is low [35, 36], and it is currently left to the diagnostic criteria of individual centers, such as with the immunological testing using the Luminex assay [37, 38]. The principal clinical issue in AMR is donor-specific anti-HLA antibodies (DSA) [4]. In addition, antibodies to non-HLA antigens have also been shown to be associated with CLAD development [39, 40], and considered therapies in lung transplantation (Fig. 22.5) [41].

Anti-HLA DSAs are IgG antibodies and are present prior to transplantation (preformed anti-HLA DSA) or result from post-transplant sensitization (de-novo DSA). Antibodies against MHC/HLA class II DQ antigens are particularly common [42, 43].

Those preformed anti-HLA DSAs are present because the recipient has been sensitized preoperatively by blood transfusion, pregnancy, or because of re-transplantation [44]. This can cause hyperacute rejection that occurs within minutes to hours after transplantation. Clinically, patients currently undergo anti-HLA antibody screening at transplant registration. In addition, with early globulin therapy and plasma exchange therapy, this rejection is prevented mostly [45].

When DSA develops in a patient, it appears mostly by 14th postoperative day [4]. The incidence of DSA in the early postoperative period (within 90 days) is reported to be 25–56% [4, 46]. Interestingly, the presence of DSA correlates with clinically diagnosed acute rejection, but not with biopsy-diagnosed acute rejection

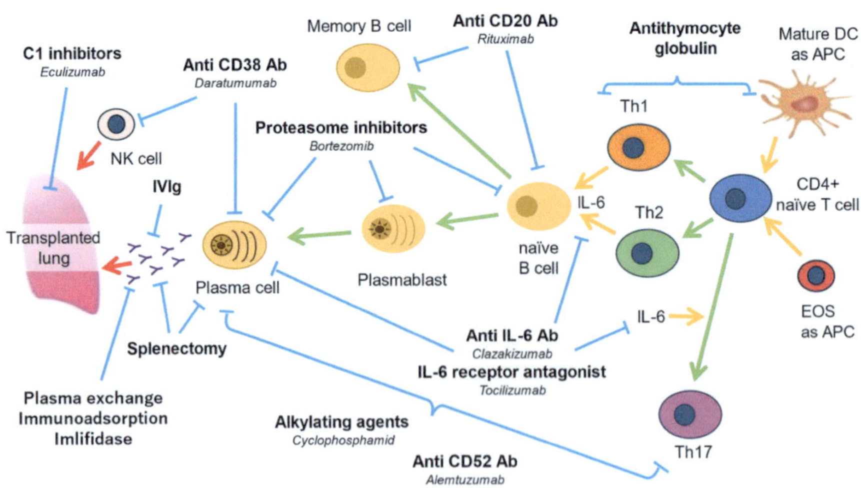

Fig. 22.5 Overview of antibody-mediated rejection and their discussed therapies in lung transplantation

[4]. This may be related to the fact that biopsy diagnoses principally cellular acute rejection [47]. In addition, the presence or absence of DSA has been associated with graft survival, engraftment, and the development of CLAD [4, 48], although a study reported no correlation between CLAD and DSA class I [38]. It may depend on the diagnostic criteria. The consensus diagnostic criteria are needed.

22.6 Biomarker

Currently, various cytokines are candidates for immune-related biomarkers for the diagnosis of acute rejection and CLAD. Of particular interest are TNF-α, TGF-β, and MCP-1, which can be found in both peripheral blood and bronchoalveolar lavage fluid (BALF) [49]. IL-26 in BALF has also been reported to be elevated in CLAD development [49]. Donor-derived cell-free DNA is also of interest as a new biomarker [51, 52]. It has been reported to be a marker for moderate or severe acute rejection, but unfortunately has not been mentioned as a marker for mild acute rejection. In addition, it is still not easy to distinguish acute rejection from infection and other conditions [50].

22.7 Animal Model

Although a rat lung transplant model had already been published by Mizuta et al. [53], it was not suitable for analyzing rejection mechanisms and developing a BO model because the reproducibility of the model was unstable and the number of genetically modified strains was not as abundant, comparing with mouse strains. Since the publication of the mouse orthotopic transplantation technique in 2007 [54], various inbred line combinations have been attempted. Acute rejection is omitted in this chapter because it is only necessary to perform transplantation in a MHC mismatch combinations. Here it is referred to as mouse models of CLAD.

Currently, there are three major combinations: first is major mismatch models, in which daily postoperative immunosuppressive therapy results in BO-like fibrotic stenotic lesions in 20–80% of the transplanted mice [55, 56]. These models have complete MHC class I and class II mismatches and are considered the most accurate representation of clinical lung transplantation. However, these are quite challenging for clinical surgeons, considering that immunosuppressive drugs must be administered daily postoperatively.

Next is minor mismatch models. The main model is the combination of C57BL/10 (B10) and C57BL/6 (B6), with 45–60% of mice developed BO [57, 58]. Recent studies have indicated that inbred mice are not completely homozygous [59], and since there is no MHC mismatch between B6 and B10, it is likely that acute rejection and the BO are caused by such genetic mismatch, i.e., the BO formation is based on an indirect allogeneic recognition response other than the MHC class recognition. B6, a genetically modified mouse that is highly susceptible to the disease, is used. We have reported that its development can be controlled by the administration of immunosuppressive drugs [58]. However, a disadvantage is that it is unclear which indirect allogeneic recognition response engages.

Lastly, models of moderate mismatch, in which an F1 mouse is created by crossing two inbred lines and its lungs are transplanted into mice of the original inbred line [60]. A BO model of this mismatch is, in which lungs from B6D2F1/J, the F1 of B6 and DBA/2 J, are transplanted into DBA/2 J, and the RAS model, in which B6D2F1/J to B6 [60, 61]. Although there are difficulties in obtaining F1 mice, this model is very interesting because it does not require the use of immunosuppressive drugs and it is clear that the CLAD occurred due to differences in its MHC mismatch.

As limitations, mice don't have respiratory bronchioles, and their terminal bronchioles are directly connected to the alveoli, which is an anatomical difference from human anatomy [62]. In addition, the fact that there are a variety of models means that the optimal mouse model has not yet been obtained. It is necessary to choose the combination that best suits the purpose of the research. Large animals, especially pigs, are more closely related to humans than rodents, and their lung structure is similar to humans. In addition, a reproducible model using genetically defined miniature pigs has been published [63].

22.8 On Going Studies

One of the current research projects in this area focuses on whether drugs with anti-inflammatory effects other than immunosuppressants can prevent risk factors such as acute rejection and ischemia-reperfusion injury, in addition to searching for drugs that can prevent BO formation and the mechanism in the mediation between them. As a recent finding, α1-antitrypsin was found to play a role in preventing acute rejection in a mouse orthotopic lung transplantation model [64]. Another study showed that hemopexin administration can suppress ischemia-reperfusion injury in lung preservation [22]. I hope that these studies with the application of such immunosuppressive-independent anti-inflammatory drugs after transplantation can be extended and support the investigation of the mechanism of BO formation to improve the survival rate of transplanted organs.

22.9 Summary

There are many other areas of transplantation immunology in addition to those mentioned above, and each is being studied in its own field, so it is difficult to give a general future perspective. Here, I would like to mention some of my personal research themes and perspectives. There are various risk factors for BO(S), but they are all acute inflammation. Even after acute inflammation settles, inflammation might still persist in the bronchial wall and alveolar interstitium due to infiltration of inflammatory cells, but the mechanism leading to chronic inflammation and BO formation from these acute inflammations has not yet been clarified. The greatest risk factor is acute rejection. However, post-lung transplant patients have already received the maximum dose or at least a higher dose of immunosuppressive drugs than other solid organ transplant patients. Therefore, it is difficult to administer more immunosuppressives in view of side effects. For solutions, two approaches are possible: One is to use anti-inflammatory therapy that does not depend on immunosuppressive drugs. The other is to study the relationship between acute inflammation and BO(S) and suppress the mechanism.

References

1. Ferreira LD, Goff C, Kamepalli S, et al. Survival benefit of solid-organ transplantation: 10-year update. Dig Dis Sci. 2023;68(9):3810–7.
2. Shah RJ, Diamond JM. Update in chronic lung allograft dysfunction. Clin Chest Med. 2017;38(4):677–92.
3. Shtraichman O, Diamond JM. Emerging biomarkers in chronic lung allograft dysfunction. Expert Rev Mol Diagn. 2020;20(5):467–75.
4. Ius F, Sommer W, Tudorache I, et al. Early donor-specific antibodies in lung transplantation: risk factors and impact on survival. J Heart Lung Transplant. 2014;33(12):1255–63.
5. Heise EL, Chichelnitskiy E, Greer M, et al. Lung transplantation despite preformed donor-specific antihuman leukocyte antigen antibodies: a 9-year single-center experience. Am J Transplant. 2023;23(11):1740–56.
6. White SR, Floreth T, Liao C, Bhorade SM. Association of soluble HLA-G with acute rejection episodes and early development of bronchiolitis obliterans in lung transplantation. PLoS One. 2014;9(7):e103643.
7. Pastva AM, Wright JR, Williams KL. Immunomodulatory roles of surfactant proteins A and D: implications in lung disease. Proc Am Thorac Soc. 2007;4(3):252–7.
8. Sahu SK, Maurya RK, Kulkarni HS. The role of complement component C3 in protection against pseudomonas pneumonia-induced lung injury. DNA Cell Biol. 2024;43(4):153–7.
9. Desai JV, Kumar D, Freiwald T, et al. C5a-licensed phagocytes drive sterilizing immunity during systemic fungal infection. Cell. 2023;186(13):2802–2822.e22. https://doi.org/10.1016/j.cell.2023.04.031.
10. Iske J, Wiegmann B, Ius F, et al. Immediate major dynamic changes in the T- and NK-cell subset composition after cardiac transplantation. Eur J Immunol. 2023;53(7):e2250097.
11. Snyder ME, Finlayson MO, Connors TJ, et al. Generation and persistence of human tissue-resident memory T cells in lung transplantation. Sci Immunol. 2019;4(33):eaav5581.
12. Nicosia M, Fairchild RL, Valujskikh A. Memory T cells in transplantation: old challenges define new directions. Transplantation. 2020;104(10):2024–34.
13. Zazara DE, Belios I, Lücke J, et al. Tissue-resident immunity in the lung: a first-line defense at the environmental interface. Semin Immunopathol. 2022;44(6):827–54.
14. Shepherd HM, Gauthier JM, Li W, et al. Innate immunity in lung transplantation. J Heart Lung Transplant. 2021;40(7):562–8.
15. Brouland JP, Egan T, Roussi J, et al. In vivo regulation of von Willebrand factor synthesis: von Willebrand factor production in endothelial cells after lung transplantation between normal pigs and von Willebrand factor-deficient pigs. Arterioscler Thromb Vasc Biol. 1999;19(12):3055–62.
16. Porrett PM, Yuan X, LaRosa DF, et al. Mechanisms underlying blockade of allograft acceptance by TLR ligands. J Immunol. 2008;181(3):1692–9.
17. Verleden GM, Glanville AR, Lease ED, et al. Chronic lung allograft dysfunction: definition, diagnostic criteria, and approaches to treatment-a consensus report from the Pulmonary Council of the ISHLT. J Heart Lung Transplant. 2019;38(5):493–503.
18. Burke CM, Theodore J, Dawkins KD, et al. Post-transplant obliterative bronchiolitis and other late lung sequelae in human heart-lung transplantation. Chest. 1984;86(6):824–9.

19. Cooper JD, Billingham M, Egan T, et al. A working formulation for the standardization of nomenclature and for clinical staging of chronic dysfunction in lung allografts. International Society for Heart and Lung Transplantation. J Heart Lung Transplant. 1993;12(5):713–6.
20. Nathan SD, Barnett SD, Wohlrab J, et al. Bronchiolitis obliterans syndrome: utility of the new guidelines in single lung transplant recipients. J Heart Lung Transplant. 2003;22(4):427–32.
21. Arjuna A, Olson MT, Walia R, et al. An update on current treatment strategies for managing bronchiolitis obliterans syndrome after lung transplantation. Expert Rev Respir Med. 2021;15(3):339–50.
22. Nakagiri T, Köhler NR, Janciauskiene S, et al. Hemopexin alleviates sterile inflammation in ischemia-reperfusion-induced lung injury. Front Immunol. 2024;15:1451577.
23. Napoli C, Benincasa G, Fiorelli A, et al. Lung transplantation: current insights and outcomes. Transpl Immunol. 2024;85:102073.
24. Nakagiri T, Inoue M, Minami M, et al. Immunology mini-review: the basics of T(H)17 and interleukin-6 in transplantation. Transplant Proc. 2012;44(4):1035–40.
25. Koutsokera A, Levy L, Pal P, et al. Acute cellular rejection: is it still relevant? Semin Respir Crit Care Med. 2018;39(2):181–98.
26. Yoshimoto T, Yasuda K, Tanaka H, et al. Basophils contribute to T(H)2-IgE responses in vivo via IL-4 production and presentation of peptide-MHC class II complexes to CD4+ T cells. Nat Immunol. 2009;10(7):706–12.
27. Nakayama T, Hirahara K, Onodera A, et al. Th2 cells in health and disease. Annu Rev Immunol. 2017;35:53–84.
28. Nakagiri T, Inoue M, Morii E, et al. Local IL-17 production and a decrease in peripheral blood regulatory T cells in an animal model of bronchiolitis obliterans. Transplantation. 2010;89(11):1312–9.
29. Goldman M, Le Moine A, Braun M, et al. A role for eosinophils in transplant rejection. Trends Immunol. 2001;22(5):247–51.
30. Nakagiri T, Warnecke G, Avsar M, et al. Lung function early after lung transplantation is correlated with the frequency of regulatory T cells. Surg Today. 2012;42(3):250–8.
31. Ius F, Salman J, Nakagiri T, et al. Increased frequency of CD4+ CD25high CD127low T cells early after lung transplant is associated with improved graft survival – a retrospective study. Transpl Int. 2020;33(5):503–16.
32. Khan MA, Lau CL, Krupnick AS. Monitoring regulatory T cells as a prognostic marker in lung transplantation. Front Immunol. 2023;14:1235889.
33. Meloni F, Morosini M, Solari N, et al. Peripheral CD4+ CD25+ Treg cell expansion in lung transplant recipients is not affected by calcineurin inhibitors. Int Immunopharmacol. 2006;6(13–14):2002–10.
34. Salman J, Ius F, Nakagiri T, et al. Association of Higher CD4+ CD25high CD127low , FoxP3+ , and IL-2+ T cell frequencies early after lung transplantation with less chronic lung allograft dysfunction at two years. Am J Transplant. 2017;17(6):1637–48.
35. Levine DJ, Glanville AR, Aboyoun C, et al. Antibody-mediated rejection of the lung: a consensus report of the International Society for Heart and Lung Transplantation. J Heart Lung Transplant. 2016;35(4):397–406.
36. Roux A, Levine DJ, Zeevi A, et al. Banff lung report: current knowledge and future research perspectives for diagnosis and treatment of pulmonary antibody-mediated rejection (AMR). Am J Transplant. 2019;19(1):21–31.
37. Lachmann N, Todorova K, Schulze H, et al. Luminex(®) and its applications for solid organ transplantation, hematopoietic stem cell transplantation, and transfusion. Transfus Med Hemother. 2013;40(3):182–9.
38. Brugière O, Suberbielle C, Thabut G, et al. Lung transplantation in patients with pretransplantation donor-specific antibodies detected by Luminex assay. Transplantation. 2013;95(5):761–5.

39. Reinsmoen NL, Mirocha J, Ensor CR, et al. A 3-center study reveals new insights into the impact of non-HLA antibodies on lung transplantation outcome. Transplantation. 2017;101(6):1215–21.
40. Xu Q, Elrefaei M, Taupin JL, et al. Chronic lung allograft dysfunction is associated with an increased number of non-HLA antibodies. J Heart Lung Transplant. 2024;43(4):663–72.
41. Böhmig GA, Eskandary F, Doberer K, et al. The therapeutic challenge of late antibody-mediated kidney allograft rejection. Transpl Int. 2019;32(8):775–88.
42. Brugière O, Roux A, Le Pavec J, et al. Role of C1q-binding anti-HLA antibodies as a predictor of lung allograft outcome. Eur Respir J. 2018;52(2):1701898.
43. Iasella CJ, Ensor CR, Marrari M, et al. Donor-specific antibody characteristics, including persistence and complement-binding capacity, increase risk for chronic lung allograft dysfunction. J Heart Lung Transplant. 2020;39(12):1417–25.
44. Aburahma K, de Manna ND, Kuehn C, et al. Pushing the survival bar higher: two decades of innovation in lung transplantation. J Clin Med. 2024;13(18):5516.
45. Ius F, Sommer W, Kieneke D, et al. IgM-enriched human intravenous immunoglobulin-based treatment of patients with early donor specific anti-HLA antibodies after lung transplantation. Transplantation. 2016;100(12):2682–92.
46. Hachem RR, Yusen RD, Meyers BF, et al. Anti-human leukocyte antigen antibodies and preemptive antibody-directed therapy after lung transplantation. J Heart Lung Transplant. 2010;29(9):973–80.
47. Stewart S, Fishbein MC, Snell GI, et al. Revision of the 1996 working formulation for the standardization of nomenclature in the diagnosis of lung rejection. J Heart Lung Transplant. 2007;26(12):1229–42.
48. Patel N, Snyder LD, Finlen-Copeland A, et al. Is prevention the best treatment? CMV after lung transplantation. Am J Transplant. 2012;12(3):539–44.
49. Silva T, Voisey J, Hopkins P, Apte S, Chambers D, O'Sullivan B. Markers of rejection of a lung allograft: state of the art. Biomark Med. 2022;16(6):483–98.
50. Magnusson JM, Ericson P, Tengvall S, et al. Involvement of IL-26 in bronchiolitis obliterans syndrome but not in acute rejection after lung transplantation. Respir Res. 2022;23(1):108.
51. Sebastian A, Silvy M, Coiffard B, et al. A review of cell-free DNA and epigenetics for non-invasive diagnosis in solid organ transplantation. Front Transplant. 2024;3:1474920.
52. De Vlaminck I, Valantine HA, Snyder TM, et al. Circulating cell-free DNA enables noninvasive diagnosis of heart transplant rejection. Sci Transl Med. 2014;6(241):241ra77.
53. Mizuta T, Kawaguchi A, Nakahara K, et al. Simplified rat lung transplantation using a cuff technique. J Thorac Cardiovasc Surg. 1989;97(4):578–81.
54. Okazaki M, Krupnick AS, Kornfeld CG, et al. A mouse model of orthotopic vascularized aerated lung transplantation. Am J Transplant. 2007;7(6):1672–9.
55. De Vleeschauwer S, Jungraithmayr W, Wauters S, et al. Chronic rejection pathology after orthotopic lung transplantation in mice: the development of a murine BOS model and its drawbacks. PLoS One. 2012;7(1):e29802.
56. Yamada Y, Windirsch K, Dubs L, et al. Chronic airway fibrosis in orthotopic mouse lung transplantation models-an experimental reappraisal. Transplantation. 2018;102(2):e49–58.
57. Suzuki H, Fan L, Wilkes DS. Development of obliterative bronchiolitis in a murine model of orthotopic lung transplantation. J Vis Exp. 2012;65:3947.
58. Nakagiri T, Ahrens L, Lienenklaus S, et al. Radiological and pathological findings in a minor-mismatch mouse orthotopic lung transplant model under immunosuppression. Int J Org Transplant Med. 2021;12:1–11.
59. Chebib J, Jackson BC, López-Cortegano E, et al. Inbred lab mice are not isogenic: genetic variation within inbred strains used to infer the mutation rate per nucleotide site. Heredity (Edinb). 2021;126(1):107–16.
60. Mimura T, Walker N, Aoki Y, et al. Local origin of mesenchymal cells in a murine orthotopic lung transplantation model of bronchiolitis obliterans. Am J Pathol. 2015;185(6):1564–74.

61. Misumi K, Wheeler DS, Aoki Y, et al. Humoral immune responses mediate the development of a restrictive phenotype of chronic lung allograft dysfunction. JCI Insight. 2020;5(23):e136533.
62. Basil MC, Morrisey EE. Lung regeneration: a tale of mice and men. Semin Cell Dev Biol. 2020;100:88–100.
63. Sahara H, Shoji T, Ng CY, et al. The role of indirect recognition of MHC class I and II allopeptides in a fully mismatched miniature swine model of lung transplantation. Transplant Proc. 2006;38(10):3253–5.
64. Nakagiri T, Wrenger S, Sivaraman K, et al. α1-Antitrypsin attenuates acute rejection of orthotopic murine lung allografts. Respir Res. 2021;22(1):295.

Immunological Transplantation Tolerance: Availability of Rat Transplant Models for Clinical Application

23

Toshinori Ito

Abstract

Induction of immune tolerance to the transplanted organ is the ultimate goal of organ transplantation. If this can be achieved, the use of permanent immunosuppressive drugs is avoided, and consequently the risk of complications such as opportunistic infection is avoided. However, whether tolerance can be induced depends on the organ. The liver is the organ in which tolerance is most easily achieved. On the other hand, pancreas, small intestine, and skin, which are highly immunogenic organs, are known to be extremely difficult. Heart and kidney are somewhere in between. In the case of pancreas transplantation, autoimmune reactions must be controlled in addition to rejection. Basic experimental studies are essential for the induction of immune tolerance. These experiments often require the use of inbred small animals, especially rats, which are relatively easy to transplant. To date, we have attempted to induce immune tolerance using various rat transplantation models.

Keywords

Immunological tolerance · Major histocompatibility complex · Immunogenicity · Active immunological enhancement · Intrathymic injection · Autoimmune recurrence · Graft versus host disease

T. Ito (✉)
Osaka Center for Cancer and Cardiovascular Disease Prevention, Osaka, Osaka, Japan
e-mail: juki@osaka-ganjun.jp

H. Matsuda et al. (eds.), *Heart and Lung Transplantation*,
https://doi.org/10.1007/978-981-96-8810-4_23

23.1 Introduction

The ultimate goal for organ transplantation is to achieve donor-specific immune tolerance. If this is successfully achieved, it will be possible to discontinue the use of permanent immunosuppressive agents.

It has been previously known that the use of donor antigens in combination with immunosuppressive agents could prolong graft engraftment at the same time of transplantation. In the 1980s, for example, an attempt was made to prolong graft survival by transfusion of donor blood prior to transplantation (DST: donor-specific transfusion) in living donor renal transplantation, together with immunosuppressive drugs. This was also the time when cyclosporine (CsA) was introduced and various efforts were made to further prolong the survival of the transplanted kidney. In extreme cases, bone marrow transplantation (BMT), in which the recipient's hematopoietic system is completely replaced by the donor's, can be used as an alternative to organ transplantation from the same donor. When an organ transplant is performed from the same donor, the donor-replaced hematopoietic system may be immunologically tolerant to the transplanted organ without any type of rejections in the recipient's body.

23.2 Active Immunological Enhancement

As described above, many attempts have been made to combine hematopoietic-derived donor antigens with immunosuppressive agents for active immunological enhancement.

First of all, in an inbred rat heart transplant combination (BUF; $RT1^b$ to WF; $RT1^u$), we administered donor soluble antigen (extracted from splenocytes with 3 M KCL) and cyclosporine for 3 days (−1, 0, +1) before and after the transplantation procedure followed by 2 cycles of cyclosporine administration (7, 8, 9; 15, 16, 17, day), resulting in a significant graft prolongation [1].

In this study, the mechanism was assessed using LDA (limiting dilution analysis) to evaluate donor-specific cytotoxic T cell (Tc) clone size, namely precursor cell frequency (fTcp).

The fTcp on day 10 post-transplant was reduced, and a further significant reduction was observed on day 30. This decrease was considered to be a result of suppression of donor antigen-specific proliferation by suppressor T cells ($CD4^+T$, $CD8^+T$).

Rejection in organ transplantation is generally known to be due to the differences in histocompatibility antigens (MHC & mH) between donor and recipient, as well as by differences in the immune response genes (*Ir* genes) of the recipient.

We investigated the differences in immune responses in heart transplantation systems using recombinant inbred rats. Rat MHC-RT1.A/C and B/D locuses correspond to class I and II MHC, respectively.

The heart grafts from R8 ($RT1.A^aB^uD^uC^u$) to PVG.U ($RT1.A^uB^uD^uC^u$), which differ only in the class I MHC antigen (RT1.A locus under $RT1^u$ background) were rejected, but the transplant from PVG.R1 ($RT1.A^aB^cD^cC^c$) to PVG ($RT1.A^cB^cD^cC^c$), which differ only in the class I MHC antigen (RT1.A locus under $RT1^c$ background) showed prolonged engraftment (>100 days) [2]. The former is a high responder system and all other organs such as liver and kidney are rejected, whereas the latter is a low responder system and organs other than pancreas and skin are not rejected. No differences in donor-specific fTcp in splenocytes were observed before transplantation both in high responder and low responder systems. However, on the fifth day after heart transplantation, the fTcp of the former showed an increase in clone size, while that of the latter did not show an increase in clone size, which correlated with transplantation outcome.

We examined the active immunological enhancement model by a newly developed immunosuppressive agent (FK506; tacrolimus) in donor BMT using an inbred rat combination (BUF; $RT1^b$ to LEW; RT1 [1, 3]. The results of this study showed that BMT on the day of transplantation and the second cycle were significantly enhanced. The transplanted hearts were significantly enhanced for prolonged periods (>100 days) after BMT on the day of transplantation and 2 cycles of FK506 −1, 0, 1; 9, 10, 11). In addition to fTcp by LDA, a newly developed system for measuring the precursor frequency of IL-2-producing helper T cells (fThp) [4] was also established and analyzed. At 10 days after transplantation, fThp was lower in the BMT + FK506 group than in the control group. However, fTcp was slightly higher, suggesting that the Tcp clone was still maintained at this time. At 50 days after transplantation, however both fThp and fTcp were low and the clone size of both was reduced, which the involvement of $CD4^+$ suppressor T cell was suggested by the mixed lymphocyte culture (MLR) results.

23.3 Induction of Immune Tolerance by Intrathymic Injection (IT) of Donor Bone Marrow Cells into the Thymus

We investigated a method of inducing immune tolerance by intrathymic injection of donor antigens into the thymus. The thymus is an organ with immunological privileges similar to the eye, brain, and reproductive organs (testis and uterus). For example, a fetus is a foreign body to a pregnant woman, but is not rejected. Therefore, such organs are less prone to inflammation and are isolated from the immune system.

In a rat heart transplant model from BUF ($RT1^b$) to WF ($RT1^u$), donor bone marrow cells were injected into the recipient thymus on the day of transplantation, and FK506 (tacrolimus; −1, 0, +1) and ALS (antilymphocyte serum, −1) were administered perioperatively [5]. Thus, the heart grafts prolonged more than 210 days. Further, skin challenge (skin grafting) at 130 days after transplantation resulted in long-term engraftment (>120 days) of the donor BUF skin, but the third party LEW skin was rejected, indicating that antigen-specific immune tolerance had been induced.

23.4 Immunogenicity of the Pancreas

It is well known that pancreatic grafts are very susceptible to allograft rejection because of the strong immunogenicity of the pancreas itself. There seems to be a hierarchy of organ- and tissue-dependent immunogenicity, the degree of which reflects the outcome of transplanted organ and tissue, that is, rejection or acceptance. In some small animal studies with matched genetic backgrounds, the most likely rejection order is skin > pancreas/small intestine > > heart > kidney > liver. This phenomenon may be due to differences in the organ and tissue distribution of MHC alloantigens, or the existence of organ- and tissue-specific antigens.

The strong immunogenicity of the transplanted pancreas was examined using a recombinant inbred rat model in which only the class I MHC (RT1.A) antigens differed. In low responder combination, PVG.R1 (RT1.$A^aB^cD^cC^c$) to PVG (RT1.$A^cB^cD^cC^c$), heart grafts could prolong (>100 days), but pancreatic grafts were rejected within a mean survival time of 21.4 days [6]. An MLR proliferative response against donor R1 was observed in pancreas transplant (PTx) recipients, but not in heart transplant (HTx) recipients. The major responder was $CD4^+$T cells, but not $CD8^+$ T cells.

Further analyses were performed by LDA to estimate the precursor frequencies of IL-2-producing Th cells and Tc cells, fThp and fTcp, respectively. PVG recipients with PTx had significantly higher fThp (1:5030) than those with HTx (1:17,326). In contrast, there was no difference in fTcp between PTx (1:1848) and HTx (1:2215) recipients. Further, in a CDC (complement-dependent cytotoxicity) assay, high titers of antibodies directed at class I MHC alloantigens were found in the sera of PTx recipients, but not in HTx recipients.

Taken together, these results suggest that Tc cells do not seem to be responsible for the of R1 pancreatic grafts in PVG recipients, but rather that the rejection may be mediated by $CD4^+$T cells and complement-fixing antibodies against class I MHC alloantigens, although adoptive transfer experiments using $CD4^+$ T cells or sera should be performed to investigate the underlying mechanism of rejection. It seemed necessary to consider not only cellular immunity but also humoral immunity in pancreatic transplantation.

23.5 Control of Autoimmune Recurrence in the Grafted Pancreas

In pancreas transplantation, the subject has type 1 diabetes mellitus (IDDM), and a recurrence of autoimmune mechanisms in the transplanted pancreas, namely "insulitis" can lead to graft failure. This was previously reported by a group at the University of Minnesota who performed pancreas transplants between monozygotic twins without the use of immunosuppressive drugs. Therefore, in addition to rejection, autoimmune reactions must also be controlled in pancreas transplantation. Although it is usually possible to examine rejection in inbred transplantation, the mechanism of autoimmune recurrence in grafted pancreas cannot be elucidated.

Thus, we decided to use an inbred model of BB (BioBreeding)–DP (diabetic prone) rat, a model of spontaneous type 1 diabetes. BB-DP rats are essentially immune deficient, having a total deficit of T cells with RT6 alloantigens, which is only expressed on rat mature T cells and consists of two subtypes, RT6.1 and RT6.2. For example, DP rats carry the RT6.1 gene, but do not express RT6.1 alloantigen, while WF rats express RT6.2 alloantigen. In a pancreas transplantation model from WF ($RT1^u$, RT6.2) to BB-DP ($RT1^u$, RT6.1), no rejection occurred, but insulitis led to diabetes and death within about 2 months due to immunodeficiency.

Here, anti-adhesion molecule antibodies (anti-ICAM-1/LFA-1 antibody) did not cause diabetes and survived for a long period of time (>100 days) [7]. As a mechanism, donor-derived $RT6.2^+$ T cells appeared at a high rate in the periphery (approximately 34% of splenic T cells), resulting in macrochimerism as shown in Fig. 23.1. As a result, the immunodeficiency was improved and insulitis was suppressed.

We investigated whether a similar phenomenon could be observed in islet transplantation. However, islet transplantation did not induce immune tolerance [8]. The difference may be due to the fact that pancreas transplantation brings in lymphoid tissue in the peripancreatic lymph nodes and in the duodenum of the graft. A report from another institution. In the NOD mouse model of type 1 diabetes mellitus, NKT cells, which possess both T cell and NK cell receptors, were adopted into the pancreas at an early stage of the disease, resulting in the suppression of onset of diabetes [9, 10]. We therefore investigated NKT cells in our model as well. The diabetes relapsed when the pancreas alone removed from the peripancreatic lymph nodes and duodenum of the graft was transplanted. Therefore, it was suggested that the

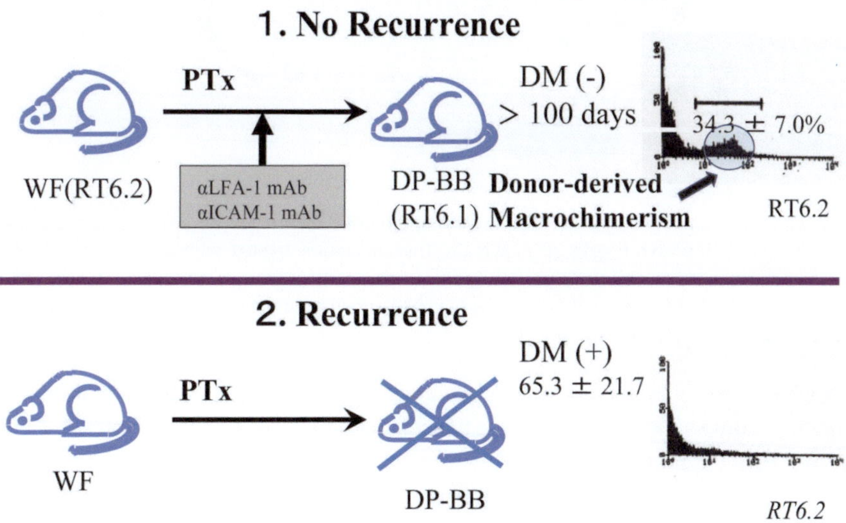

Fig. 23.1 IDDM recurrent model in pancreas transplantation using BB rats. Anti-adhesion molecule antibodies (anti-ICAM-1/LFA-1 antibody) did not cause diabetes and survived for a long period of time (>100 days). As a mechanism, donor-derived $RT6.2^+$ T cells appeared at a high rate in the periphery (approximately 34% of splenic T cells), resulting in macrochimerism

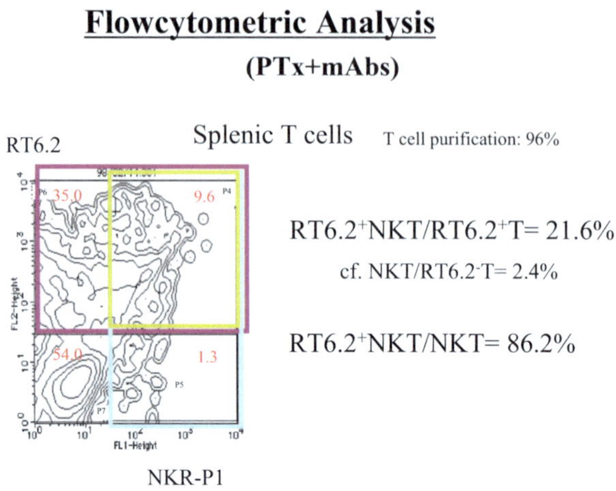

Fig. 23.2 Flow cytometric analysis of splenic T cells in the nonrecurrent BB rat (WF-to-DP) 60 days after grafting. In the splenic T (Ig$^-$) cells depleted of Ig$^+$ cells, macrochimerism due to donor-derived RT6.2$^+$ T cells was 44.4%. Further, there were 21.2% NKT cells in this population

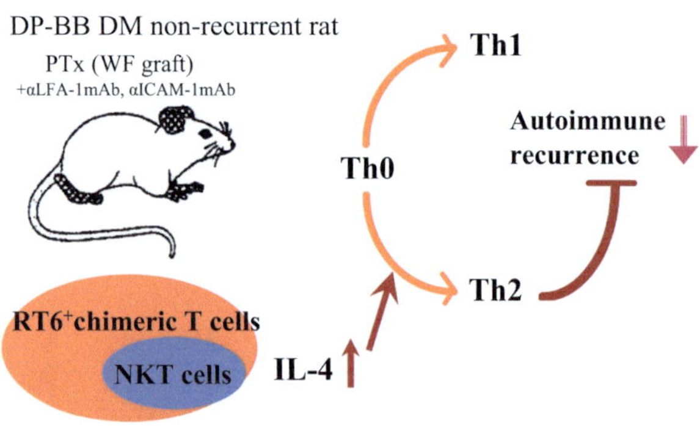

Fig. 23.3 Immunoregulatory mechanism of autoimmune recurrence by a macrochimerisim of donor-derived RT6$^+$ NKT cells in pancreatic transplantation treated with anti-ICAM-1/LFA-1 mAbs. Letting T-helper cell function shift to Th2 from Th0 by primarily secreting IL-4, RT6$^+$ NKT cells derived from pancreaticodudenal graft may have an important immune-regulatory function of preventing IDDM recurrence

lymphoid tissue in the pancreaticoduodenal graft contains cells that modulate immune-competence. Therefore, the pancreaticoduodenal graft IELs (intestinal epithelial lymphocytes) and peripancreatic lymph nodes contained a high percentage of NKT cells (20% and 17%, respectively). In addition, more than 80% of the NKT cells were chimeric RT6.2$^+$ T cells (Fig. 23.2) [11]. Further, IL-4 was highly secreted as a serum cytokine in the immune tolerance model. These results suggest that the graft-derived NKT cells secreted IL-4, which shifted the Th1/Th2 balance to Th2, suppressed the recurrence of type 1 diabetes, and the appearance of chimeric T cells contributed to the improvement of immune function, as shown in Fig. 23.3.

23.6 Induction of Immune Tolerance by Gene Transfer into Pancreatic Grafts

We attempted to prolong graft engraftment by introducing a gene that regulates alloimmune responses into transplanted pancreatic grafts during cold storage. This is a strategy to achieve local immunosuppression of the graft and limit the use of systemic immunosuppressive drugs. In a rat pancreaticoduodenal transplantation model from BN to LEW, the CTLA4Ig gene was transfected with an adenovirus vector via the graft artery.

CTLA4 is an immune checkpoint receptor that negatively regulates immune responses. Currently, an antibody that inhibits CTLA4 (ipilimumab) is used for immunotherapy of cancer together with an anti-PD-1 antibody (nivolumab). In addition to the CTLA4Ig gene transfer, FK506 is used in the perioperative period for 3 days (−1, 0, +1), resulting in long-term (> 100 days) graft survival [12]. The mechanism of this phenomenon was a significant increase in regulatory T cells (Treg, $CD4^{+}CD25^{+}$T cells) in the immune-tolerant rats.

23.7 Induction of Immune Tolerance by Gene Transfer in Islet Transplantation

We examined the effect of CTLA4Ig gene transfer in islet transplantation from BN into LEW rats in the subrenal capsule [13]. Ex vivo, islet transplantation was slightly prolonged (mean 6.7 days to 8.6 days) compared to the control group, but the perioperative treatment of FK506 for 3 days (−1, 0, +1) prolonged graft survival up to 33 days.

In comparison to the organ (pancreas), induction of tolerance in islets seems to be more difficult. Therefore, systemic gene transfer induces a prolonged effect of islet grafts up to 15 days. However, in all cases when FK506 is used in combination with the islets, islet grafts could survive more than 100 days. Thus, the second challenge transplantation of islets or heart was performed on day 100 posttransplant in the long survivors. The islets were rejected, but half of the transplanted hearts showed long-term engraftment. Thus, islets were corroborated to be highly immunogenic.

23.8 Induction of Immune Tolerance by Hybrid Islet Transplantation in Islet Transplantation

In clinical islet transplantation, multiple donors are required for each recipient. In the limited number of potential donors, various efforts are being made to achieve a one-donor-one recipient concept. We investigated whether the maintenance and improvement of insulin-secreting ability of transplanted pancreatic islets in mice (BALB/cA to C57BL/6 J) could be achieved by combining marginal number of 200 islets together with adipose-derived stem cells (ADSCs: 2×10^5) derived from donors [14]. As a result, we obtained a prolonged islet engraftment time (average 13 days) equivalent to that of 400 islet transplants. The 200 islets alone did not improve diabetes mellitus. The glucose tolerance test performed 7 days after islet transplantation showed significantly better results than islet transplantation alone. Recipient-derived ADSCs were also examined. The same effect as that of donor-derived ADSCs was observed.

There are several advantages of using ADSCs. (1) Easy to obtain and large doses can be secured. (2) Excellent regenerative and angiogenic capabilities. (3) Immunomodulation ability. Therefore, it is thought that the successful use of ADSCs may contribute to the shortage of donors by enabling one donor-one recipient even with a small number of islets.

23.9 Mechanism of Spontaneous Immunological Tolerance in Liver Transplantation

We compared the differences between low responder (BN to LEW) and high responder (DA to LEW) systems in which rejection does occur between inbred rats. Passenger leukocytes in grafts are known to be usually involved in graft rejection, but it has been reported that they may contain immune regulatory cells that lead to tolerance. We focused on NKT cells, which are abundant in bone marrow and liver as candidates. We previously showed that NKT cells suppressed the mechanism of autoimmune recurrence by administration of anti-adhesion molecule antibodies in BB rat pancreatic transplantation system.

To confirm the involvement of NKT cells, irradiated liver grafts were reconstructed with BN splenocytes or NKT-depleted BN splenocytes and then transplanted. The former showed a significant prolongation of liver engraftment, whereas the latter was rejected in the acute fashion. Furthermore, cytokine profiles of culture supernatants of Ig^{-}GICs (Ig^{-}graft-infiltrating cells) obtained from transplanted livers showed secretion of IL-10 and TGF-β in the low responder group and IFN-γ in the high responder group [15, 16].

Therefore, donor-derived NKT cells may be involved in spontaneous tolerance in low responder.

23.10 Regulation of GVHD and HVGD by Novel Immunosuppressive Agents in Small Intestine Transplantation

The small intestine, like the pancreas, is known to be a highly immunogenic organ and susceptible to rejection. In addition, since lymphoid tissue is abundant in the graft, immune cells of the graft recognize the recipient host as foreign and attack GVHD and HVGD as in the case of bone marrow transplantation.

FTY720 (fingolimod), a sphingosine 1-phosphate receptor modulator, is a novel immunosuppressant (modulator) isolated and synthesized from the insect parasite

Cordyceps sinensis. It has a completely different mechanism of action from conventional immunosuppressive agents, and has no effect on T cell activation, proliferation, or differentiation. Thus, opportunistic infections seen with conventional immunosuppressive agents may be avoided. The mechanism of immunosuppression is by promoting homing of lymphocytes in the peripheral blood to secondary lymphoid tissues, such as peripheral lymph nodes, mesenteric lymph nodes, and Peyer's patches, and by retaining them in secondary lymphoid tissues (sequestration). This has been reported to reduce lymphocyte infiltration into grafts and inflammatory sites.

We used a model of ectopic small intestine transplantation from WF to F1 (WF × ACI) rats in which only GVHD occurs without rejection [17]. In the untreated group of recipients who underwent small intestine transplantation, all recipients died of GVHD within an average of 16 days. In this study, FTY720 was administered daily for 2 weeks to this group. GVHD histopathology of target organs (liver and skin) was significantly improved and the recipients survived for a long period (>100 days). The T cells from the donor in the target organs are homed to the secondary lymphoid tissues of the donor (graft) and retained there, rather than to the recipient. Therefore, we hypothesized that FTY720 could prevent activated donor-derived T cells from recirculating and reaching the target organs, thereby avoiding GVHD. In addition, FY720 also suppressed IFNγ production in target organs.

23.11 Conclusion

We have attempted to induce immune tolerance by the different methods using various rat transplantation models. There is a hierarchy of organ-dependent immunogenicity which may be due to differences in the organ of MHC alloantigen or the existence of organ-specific antigens. The liver is the most tolerogenic, followed by the kidney and heart. In contrast, skin is the most immunogenic. Pancreatic or intestinal grafts are also immunogenic, ranked next to skin. The method of immune induction must be selected according to the organ to be transplanted.

With approaches and applications of the new fields of genomics and active immunologic manipulations, it may be expected that near-tolerance in the clinical situation can be achieved with nontoxic drugs even in the immunogenic organ transplantation.

Acknowledgments I would like to thank all the following doctors and researchers who were involved in our study. Stanislaw Stepkowski, PhD, Barry Kahan, MD, Akira Ito, MD, Shigetaka Yamamoto, MD, Fumihiro Uchikoshi, MD, Masayuki Tori, MD, Gang Miao, MD, Yusuke Akamaru, MD, Yoshiaki Ohmura, MD, Atsushi Ohkawa, MD, Tetsuma Kiyomoto, MD, Jinghai Song, MD, Masumi Nozawa, MD, and Hikaru Matsuda, MD.

References

1. Ito T, Stepkowski SM, Kahan BD. Soluble antigen and cyclosporine-induced specific unresponsiveness in rats. Frequency of alloantigen-specific T cytotoxic cells in normal, sensitized and unresponsive rats. Transplantation. 1990;49:422–8.
2. Stepkowski SM, Ito T. Frequency of alloantigen-specific T cytotoxic cells in high- and low responder recipients of class MHC-I disparate heart allografts. Transplantation. 1990;50:112–9.
3. Ito T, Shirakura R, Nakata S, et al. Bone marrow cells and FK506-induced donor specific unresponsiveness in rat heart allografts. Transplant Proc. 1991;23(6):3297–9.
4. Ito T, Stepkowski SM, Shirakura R, et al. Role of IL-2 producing $CD4^{+}T$ cells in acute rejection of class I MHC disparate rat heart allografts. Transplant Proc. 1993;25(1):885–7.
5. Ito A, Ito T, Kamiike W, et al. Donor-specific tolerance by perioperative intrathymic injection of bone marrow cells in rat cardiac allograft model. – the use of FK506 can shorten the necessary duration of pretransplant intrathymic conditioning. Transplantation. 1997;64(5):752–7.
6. Yamamoto S, Ito T, Nakata S, et al. Rejection mechanism of rat pancreaticoduodenal allografts with a class I MHC disparity. Transplantation. 1994;57:1217–22.
7. Uchikoshi F, Ito T, Kamiike W, et al. Restoration of immune abnormalities in diabetic BB rats after pancreas transplantation. I. Macrochimerism of donor graft-derived $RT6^{+}$ T cells responsible for restoration of immune responsiveness and suppression of autoimmune reaction. Transplantation. 1996;61:1629–36.
8. Uchikoshi F, Ito T, Kamiike W, et al. Pancreas transplantation, but not islet transplantation, protects graft recurrence of IDDM in diabetic BB rats. Transplant Proc. 1997;29:753–5.
9. Gombert JM, Herbelin A, Tancrede-Bohin E, et al. Early quantitative and functional deficiency of $NK1^{+}$-like thymocytes in NOD mouse. Eur J Immunol. 1996;26:2989–98.
10. Hammond KJL, Poulton LD, Palmisano LJ, et al. T cell receptor $(TCR)^{+}$CD4-CD8- (NKT) thymocytes prevent insulin-dependent diabetes mellitus in nonobese (NOD)/LT mice by the influence of interleukin (IL)-4 and/or IL-10. J Exp Med. 1998;187:1047–56.
11. Tori M, Ito T, Kitagawa-Sakakida S, et al. Importance of donor-derived lymphocytes in the protection of pancreaticoduodenal or islet grafts from recurrent autoimmunity. A role for $RT6^{+}NKR\text{-}P1^{+}$ T cells. Transplantation. 2000;70:32–8.
12. Miao G, Ito T, Uchikoshi F, et al. Development of donor-specific immunoregulatory T cells after local CTLA4Ig gene transfer to pancreatic allograft. Transplantation. 2004;78:59–64.
13. Akamaru Y, Ito T, Uchikoshi F, et al. Ex vivo and systemic transfer of adenovirus-mediated CTLA4-Ig gene combined with a short course of FK506 therapy prolongs islet graft survival. Transplant Immunol. 2003;11(1):91–100.
14. Ohmura Y, Tanemura M, Kawaguchi N, et al. Transplantation of pancreatic islets at marginal mass combined with adipose tissue-derived stem cells enhances the survival and insulin-function of islet grafts in diabetic mice. Transplantation. 2010;90(12):1366–73.
15. Ohkawa A, Ito T, Yumiba T, et al. Immunological characteristics of intragraft $NKR\text{-}P1^{+}$ $TCR\alpha\beta^{+}$ T (NKT) cells in rat hepatic allografts. Transplant Proc. 1999;31:2699–700.
16. Kiyomoto T, Ito T, Uchikoshi F, et al. The potent role of graft-derived $NKT\text{-}P1^{+}TCR\alpha\beta^{+}T$ (NKT) cells in the spontaneous acceptance rat liver allografts. Transplantation. 2005;80:1749–55.
17. Song J, Ito T, Matsuda T, et al. Inhibition of donor-derived T cells trafficking into target organs by FYT720 during acute graft-versus-host disease in small bowel transplantation. Clin Exp Immunol. 2006;146:85–92.

Aiming for the Clinical Application of Xenotransplantation

24

Shuji Miyagawa, Akira Maeda, Katsuyoshi Matsunami, Hiroshi Eguchi, and Hiroomi Okuyama

Abstract

Recently, xenotransplantation has been introduced in humans using genetically modified pigs in the United States. Although data of its results remains scarce, they undoubtedly harken the arrival of a new era. Our research on xenotransplantation began in 1986, demonstrating that the cause of hyperacute rejection was species-specificity in the complement system. Since then, the existence of xenoglycoantigens has become clear, and α-Gal, H-D, and Sda have been identified and knocked out worldwide. Gradually, attention has started to be paid not only to the movement of adaptive immune cells but also to the movement of innate immune cells, and efforts are being made to establish methods to control them. Preclinical research has built on this fundamental research across the world, producing results that will allow clinical trials to begin. In addition to the importance of research, this work also highlights the legislative progress being made in Japan for the use of animal models in clinical research. With the production of several transgenic and knockout pigs, we are currently in the process of forming a consortium in Japan and pushing for legal reform in an effort to allow pigs to be used in clinical studies.

S. Miyagawa (✉) · A. Maeda · H. Eguchi · H. Okuyama
Department of Pediatric Surgery, The University of Osaka Graduate School of Medicine, Suita, Osaka, Japan
e-mail: miyagawa@pedsurg.med.osaka-u.ac.jp; zul06720@nifty.com; hiroshieguchi@hotmail.com; okuyama@pedsurg.med.osaka-u.ac.jp

K. Matsunami
Graduate School of Biomedical and Health Sciences (Pharmaceutical Sciences), Hiroshima University, Hiroshima, Japan
e-mail: matunami@hiroshima-u.ac.jp

H. Matsuda et al. (eds.), *Heart and Lung Transplantation*,
https://doi.org/10.1007/978-981-96-8810-4_24

Keywords

Xenotransplantation · GE-pigs · Preclinical study · Complement · Carbohydrate antigens · HLA class Ib · Monocyte/macrophages · Neutrophil · PERV · Xenoheart transplantation

24.1 Introduction

By the end of 2021, clinical trials of xenotransplantation had begun in the United States. Eight pig kidney and two pig heart transplants were performed on brain-dead patients in a short period of time [1]. In 2022, a pig heart transplant was also performed, with the patient surviving for 60 days [2]. In 2024, the practice of pig kidney transplantation started. These studies have proven that the use of gene-edited (GE) pigs can help to avoid hyperacute rejection, previously impossible, and is undoubtedly the result of many years of xenotransplantation research. This undoubtedly provides a sense of arrival into a new era [3, 4]. In Japan, although this field has not received much attention, the early work of many researchers has greatly contributed to this advance.

In this article, we briefly summarize the research that our group has conducted so far that has been fundamental to the clinical application of xenotransplantation, focusing on research that is closely linked to clinical practice, along with trends in each country.

24.2 Basic Research

Complement Control

Our research on xenotransplantation began in 1986 by elucidating the mechanisms underlying hyperacute rejection. Using a heterotopic heart transplant system from guinea pigs to rats, we demonstrated that this reaction involves an alternative complement pathway and is caused by species specificity between the complement and complement regulatory proteins (CRPs) [5, 6]. Next, we focused on membrane-type human CRPs, such as MCP (CD46) [7], DAF (CD55) [8], CD59, and their hybrids [9, 10] and used swine endogenous cells (SEC) to verify the cytotoxic inhibitory function of each CRP on pig cells [11, 12]. In this study, we optimized the codons of mammalian cDNA. We also investigated the relationship between CRP levels and viral receptors [9]. Moreover, we converted serum CRPs into membrane-type CRPs, expressed them in pig cells, and examined their anticomplement function. Initially, we identified C4bp [13, 14], CR1 [15], factor H [16], factor I [16], delta99aaC1-INH [17–20], and gC1 of the Heles virus [21]. We also identified porcine C1-INH [22] and factor I [22] and compared their functions with those in humans. In addition, we measured the hemolytic activity of monkey [23] and porcine complement [24, 25].

Control of Carbohydrate Antigens

In 1994, DAF transgenic (TG) pigs were developed in an attempt to address and overcome hyperacute rejection [26]. This work highlighted the role of delayed rejection, a phenomenon that has since come to the fore, with large amounts of antibody deposition observed in the grafts [27]. As a result, species-specific carbohydrate antigens, such as the α-Gal epitope [28], became the focus of attention. Research conducted on knockout (KO) of the α-Gal antigen gene (GGTA1) was initially impossible, and other methods to reduce α-Gal were used [29]. In 1995, the gene transfer of α1,2 fucosyltransferase (α1,2FT) into pig cells was found to suppress α-Gal expression by competitive inhibition in the Golgi apparatus [30]. In response to this finding, we found that α2,3 sialyltransferase (α2,3ST) [31] and α2,6 sialyltransferase (α2,6ST) [32] at al [33]. were more effective at reducing antigenicity to pig cells than α1,2FT. In addition, we also verified a method of remodeling N-glycan synthesis using N-acetylglucosaminyltransferase III (GnT-III) to reduce the antigenicity [34]. N-Glycans exhibit strong antigenicity against interspecies glycan antigens [35, 36]. Subsequently, GnT-III-TG pigs were developed [37, 38]. Although KO in pigs was once thought to be impossible, a report on Dolly sheep prompted somatic cell nuclear transfer using fetal fibroblasts to be attempted in pigs.

As a result, in 2002, homozygous α-Gal-KO pigs were created [39]. Subsequently, we successfully created α-Gal-KO pigs in 2005 [40]. From this point on, the issue became the fact that 10–30% of non-Gal antigens remained on the cell surface of pigs even after α-Gal KO [41]. The Hanganutziu-Deicher (H-D) antigen (NeuGc: CMAH) [42] was identified as one of the most important epitopes. Porcine CMAH was elucidated and insights were gained on exon-3 and -8 [43]. Porcine CMAH was knocked down (KD) [44] or KO *in vitro* using CRISPR/Cas9 to verify its effects [45]. In collaboration with a group from Meiji University, we produced CMAH knockout pigs using the TALEN method [46]. Next, the third glycan, pig Sda antigen (β4GalNT2) [47, 48], was discovered in 2014 by analyzing antibodies produced in monkeys transplanted pig hearts. However, the Sda antigen was originally a blood-type antigen. We tested the serum of 6–7 researchers in our group, and only one of them reacted to this antigen. Pig β4GalNT2 may have another function from those of humans. As a result, pigs in which these glycan genes were knocked out were created [27].

Control of NK Cells

Natural killer (NK) cell activity is strongly associated with rejection during xenotransplantation from hamsters to rats. Therefore, we approached this issue from the perspective of glycobiology [49] and MHC class Ib (HLA-G [50] and HLA-E [51]) recognition.

First, we verified and reported that the aggression of NK cells against pig cells was reduced when α-Gal on pig cells was reduced [52]. On the other hand, negative results were obtained on the recognition of α-Gal by NK cells, although it was later reported that NK cells can recognize α-Gal via CD161 [53]. Additionally, HLA-G is easily expressed in SECs and suppresses NK cell-dependent cytotoxicity. However, HLA-E expression was insufficient. Therefore, we developed a mutant with high expression of HLA-E mutant: HLA-Ev147 [54–56]. We also investigated whether DAF directly controlled NK cells [57].

Control of Monocytes/Macrophages (Mo/Ma)
The so-called "Don't eat me signal" is well known for avoiding attacks by Mo/Ma and is related to the relationship between CD47 and SIRPα. We identified several other molecules that control the attacks by Mo and Ma in pig cells. First, we examined the expression of NKG2A in Mo/Ma and confirmed that the HLA-E ligand has an inhibitory function against Mo/Ma [58]. Moreover, we confirmed the expression of ILT-2/ILT-4 and reported that the ligand HLA-G1 [59] controls the Mo/Ma ratio in the same way [60]. We also studied CD200 [61], TIGIT [62], and CD177 [63], and verified their regulatory functions against Mo/Ma in SEC. Furthermore, we developed a hybrid molecule, CL-SP-D/-A [64, 65], in which the pulmonary surfactant SP-D/-A was bound to CL-P1, and checked its regulatory function against Mo/Ma on SEC. These molecules bind to SIRPα and show a more efficient reaction than CD47. We also reported that changes in carbohydrate antigens on SECs, such as the overexpression of α2,6 sialic acid, are also effective in regulating Mo/Ma [66–69].

Regulation of Neutrophils
Neutrophils, originally known as "microphages," are cells of the innate immune system that are more specialized in attacking invading foreign bodies. Neutrophils are essential for regulating the cells of the innate immune system in xenotransplantation, and current research is seeking to understand how to control them. To date, we have verified that CD31 [70], CD177 [71], CD200 [72], CD47 [73], and CL-SP-D [73] exhibit regulatory functions in neutrophils.

Anti-apoptosis and Anti-inflammatory Properties
HO-1 and A20 are candidates for gene transfer into pigs, with HO-1 having been transferred into the "10-GE pig" used in clinical trials. We identified several molecules and cloned the sequences of a porcine serine proteinase inhibitor (PI-9) [74] and porcine FLIPs [75].

Role of T Cells
To understand the role of T cells, we first identified basic pattern of T cell infiltration into allografts [76, 77], and confirmed the importance of CD4+ T cells in a concordant model [78, 79], and then investigated how FasL regulates CD8+ T cells [80].

24.3 Creating Genetically Modified Pigs

The greatest advances in the past decade have been in gene targeting technology. The first was the development of the ZFN method, followed by the creation of the TAREN and CRISPR methods. The CRISPR method includes not only Cas9 but Cas3 as well [81]. These methods have revolutionized certain aspects of gene targeting technologies. In addition to α-Gal-KO, CMAH(NeuGc)-KO, and β4GalNT2-KO, SLA classI-KO have been established in combination with human gene transfer in many research institutions. In addition, the 2A peptide technology that connects two independent molecules is widespread. Furthermore, the knock-in (KI) of the ROSA locus of the pig genome for stable expression of the introduced gene has attracted attention. We are actively engaged in this field, starting with the creation of a Cre recombinase that matches the mammalian codon usage, and used this method with several cDNAs [82, 83]. In fact, we have cloned several porcine genes related to homologous recombination [84, 85].

In collaboration with Meiji University, we created GGTA1/CMAH double-KO pigs in 2014 [46], as described below. Furthermore, we have reported on the effects of the CRISPR/Cas3 method on α-Gal [81].

Pig Islets for Clinical Use

We began our research using adult pig islets (API) and neonatal pig islet-like cell clusters (NPCC) and investigated the response of pig API to the human complement system. As a result, API were found to directly activate alternative pathways [86, 87].

We extracted API from GnT-III-TG pigs, investigated the properties of their glycans, and transplanted them into monkeys to examine the rejection reaction and verify the effectiveness of GnT-III gene transfer [88].

First, surface glycan antigen analysis by lectin array showed that wild-type API was rich in high mannose-type N-glycans, and the expression of terminal α-GalNAc (Tn antigen) was reduced with the disappearance of α-Gal [89–91]. On the other hand, NPCC was found to be highly enriched in α2,6NeuNAc compared to API [92].

Next, further analyses were performed using HPLC and MALDI-TOF-MS. The general characteristics were the same as those of the lectin array data [93, 94]. Furthermore, LC-MS-based structural analysis (O'Neil) was added to the API [95].

Preclinical Study

Remarkable progress has been made in preclinical xenotransplantation experiments in recent years. Surprisingly, a group at the University of Maryland (USA) conducted the heterotopic transplantation of GE pig hearts into the abdomens of monkeys and reported survival rates of almost 2.5 years [96]. The pigs were Gal-KO and DAF&TM-TG mice. However, in the case of orthotopic heart transplantation, the results were not as good due to the fact that the sizes of the GE pigs initially produced did not match those of the experimental monkeys. However, a German group used pigs with growth hormone receptor (GHR) KO, which, by skillfully controlling blood pressure, survived for more than six months for the first time. This led to clinical pig-heart transplantation at the University of Maryland. Similarly, at Harvard University, genetically modified pig kidneys have been functioning in monkeys for more than two years, leading to clinical trials [97]. At the same time, pancreatic islet cells were engrafted for more than 600 days using the wild-type adult pig islets (API) with only immunosuppressants. This finding suggests that long-term engraftment can be achieved by combining GE pigs with immunoisolation membranes.

We previously observed an extension of engraftment by the heterotopic transplantation of DAF pig hearts [98]. We successfully transplanted islets under the renal capsules of monkeys without immunosuppressant administration. Moreover, in a joint study with the Department of Dermatology at Sapporo Medical University, we simultaneously engrafted pig skin expressing DAF and GnT-III in monkeys for 31 days by administering the immunosuppressant FK [99].

To date, there have been few reports on these preclinical experiments in Japan owing to research funding restrictions.

Zoonotic Disease: PERV

In 1997, a study found that porcine endogenous retroviruses (PERVs) could infect human cells *in vitro*, drawing attention to PERVs. However, to date, no cases of infection have been reported. Currently, there have been successful attempts to knock out all PERVs from the pig genome using the CRISPR/Cas9 technology [100], including efforts to knock out only the highly infectious PERV-C. To produce GE pigs that do not develop PREV, we were the first to verify the importance of high-mannose-type glycans among the N-glycans of the ligands on the surface of PERV [101–104]. In addition, we verified that the PI-anchor-type molecules, DAF and CD59, increased the resistance of PERVs to human serum [105]. Furthermore, we reported that the molecular size of CRP on PERV and the characteristics of the transfer membrane were related to infectivity [106, 107]. In 2003, we first reported the inhibitory effect of siRNAs on PERV infectivity [108, 109].

Consortium and Venture

In 1996, we formed a consortium with four internal departments–Osaka University, Osaka Adult Disease Center, and Nippon Ham Central Research Institute–funded by the National Institute of Biomedical Engineering, Ministry of Agriculture, Forestry, and Fisheries, and started to create transgenic pigs. We generated a TG pig line by linking DAF to the promoter (pGL-3) of porcine MCP (equivalent to MCP) [98, 110]. The characteristic feature of this DAF pig is that it is expressed ubiquitously, and its expression in the vascular endothelium is approximately twice that of humans in heterozygous pigs. We also generated a TG pig for the glycosyltransferase GnT-III. The characteristic feature of this line was that it was also expressed ubiquitously, and its expression in the vascular endothelium was high [37]. Subsequently, unsuccessful attempts were made to create α2,3ST pigs.

From 2000 to 2006, we established the Animal Engineering Research Institute (AERI), a venture capital company, with support from Nippon Ham, Inc. and Nipro, Inc. Just after the report of Dolly the sheep in 1996, we attempted to create α-Gal-KO pigs using fetal pig fibroblasts; however, this took a relatively long time to achieve. Finally, in May 2004, we created α-Gal heterozygous knockout pigs expressing DAF and GnT-III using conventional targeting vectors and nuclear transfer technology [40]. Then, in 2006, we created α-Gal homozygous KO pigs. At this point, we were finally able to catch up with the research community in other parts of the world.

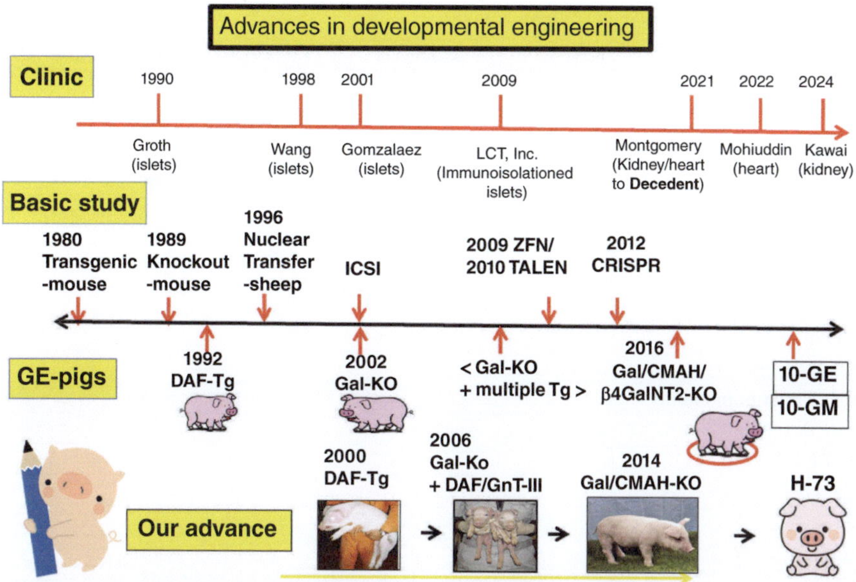

Fig. 24.1 Advances in the developmental engineering for transgenic pigs

We continued our collaborative research with Meiji University, and in 2014, we completed a double KO pig in which α-Gal (GGTA1) was knocked out using the ZFN method and H-D antigen was also using the TAREN method [46].

As a summary, the advances in developmental engineering targeted to transgenic pigs for xenotransplantation to humans during the last over 30 years are illustrated by comparing the steps in the field of basic study, GE-pigs, and clinical application adding the process in our team in the bottom (Fig. 24.1). In addition, in the spring of 2022, Osaka University, the National Cerebral and Cardiovascular Institute, Meiji University, Setsunan University, and PorMedTeck launched a xenotransplantation consortium. They are currently working towards developing a multi-molecule co-expressing pig model (Table 24.1).

Legal Arrangements in Japan

In Japan, the "Pig Cell (Islet) Transplantation Act" was enacted in 2014, and the "Guidelines for Xenotransplantation" were revised in 2016. As a result, clinical trials of porcine islet transplantation can be formally started under specific conditions.

In response to the introduction of xenotransplantation in the United States, legal regulations regarding the transplantation of hearts and kidneys from genetically modified pigs have been under consideration in Japan since 2022, with the relevant guidelines being enacted in 2024 ("Guidelines for risk management of xenograft-derived infections associated with xenotransplantation (draft)" (PDF: 679 KB)). Although the legal restrictions are as strict as those in the United States, it can be said that legal regulations allowing pig organ transplantation have been established.

Table 24.1 Representative gene-modified pigs

Gene	Revivicor	eGenesis	LifeStock	PorMedTech
–	10GE	10GM		Heisei-73
GGTA1	●	●	●	●
CMAH	●	●	●	●
β2GalNT2	●	●		●
GHR	●			
RERV		●		
CD46(MCP)	○	○	○	○
CD55(DAF)	○	○	○	○
CD59			○	○
C1-INH				○
TM(Thrombomodulin)	○	○		○
EPCR	○	○		○
TFPI				○
CD47	○	○		○
HLA-E				○
B2m				○
CD39				○
HO-1	○	○	○	
A20(TNFAIP3)		○	○	

● knockout, ○ transgenic

References

1. Loupy A, Goutaudier V, et al. Immune response after pig-to-human kidney xenotransplantation: a multimodal phenotyping study. Lancet. 2023;402(10408):1158–69.
2. Griffith BP, Goerlich CE, et al. Genetically modified porcine-to-human cardiac xenotransplantation. N Engl J Med. 2022;387(1):35–44.
3. Miyagawa S, Yamamoto A, et al. Complement regulation in the GalT KO era. Xenotransplantation. 2010;17(1):11–25.
4. Miyagawa S, Maeda A, et al. Complement regulation in the triple-KO era. Front Immunol. 2022;13:860165. https://doi.org/10.3389/fimmu.2022.860165.
5. Miyagawa S, Hirose H, et al. The mechanism of discordant xenograft rejection. Transplantation. 1988;46(6):825–30.
6. Miyagawa S, Shirakura R, et al. Prolonging discordant xenograft survival with anticomplement reagents K76COOH and FUT175. Transplantation. 1993;55(4):709–13.
7. Miyagawa S, Mikata S, et al. The regulation of membrane cofactor protein (CD46) expression by the 3′untranslated region in transgenic mice. Biochem Biophys Res Commun. 1997;233(3):829–33.
8. Miyagawa S, Fukuta D, et al. Effect of tandem forms of DAF(CD55) on complement-mediated xenogeneic cell lysis. Xenotransplantation. 2006;13(5):433–9.
9. Miyagawa S, Shirakura R, et al. Effects of transfected complement regulatory proteins, MCP, DAF, and MCP/DAE hybrid, on complement-mediated swine endothelial cell lysis. Transplantation. 1994;58(7):834–40.
10. Sakai R, Maeda A, et al. Expression of a synthetic gene of CTDM by transgenic animals. Transplant Proc. 2016;48(4):1279–81.

11. Miyagawa S, Shirakura R, et al. Test for ability of decay-accelerating factor(DAF, CD55) and CD59 to alleviate complement-mediated damage of xeno-erythrocytes. Scand J Immunol. 1993;38(1):37–44.
12. Miyagawa S, Mikata S, et al. C5b-8 step lysis of swine endothelial cells by human complement and functional feature of transfected CD59. Scand J Immunol. 1996;43(4):361–6.
13. Mikata S, Miyagawa S, et al. Regulation of complement-mediated swine endothelial cell lysis by a surface-bound form of human C4b binding protein. Transplantation. 1998;65(3):363–8.
14. Mikata S, Miyagawa S, et al. A monomeric human C4b-binding protein (C4bp) more efficiently inactivates C3b than natural C4bp: participation of C-terminal domains in factor I-cofactor activity. Mol Immunol. 1998;35(9):537–44.
15. Mikata S, Miyagawa S, et al. Prevention of hyperacute rejection by phosphatidylinositol-anchored mini-complement receptor type 1. Transpl Immunol. 1998;6(2):107–10.
16. Yoshitatsu M, Miyagawa S, et al. Function of human factor H and I on xenosurface. Biochem Biophys Res Commun. 1999;265(2):556–62.
17. Matsunami K, Miyagawa S, et al. A surface-bound form of human C1 esterase inhibitor improves xenograft rejection. Transplantation. 2000;69(5):749–55.
18. Fukuta D, Miyagawa S, et al. Effect of Various forms of C1 esterase inhibitor (C1-INH) and DAF on complement mediated xenogeneic cell lysis. Xenotransplantation. 2003;10(2):132–41.
19. Fukuta D, Miyagawa S, et al. Effect of hybrid complement regulatory proteins on xenogeneic cells. Biochem Biophys Res Commun. 2003;306(2):476–82.
20. Fukuta D, Miyagawa S, et al. The heavy chain is not required for the serine protease function of the membrane bound form of factor I on a xeno-surface. Transpl Immunol. 2004;12:109–14.
21. Matsunami K, Miyagawa S, et al. Regulation of complement-mediated swine endothelial cell lysis by herpes simplex virus glycoprotein, gC1. J Biochem. 2002;131(5):745–9.
22. Kobayashi C, Matsunami K, et al. Features of a newly cloned pig C1 esterase inhibitor. J Biochem. 2006;140(3):421–7.
23. Nakahata K, Matsunami K, et al. Analysis of the serine protease function of porcine factor I produced by liver cells for xenotransplantation. Transpl Immunol. 2008;19(1):30–6.
24. Xu H, Kitano E, et al. Studies of monkey complement: measurement of cynomolgus monkey CH50, ACH50, C4, C2 and C3. Xenotransplantation. 2008;15(1):14–9.
25. Sakai R, Kitano E, et al. Studies of innate immune systems against human cells. Transpl Immunol. 2017;40:66–71.
26. White DJ, Cozzi E, et al. The control of hyperacute rejection by genetic engineering of the donor species. Eye (Lond). 1995;9(Pt 2):185–9.
27. Miyagawa S. Xenotransplantation and glycomedicine. In: Kamerling JP, editor. Comprehensive glycoscience. from chemistry to systems biology, Cell glycobiology and development, vol. 4. 2nd ed. Elsevier; 2021.
28. Galili U, Clark MR, et al. Evolutionary relationship between the natural anti-Gal antibody and the Gal alpha 1-3Gal epitope in primates. Proc Natl Acad Sci USA. 1987;84(5):1369–73.
29. Miyagawa S, Maeda A. Glycoprotein alpha 1,3-galactosyltransferase 1, pseudogene (GGTA1P). In: Handbook of Glycosyltransferases and related genes. 2nd ed. Springer; 2014. p. 109–20.
30. Sandrin MS, Fodor WL, et al. Enzymatic remodelling of the carbohydrate surface of a xenogenic cell substantially reduces human antibody binding and complement-mediated cytolysis. Nat Med. 1995;1(12):1261–7.
31. Tanemura M, Miyagawa S, et al. Reduction of the major swine xenoantigen, the α-galactosyl epitope by transfection of the α2,3-sialyltransferase gene. J Biol Chem. 1998;273(26):16421–5.
32. Koma M, Miyagawa S, et al. Reduction of the major xenoantigen on glycosphingolipids of swine endothelial cells by various glycosyltransferases. Glycobiology. 2000;10(7):745–51.
33. Koma M, Miyagawa S, et al. The Possibility of reducing of xenoantigen levels with a novel gal 3′-sulfotransferase (GP3ST). J Biochem. 2002;131(4):517–22.

34. Tanemura M, Miyagawa S, et al. Significant downregulation of the major swine xenoantigen by N-acetylglucosaminyltransferase III gene transfection. Biochem Biophys Res Commun. 1997;235(2):359–64.
35. Miyagawa S, Tanemura M, et al. Masking and reduction of the galactose-α 1,3-galactose (α-Gal) epitope, the major xenoantigen in swine, by the glycosyltransferase gene transfection. Biochem Biophys Res Commun. 1999;264(3):611–4.
36. Koyota S, Ikeda Y, et al. Down-regulation of the alpha-Gal epitope expression in N-glycans of swine endothelial cells by transfection with the N-acetylglucosaminyltransferase III gene. Modulation of the biosynthesis of terminal structures by a bisecting GlcNAc. J Biol Chem. 2001;276(35):32867–74.
37. Miyagawa S, Murakami H, et al. Remodeling of the major pig xenoantigen by N-acetylglucosaminyltransferase III in transgenic pig. J Biol Chem. 2001;276(42):39310–9.
38. Matsunami K, Miyagawa S, et al. Molecular cloning of pigGnT-I and I.2: an application to xenotransplantation. Biochem Biophys Res Commun. 2006;343(3):677–83.
39. Dai Y, Vaught TD, et al. Targeted disruption of the alpha1,3-galactosyltransferase gene in cloned pigs. Nat Biotechnol. 2002;20(3):251–5.
40. Takahagi Y, Fujimura T, et al. Production of alpha 1,3-galactosyltransferase gene knockout pigs expressing both human decay-accelerating factor and N-acetylglucosaminyltransferase III. Mol Reprod Dev. 2005;71(3):331–8.
41. Sakai R, Watanabe M, et al. Immunological response of pigs anti-human cell, included issues such as the production of natural antibodies in newborn. Transplant Proc. 2018;50(9):2839–41. https://doi.org/10.1016/j.transproceed.
42. Irie A, Koyama S, et al. The molecular basis for the absence of N-glycolylneuraminic acid in humans. J Biol Chem. 1998;273(25):15866–71.
43. Ikeda K, Yamamoto A, et al. A cloning of cytidine monophospho-N-acetylneuraminic acid hydroxylase from porcine endothelial cells. Transplant Proc. 2012;44(4):1136–8.
44. Yamamoto A, Ikeda K, et al. Trial using pig cells with the H-D antigen knocked down. Surg Today. 2013;43(7):782–6.
45. Sakai R, Esaki Y, et al. Knockout of cytidine monophospho-N-acetylneuraminic acid (CMP-NeuAc) hydroxylase from porcine endothelial cells by a CRISPR system. Transplant Proc. 2016;48(4):1320–2.
46. Miyagawa S, Matsunari H, et al. Generation of α1,3-galactosyltransferase and cytidine monophospho-N-acetylneuraminic acid hydroxylase gene double-knockout pigs. J Reprod Dev. 2015;61(5):449–57.
47. Byrne GW, Du Z, et al. Cloning and expression of porcine β1,4 N-acetylgalactosaminyl transferase encoding a new xenoreactive antigen. Xenotransplantation. 2014;21(6):543–54.
48. Lo PC, Eguchi H, et al. Reaction to the porcine cells with or without b4GalNT2. Transplant Proc. 2020;52(6):1916–8.
49. Miyagawa S, Nakai R, et al. Co-effect of HLA-G1 and glycosyltransfeses in reducing NK cell-mediated pig endothelial cell lysis. Transplant Immunol. 2003;11(2):147–53.
50. Matsunami K, Miyagawa S, et al. The possible use of HLA-G1 and G3 in the inhibition of NK cell-mediated swine endothelial cell lysis. Clin Exp Immunol. 2001;126(1):165–72.
51. Matsunami K, Miyagawa S, et al. Modulation of the leader peptide sequence of the HLA-E gene up-regulates its expression and downregulates natural killer cell-mediated swine endothelial cell lysis. Transplantation. 2002;73(10):1582–9.
52. Miyagawa S, Nakai R, et al. Regulation of natural killer cell-mediated swine endothelial cell lysis through genetic remodeling of a glycoantigen. J Biochem. 1999;126(6):1067–73.
53. Christiansen D, Mouhtouris E, et al. Recognition of a carbohydrate xenoepitope by human NKRP1A (CD161). Xenotransplantation. 2006;13(5):440–6.
54. Matsunami K, Okura E, et al. Identification of amino acid positions involved in HLA-E expression. J Biochem. 2008;143(5):641–7.
55. Matsunami K, Kusama T, et al. Involvement of position-147 for HLA-E expression. Biochem Biophys Res Commun. 2006;347(3):692–7.

56. Matsuura R, Maeda A, et al. Human HLA-Ev (147) expression in transgenic animals. Transplant Proc. 2016;48(4):1323–5.
57. Miyagawa S, Kubo T, et al. Delta-short consensus repeat 4-decay accelerate factor (DAF:CD55) inhibits complement-mediated cytolysis but not NK cell-mediated cytolysis. J Immunol. 2004;173(6):3945–52.
58. Maeda A, Kawamura T, et al. The suppression of inflammatory macrophage-mediated cytotoxicity and proinflammatory cytokine production by transgenic expression of HLA-E. Transpl Immunol. 2013;29(1–4):76–81.
59. Eguchi H, Maeda A, et al. HLA-G1, but not HLA-G3, suppresses human monocyte/macrophage-mediated swine endothelial cell lysis. Transplant Proc. 2016;48(4):1285–7.
60. Esquivel EL, Maeda A, et al. Suppression of human macrophage-mediated cytotoxicity by transgenic swine endothelial cell expression of HLA-G. Transpl Immunol. 2015;32(2):109–15.
61. Sakai R, Maeda A, et al. Human CD200 suppresses macrophage-mediated xenogeneic cytotoxicity and phagocytosis. Surg Today. 2018;48(1):119–26. https://doi.org/10.1007/s00595-017-1604-9.
62. Noguchi Y, Maeda A, et al. Human TIGIT on porcine aortic endothelial cells suppresses xenogeneic macrophage-mediated cytotoxicity. Immunobiology. 2019;224(5):605–13.
63. Kogata S, Lo PC, et al. Suppression of macrophage-mediated xenogeneic rejection by the ectopic expression of human CD177. Transpl Immunol. 2022;74:101663. https://doi.org/10.1016/j.trim.2022.101663.
64. Jiaravuthisan P, Maeda A, et al. A membrane-type surfactant protein D (SP-D) suppresses macrophage-mediated cytotoxicity in swine endothelial cells. Transpl Immunol. 2018;47:44–8. https://doi.org/10.1016/j.trim.2018.02.003.
65. Toyama C, Maeda A, et al. Suppression of xenogeneic innate immune response by a membrane-type human surfactant protein-A. Exp Ther Med. 2022;24(3):590. https://doi.org/10.3892/etm.2022.11527.
66. Maeda A, Kawamura T, et al. Regulation of macrophage-mediated xenocytotoxicity by overexpression of alpha 2,6-sialyltransferase in swine endothelial cells. Transplant Proc. 2014;46(4):1256–8.
67. Maeda A, Kawamura T, et al. Monocytic suppressor cells derived from human peripheral blood suppress xenogenic immune reaction. Xenotransplantation. 2014;21(1):46–56.
68. Maeda A, Eguchi H, et al. Monocytic MDSCs regulate macrophage-mediated xenogenic cytotoxicity. Transpl Immunol. 2015;33(2):140–5.
69. Maeda A, Kogata S, et al. The innate cellular immune response in xenotransplantation. Front Immunol. 2022;13:858604. https://doi.org/10.3389/fimmu.2022.858604.
70. Eguchi H, Maeda A, et al. Human CD200 suppresses the HL-60 mediated xenocytotoxicity. Transplant Proc. 2020;52(6):1910–2.
71. Iemitsu K, Sakai R, et al. The hybrid CL-SP-D molecule has the potential to regulate xenogeneic rejection by human neutrophils more efficiently than CD47. Transpl Immunol. 2024;84:102020. https://doi.org/10.1016/j.trim.2024.102020.
72. Wang HT, Maeda A, et al. Human CD31 on porcine cells suppress xenogeneic neutrophil-mediated cytotoxicity via the inhibition of NETosis. Xenotransplantation. 2018;25(5):e12396. https://doi.org/10.1111/xen.12396.
73. Yoneyama T, Maeda A, et al. The regulation of neutrophil extracellular trap-induced tissue damage by human CD177. Transplant Direct. 2021;7(8):e734.
74. Matsunami K, Kondo A, et al. Cloning of pig serine proteinase inhibitor 9 (PI-9) and its use in protecting against apoptosis. Transpl Int. 2007;20(5):453–9.
75. Xu H, Firdawes S, et al. Cloning and in vitro anti-apoptotic effects of pig FLIPs. Transplant Proc. 2008;40(8):2779–81.
76. Izutani H, Miyagawa S, et al. Evidence that graft coronary arteriosclerosis begins in the early phase after transplantation and progresses without chronic immunoreaction. Histopathological analysis using a retransplantation model. Transplantation. 1995;60(10):1073–9.

77. Izutani H, Miyagawa S, et al. Essential initial immunostimulation in graft coronary arteriosclerosis induction detected by retransplantation technique in rats: The participation of T Cell subsets. Transpl Immunol. 1997;5(1):11–5.
78. Matsumiya G, Shirakura R, et al. Analysis of rejection mechanism in the rat to mouse cardiac xenotransplantation. Role and characteristics of anti-endothelial cell antibodies. Transplantation. 1994;57(11):1653–60.
79. Matsumiya G, Shirakura R, et al. Role of CD4+ T cells in the rat to mouse cardiac xenotransplantation. Transpl Int. 1994;7:S654–9.
80. Kawamoto K, Tanemura M, et al. Significant inhibition of human $CD8^+$ cytotoxic T lymphocyte-mediated xenocytotoxicity by overexpression of the human decoy Fas antigen. Transplantation. 2006;81(5):789–96.
81. Miyagawa S, Watanabe M, et al. The study of the CPISPR/Cas3 system for xenotransplantation field. Transplant Proc. 2022;54(2):522–4. https://doi.org/10.1016/j.transproceed.2021.09.070.
82. Koresawa Y, Miyagawa S, et al. Synthesis of a new cre recombinase gene based on optimal codon usage for mammalian systems. J Biochem. 2000;127(3):367–72.
83. Miyagawa S, Yamada M, et al. A synthetic dDAF (CD55) gene based on optimal codon usage for transgenic animals. J Biochem. 2001;129(5):795–801.
84. Matsunami K, Otsuka H, et al. Molecular cloning of pig Rad51, Rad52 and Rad54 genes, which are involved in homologous recombination machinery. Transplant Proc. 2008;40(8):2776–8.
85. Matsunami K, Otsuka H, et al. Molecular cloning of pig Rad51, Rad52 and Rad54 genes, which are involved in homologous recombination machinery. Transplant Proc. 2008;40(8):2773–5.
86. Omori T, Nishida T, et al. A study of the xenoantigenicity of neonatal porcine islet-like cell clusters (NPCC) and the efficiency of adenovirus-mediated DAF (CD55) expression. Xenotransplantation. 2006;13(5):455–64.
87. Komoda H, Miyagawa S, et al. A study of the xenoantigenisity of adult pig islets. Xenotransplantation. 2004;11(3):237–46.
88. Komoda H, Miyagawa S, et al. Survival of adult islet grafts from transgenic pigs with N-acetylglucosaminyltransferase-III (GnT-III) in cynomolgus monkeys. Xenotransplantation. 2005;12(3):209–16.
89. Miyagawa S, Takeishi S, et al. Survey of glycoantigens in cells from a1-3galactosyltransferase knockout pig using a lectin microarray. Xenotransplantation. 2010;17(1):61–70.
90. Miyagawa S, Maeda A, et al. A lectin array analysis for wild-type and α-Gal-knockout pig islets, compared with humans. Surg Today. 2013;43(12):1439–47.
91. Nakatsu S, Takama Y, et al. A study of the glycoantigens of neonatal porcine islet-like cell clusters (NPCC) using a lectin microarray. Transplant Proc. 2012;44(4):1134–5.
92. Maeda A, Ueno T, et al. A lectin microarray study of glycoantigens in neonatal porcine islet-like cell clusters. J Surg Res. 2013;183(1):412–8.
93. Miyagawa S, Maeda A, et al. A comparison of the main structures of N-glycans of porcine islets with those from humans. Glycobiology. 2014;24(2):125–38.
94. Miyagawa S, Maeda A, et al. A structural analysis of N-glycans of neonatal porcine islet-like cell clusters (NPCC). Transpl Immunol. 2014;31(1):48–53.
95. Eguchi H, Kawamura T, et al. Supplemental analysis for N-linked sugars in adult pig islets. Transplant Proc. 2016;48(4):1302–3.
96. Mohiuddin MM, Singh AK, et al. Chimeric 2C10R4 anti-CD40 antibody therapy is critical for long-term survival of GTKO.hCD46.hTBM pig-to-primate cardiac xenograft. Nat Commun. 2016;7:11138.
97. Anand RP, Layer JV, et al. Design and testing of a humanized porcine donor for xenotransplantation. Nature. 2023;622(7982):393–401.
98. Murakami H, Nagashima H, et al. Transgenic pigs expressing human decay-accelerating factor regulated by porcine MCP gene promoter. Mol Reprod Dev. 2002;61(3):302–11.
99. Fujita T, Miyagawa S, et al. Skin graft of double transgenic pigs of N-acetylglucosaminyltransferase III (GnT-III) and DAF (CD55) genes survived in cynomolgus monkey for 31 days. Transpl Immunol. 2004;13(4):259–64.

100. Yang L, Güell M, et al. Genome-wide inactivation of porcine endogenous retroviruses (PERVs). Science. 2015;350(6264):1101–4.
101. Hazama K, Miyagawa S, et al. The significance of N-linked glycosylation in pig endogenous retrovirus (PERV) infectivity. Biochem Biophys Res Commun. 2003;310(2):327–33.
102. Miyagawa S, Nakatsu S, et al. A novel strategy for preventing PERV transmission to human cells by remodeling the viral envelope glycoprotein. Xenotransplantation. 2006;13(3):258–63.
103. Kurihara T, Miyazawa T, et al. Sensitivity to human serum of gammaretroviruses produced from pig endothelial cells transduced with glycosyltransferase genes. Xenotransplantation. 2003;10(6):562–8.
104. Yamamoto A, Nakatsu S, et al. A Newly cloned pig dolichyl-phosphate mannosyltransferase for preventing the transmission of porcine endogenous retrovirus to human cells. Transpl Int. 2010;23(4):424–31.
105. Hazama K, Miyagawa S, et al. The effect of expression of complement regulatory protein on pig endothelial cells to pig endogenous retrovirus (PERV) lyses by human sera. Transplant Proc. 2005;37(1):503–5.
106. Yamamoto A, Kobayashi C, et al. Expression of complement regulatory protein on porcine endogenous retrovirus (PERV) depends on molecular size. Transpl Immunol. 2010;23(1–2):71–6.
107. Okura E, Ishimaru A, et al. Differential human serum-mediated neutralization of PERV released from pig cells transfected with variants of hDAF. Xenotransplantation. 2008;15(6):365–73.
108. Miyagawa S, Takama Y, et al. Carbohydrate antigens. Curr Opin Organ Transplant. 2012;17(2):174–9.
109. Miyagawa S, Nakatsu S, et al. Prevention of PERV infections in pig to human xenotransplantation by the RNA interference silences gene. J Biochem. 2005;137(4):503–8.
110. Murakami H, Takahagi Y, et al. Porcine MCP gene promoter directs high level expression of human DAF (CD55) in transgenic mice. Immunobiology. 2000;201(5):583–97.

MIX
Papier aus verantwortungsvollen Quellen
Paper from responsible sources
FSC® C105338

If you have any concerns about our products,
you can contact us on
ProductSafety@springernature.com

In case Publisher is established outside the EU,
the EU authorized representative is:
Springer Nature Customer Service Center GmbH
Europaplatz 3, 69115 Heidelberg, Germany

Printed by Libri Plureos GmbH
in Hamburg, Germany